Lower Your Sodium Intake, Lower Your Blood Pressure!

Studies show that as many as 60 percent of people with hypertension can lower their blood pressure by eating less salt. Experts estimate that if everyone ate less than 2,000 milligrams of sodium a day, blood pressure would not increase as people grow older. In addition, the risk of early death would be reduced by 23 percent for stroke, 16 percent for coronary heart disease, and 13 percent for all other causes. Be an educated consumer: the life you save may be your own! Let *THE SODIUM COUNTER* be your guide.

Annette B. Natow, Ph.D., R.D., and Jo-Ann Heslin, M.A., R.D., are the authors of fifteen books on nutrition, including *The Cholesterol Counter, The Fat Counter, The Diabetes Carbohydrate and Calorie Counter, The Fat Attack Plan, The Iron Counter,* and *The Pregnancy Nutrition Counter* (all available from Pocket Books). Both are former faculty members of Adelphi University and State University of New York, Downstate Medical Center. They are editors of *The Journal of Nutrition for the Elderly,* serve as editorial board members for *American Baby* and *Environmental Nutrition Newsletter,* and are frequent contributors to magazines and journals.

Books by Annette B. Natow and Jo-Ann Heslin

The Cholesterol Counter
The Diabetes Carbohydrate and Calorie Counter
The Fat Attack Plan
The Fat Counter
The Iron Counter
Megadoses
No-Nonsense Nutrition for Kids
The Pocket Encyclopedia of Nutrition
The Pregnancy Nutrition Counter
The Sodium Counter

Published by POCKET BOOKS

T·H·E
SODIUM
COUNTER

Annette B. Natow, Ph.D.,R.D.,
and Jo-Ann Heslin, M.A.,R.D.

POCKET BOOKS

New York   London   Toronto   Sydney   Tokyo   Singapore

An *Original* Publication of POCKET BOOKS

POCKET BOOKS, a division of Simon & Schuster Inc.
1230 Avenue of the Americas, New York, NY 10020

ISBN: 0-671-69566-5

First Pocket Books printing July 1993

10 9 8 7 6 5 4 3 2 1

POCKET and colophon are registered trademarks of
Simon & Schuster Inc.

Cover design by Tom McKeveny

Printed in the U.S.A.

To our families, who support us through every project: Harry, Allen, Irene, Sarah, Meryl, Laura, Marty, George, Emily, Steven, Joe, Kristen and Karen.

ACKNOWLEDGMENTS

Without the tireless cooperation of Steven and Stephen, *The Sodium Counter* would never have been completed. Our thanks to Dr. Martin Lefkowitz and Athena Stavrakos for reviewing the material. A special thanks to our editor, Sally Peters, and our agent, Nancy Trichter.

―――――――――

"So, too, the chemical elements which make up the body substance must be nicely balanced or trouble ensues. The blood maintains its neutrality, the heart its regular beat . . ."

MARY SWARTZ ROSE, PH.D.
Feeding the Family
The Macmillan Company, 1919

SOURCES OF DATA

Values in this counter have been obtained from the Composition of Foods, United States Department of Agriculture, Agricultural Handbooks: No. 8-1, Dairy and Egg Products; No. 8-2, Spices and Herbs; No. 8-3, Baby Foods; No. 8-4, Fats and Oils; No. 8-5, Poultry Products; No. 8-6, Soups, Sauces and Gravies; No. 8-7, Sausages and Luncheon Meats; No. 8-8, Breakfast Cereals; No. 8-9, Fruit and Fruit Juices; No. 8-10, Pork Products; No. 8-11, Vegetables and Vegetable Products; No. 8-12, Nut and Seed Products; No. 8-13, Beef Products; No. 8-14, Beverages; No. 8-15, Finfish and Shellfish Products; No. 8-16, Legumes and Legume Products; No. 8-17, Lamb, Veal and Game Products; No. 8-19, Snacks and Sweets; No. 8-20, Cereal Grains and Pasta; No. 8-21, Fast Foods; Supplements 1989, 1990.

Nutritive Value of Foods, United States Department of Agriculture, Home and Garden Bulletin No. 72.

J. Davies and J. Dickerson, *Nutrient Content of Food Portions* (Cambridge, UK: The Royal Society of Chemistry, 1991).

G. A. Leveille, M. E. Zabik, and K. J. Morgan, *Nutrients in Foods* (Cambridge, MA: The Nutrition Guild, 1983).

Souci, Fachmann, and Kraut, *Food Composition and Nutrition Tables* (Stuttgart: Wissenschaftliche Verlagsgesellschaft MbH, 1989).

Information from food labels, manufacturers and processors: The values are based on research conducted prior to 1992. Manufacturers' ingredients are subject to change, so current values may vary from those listed in this book.

SOURCES OF DATA

Values in this manual have been obtained from the Composition of Foods, United States Department of Agriculture, Agricultural Handbooks: No. 8-1, Dairy and Egg Products; No. 8-2, Spices and Herbs; No. 8-3, Baby Foods; No. 8-4, Fats and Oils; No. 8-5, Poultry Products; No. 8-6, Soups, Sauces and Gravies; No. 8-7, Sausages and Luncheon Meats; No. 8-8, Breakfast Cereals; No. 8-9, Fruit and Fruit Juices; No. 8-10, Pork Products No. 8-11, Vegetables and Vegetable Products; No. 8-12, Nut and Seed Products; No. 8-13, Beef Products No. 8-14, Beverages; No. 8-15, Finfish and Shellfish Products; No. 8-16, Legumes and Legume Products; No. 8-17, Lamb, Veal and Game Products; No. 8-18, Snacks and Sweets; No. 8-20, Cereal Grains and Pasta; No. 8-21, Fast Foods; Supplements 1990, 1990.

Nutritive Value of Foods, United States Department of Agriculture, Home and Garden Bulletin No. 72.

Davies and a. Dickerson, Nutrient Content of Food Portions (Cambridge, UK, The Royal Society of Chemistry, 1991).

B. A. Levelle, M. E. Zabik, and R. J. Morgan, Nutrients in Foods (Cambridge, MA, The Nutrition Guild, 1983).

Souci, Fachmann, and Kraut, Food Composition and Nutrition Tables (Stuttgart, Wissenschaftliche Verlagsgesellschaft MbH, 1989).

Information from food labels, manufacturers, and processors. The values are based on research conducted prior to 1992. Manufacturers' ingredients are subject to change, so current values may vary from those listed in this book.

INTRODUCTION

• Is salt the same as sodium?

It's easy to confuse sodium and salt. In fact, the two terms are often used interchangeably. Salt is a mixture of two minerals—sodium and chloride. If you used a teaspoon of salt, which weighs 5,000 milligrams, 2,000 of the 5,000 would be sodium and the other 3,000 milligrams would be chloride. Another way of saying this is that salt is 40 percent sodium and 60 percent chloride. The average salt intake of two to three teaspoons a day is equal to 4,000 to 6,000 milligrams of sodium.

Measuring Sodium

Teaspoons of Salt	Milligrams of Sodium
1 teaspoon	2,000
½ teaspoon	1,000
¼ teaspoon	500
⅛ teaspoon	250

Experts agree, Americans eat too much salt:

American Medical Association recommends 4,800 to 12,000 milligrams of salt a day. This equals an average of 3,300 milligrams of sodium a day.

American Heart Association recommends no more than 3,000 milligrams of sodium a day.

American Dietetic Association recommends reducing intake of sodium.

United States Departments of Agriculture and of Health and Human Services, Dietary Guidelines for Americans, recommend using salt and sodium only in moderation.

The Surgeon General's Report on Nutrition and Health recommends that sodium intake be reduced.

The National Research Council's Recommended Dietary Allowances (RDA), 10th edition, recommends a minimum of 500 milligrams a day of sodium.

National Research Council, Report of the Committee on Diet and Health, recommends limiting the total daily intake of salt to 6,000 milligrams or less, or 2,400 milligrams of sodium or less.

Salt Sources

Dr. Mark Hegstead of the Human Nutrition Research Center of the United States Department of Agriculture has stated that the amount of salt eaten by Americans is about half the toxic dose. He has said, "Common sense tells even the uninitiated that it is wise to limit salt intake. Indeed, if salt were a new food additive, it is doubtful that it would be classified as safe and certainly not at the level most of us consume."

Everyone needs to lower his or her salt intake. Americans eat 2 to 3 teaspoons (10,000 to 15,000 milligrams) of salt a day, which equals 4,000 to 6,000 milligrams of sodium. A healthier intake would be much less.

You've emptied the saltshaker. You don't use salt in cooking. You think you've beaten the salt habit. Absolutely not! *Seventy-seven percent* of your salt comes from the boxes, cans and jars you buy in the supermarket.

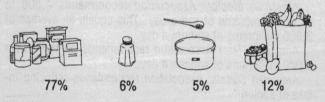

77%   6%   5%   12%

- **Don't I need to eat some sodium?**
  Every cell in your body needs sodium. Though you need

SODIUM EQUIVALENTS

Sodium can be measured in milligrams (mg) or in milli-equivalents (mEq).

To convert mg of sodium to mEq, divide the number of mg of sodium by 23.

$$506 \text{ mg of sodium} = 22 \text{ mEq}$$
$$506 \div 23 = 22$$

To convert mEq of sodium to mg, multiply the number of mEq of sodium by 23.

$$20 \text{ mEq of sodium} = 460 \text{ mg}$$
$$20 \times 23 = 460$$

Sodium Equivalents

Milligrams of Sodium (mg)	Milli-equivalents of Sodium (mEq)	Grams of Salt (g)
500	21.7	1.3
1,000	43.5	2.5
1,500	65.2	3.8
2,000	87.0	5.0

only a small amount of sodium—about 200 to 500 milligrams a day—it is almost impossible to keep your intake that low. Sodium is found in almost everything you eat. Milk, meat and vegetables contain sodium but there is often much more in processed foods. That is why most of us eat almost twenty times as much sodium as we need!

You can get all the sodium you need in a half-teaspoon of salt. You get that much without adding salt when you eat a variety of fresh foods—milk, meat, fish, poultry, bread, fruit and vegetables.

• Which foods are naturally high in sodium?

Fresh foods that come from animals like meat, fish, poultry, milk, cheese and eggs are naturally high in sodium. Organ meats like liver and shellfish are higher in sodium than other meats and fish. But you may be surprised to learn that saltwater fish like cod, mackerel and striped bass do not have more sodium than freshwater fish like trout and whitefish.

Fresh vegetables like spinach, kale, carrots, artichokes and celery have more sodium than other fresh vegetables, but even these have much less than many packaged foods. Fruits, sugar, coffee, tea, jelly, oils, grains and pasta are all very low in sodium, too.

Cereals vary, with most cooked cereals, like oatmeal, being low in sodium. Instant hot cereals and most ready-to-eat cereals contain much more. Even the water you drink can contain sodium. To find out about your water supply, check with your local water department. If you drink bottled water or mineral water, check the label.

• Why is salt bad for high blood pressure?

In places in the world where little salt is eaten, people have practically no high blood pressure. In countries like ours, where a lot of salt is used, blood pressure tends to rise. People who eat less than 8,000 milligrams of salt a day have a 20 percent chance of having high blood pressure. This risk increases to 36 percent when salt intake goes up to 13,000 milligrams or more a day.

Experts agree that there would be less high blood pressure in the second half of life if people simply ate less salt. And if you have high blood pressure, it is easier to treat when you eat less salt. Even a small reduction in salt intake makes a difference in blood pressure.

- **Is there any other reason why too much salt is bad for my health?**

Studies show that eating a lot of salt causes more calcium to be lost in the urine. This loss of calcium could be a factor in osteoporosis, a condition in which bones are reduced in strength as people age. Osteoporosis is a major cause of disability in older people, particularly in women. Eating less salt may be one way to protect against it.

People with congestive heart failure or kidney disease can make the condition worse when they eat too much salt.

- **I like the taste of salty foods. How can I ever get used to eating less salt?**

Believe it or not, you can wean yourself from a high salt diet. Babies are not born with a preference for salt, but by the time they are toddlers children prefer salted foods to unsalted ones. Scientists do not know how much of this preference is inborn and how much is learned. But we do know that this preference can be changed. It takes time to unlearn the "salt habit." You'll find that within two months of eating less salt, foods begin to taste saltier to you. And those salty foods that you used to enjoy become too salty.

- **Is it possible to lower your sodium intake too much?**

Not on a varied diet. *The Sodium Counter* shows you how much sodium is found in all the foods you eat. You'll be surprised to see how quickly the milligrams add up. *The National Research Council's Recommended Dietary Allowances* (RDA) published in 1989 gives 500 milligrams of sodium, as much as you get in a quarter teaspoon of salt, as the minimum requirement for healthy people. There are populations throughout the world that live very well on even less. These people rarely suffer from high blood pressure.

SHOPPING SENSE

What you buy is more important than how you cook. Even though sales of salt have gone down in recent years, that doesn't mean we are eating less salt. You get most of your salt from packaged foods. Convenience foods like frozen dinners, canned soups and dry soup mixes, sauces and salad dressings are some foods that usually contain large amounts of salt. Some low-salt versions of these foods are appearing on supermarket shelves. In a report recently issued by the National High Blood Pressure Education Program of the National Institutes of Health, federal health officials challenged the food industry to substantially lower the amount of salt and calories in processed foods.

Sodium watchers need to be label readers. Any food that has more than 400 milligrams of sodium per serving should be eaten less often.

A 1992 study by Food Marketing Institute found that six in ten shoppers said they had made major changes in their diets for health reasons in the last three years. Almost one-third of these supermarket shoppers reduced their salt or sodium intake and want less salt in the products they are buying. Food companies are responding to these concerns and so are the new food labeling regulations. In 1990 there were 37 percent more new foods than in the previous year that made health claims about reduced salt. The new food labeling law will allow health claims on foods that are low in salt.

Selecting Less Salt

There are good low-salt choices in the supermarket if you know where to look. It's best to wheel your cart around the outside aisles first. That's where the fresh foods are. They tend to have less sodium than the processed, packaged foods in the inside aisles. Watch out for samples in the supermarket, too! More often than not these samples are salty.

Fruits and Vegetables

Fresh, frozen and canned fruits are very low in sodium. Dried fruits have a little more, but it is a small amount. Most fresh vegetables have very little sodium; some—like spinach, kale, carrots, artichokes and celery—have a bit more but still not anywhere near the amount found in most canned or sauced frozen versions. Look at how the amount of sodium varies with the way a food is prepared.

One-Half Cup of Peas	Sodium (mg)
raw	3
cooked	2
frozen	70*
canned	186
canned, low-sodium	2
frozen in butter sauce	410

One-Half Cup of Green Beans	Sodium (mg)
fresh	3
shelf stable (see Definitions)	20
frozen	10
frozen in butter sauce	230
canned	385

*During the sorting process, frozen peas are sized in a bath of salted water, causing the peas to absorb some of the salt. That's why plain frozen peas have more sodium than other plain frozen vegetables.

Meat, Poultry, Fish

Fresh meat, poultry and finfish are all fairly low in sodium. They average less than 90 milligrams in a three-ounce portion. Shellfish have more sodium than finfish: 126 milligrams in three ounces of shrimp. Scallops have a little more: 137 milligrams.

Saltwater fish like Atlantic cod, with 66 milligrams of sodium in three ounces, do not have much more sodium than freshwater fish like catfish, with 54 milligrams in three ounces. Canned fish and meat products, like hash, have varying amounts of salt added. They are usually much higher in salt than similar home-cooked food. Cured meats like frankfurters, sausages, luncheon meats and ham can have as much as ten to fifteen times the sodium in fresh meat.

Bread, Cereals, Grains

Plain breads have moderate amounts of salt, averaging 100 to 175 milligrams a slice. Local bakery breads may have less because they often are made with fewer sodium-containing additives. Biscuits, muffins, crackers and other baked products have varying amounts of salt, often twice as much as plain bread.

Cooked cereals, pasta, rice, buckwheat groats (kasha), bulgur, and couscous contain very little sodium, less than 5 milligrams in a one-half cup serving. In ready-to-eat cereals, grains and/or noodle mixes, the sodium is much higher.

Cookies, snack cakes, pastry and other cakes have varying amounts of sodium. Coffeecakes and sweet rolls made with yeast usually contain less sodium than those made with baking powder and baking soda.

Milk, Yogurt, Cheese

Milk and yogurt naturally contain between 120 and 160 milligrams of sodium in an eight-ounce serving. Buttermilk is higher, about 257 milligrams in a cup, because salt is added.

Natural cheeses like cheddar and Swiss have less sodium than processed cheese like American and cheese spreads. Cottage cheese, both regular and low-fat, has the same amount of sodium, about 457 milligrams in a half cup serving. There are cheese products available with less salt. Choose these more often.

Snacks

Potato chips, corn chips, popcorn, nuts and other bite-sized snacks are usually very high in salt. You can find reduced salt and no-salt versions in the supermarket, or you can pop your own popcorn from scratch in the microwave or hot-air popper with no salt added at all.

Fats, Oils

Vegetable oils like corn, cottonseed, olive, soybean and canola do not have any sodium. Gourmet-type oils like walnut, hazelnut and almond are also sodium-free. Butter and margarine have about 45 milligrams of sodium in a teaspoon. Both are available in unsalted versions. Prepared salad dressings contain varying amounts of salt, from very low to very high. You can mix your own salad dressing with oil and vinegar; both are salt-free.

Condiments

Soy sauce, catsup, chili sauce and steak sauce usually contain a lot of salt. Reduced sodium versions are available. Salsa, which now is outselling catsup, is sometimes made without any added salt.

SHOPPING FOR **LESS** SALT

Consider this list as only a guide; it's important to read labels for individual brands you buy.

BUY OFTEN	BUY LESS OFTEN
fresh fruit	fruit-filled pastries
frozen fruit	fruit pie
dried fruit	
canned fruit	
fresh vegetables	canned vegetables

BUY OFTEN	BUY LESS OFTEN
frozen vegetables	frozen vegetables in sauce
plain bread, hard rolls, bagels	muffins, biscuits, croissants
milk, yogurt low sodium cheese	cheese
fresh meat, poultry	cured meats like ham, frankfurters
frozen meat	frozen meats with sauce or gravy
fresh fish	breaded and/or stuffed fresh fish smoked or pickled fish
frozen fish	breaded, battered, sauced frozen fish
pasta	pasta with sauce
unsalted butter and margarine	salted butter and margarine
rice cakes, matzos, breadsticks, baldy pretzels, pita	regular crackers, salted pretzels
cooked quick or regular hot cereal	instant hot cereal
puffed wheat, puffed rice, shredded wheat, low-sodium cereals	ready-to-eat cereals
mustard, salsa, fresh chili peppers, herbs, spices, seasoned pepper	pickles, olives, catsup, relish, salt

Reading Labels

When you want to know more about a food, look at the list of ingredients. Packaged foods have ingredient listings. Ingredients are listed according to the amounts that are in the food, in decreasing order. There's a lot of information about salt on labels, but it can be confusing. The current legal definitions for salt descriptions on food labels are as follows:

sodium-free: less than 5 mg of sodium per serving
very-low sodium: less than 35 mg of sodium per
serving
low-sodium: less than 140 mg of sodium per serving
reduced sodium: 25 percent less sodium than the
product it replaces

These definitions may change in the future, as food labeling laws are being revised.

If you see salt in the first few ingredients, as in some snacks and condiments, there is probably a lot of salt in that food. But even if salt is not one of the main ingredients listed, the food can still be high in sodium because there are many ingredients and additives that *contain* sodium.

SODIUM-CONTAINING INGREDIENTS AND ADDITIVES

ADDITIVE	USE
baking powder	used in bread and cake to make them rise
baking soda (sodium bicarbonate)	used in bread and cake to make them rise
disodium phosphate	emulsifier used in quick-cooking cereals and processed cheese
monosodium glutamate (MSG)	seasoning, flavor enhancer
salt	seasoning and preservative
sodium alginate	used in chocolate milk and ice cream to make them smooth
sodium aluminum sulfate	bleaching agent for flour
sodium ascorbate	vitamin C
sodium benzoate	preservative in soda, relishes, sauces and salad dressings

ADDITIVE	USE
sodium bisulfite	prevents discoloration in wine and beer, preservative
sodium carboxymethyl cellulose	stabilizer in frozen desserts, salad dressing and chocolate milk
sodium caseinate	improves texture of frozen desserts
sodium erythorbate	color brightener, preservative in processed meat
sodium hexametaphosphate	emulsifier used in breakfast cereals, lemon juice and ice cream
sodium hydroxide	used in processing ripe olives, fruits and vegetables to soften skins
sodium nitrite	preservative in cured meats
sodium pectinate	thickener in frozen desserts and salad dressings
sodium propionate	mold inhibitor used in bread, cake and pasteurized cheese
sodium pyrophosphate	used in tuna and instant pudding mix to improve texture
sodium saccharin	artificial sweetener
sodium sulfite	used to bleach maraschino cherries and preserve dried fruits

Some over-the-counter drugs are high in sodium. The following is a list of commonly used nonprescription medications that contain little sodium. Because drug formulations change frequently, check with your pharmacist.

LOW-SODIUM MEDICATIONS

The following nonprescription drugs have less than 5 milligrams of sodium in a dose.

PAIN RELIEVERS

Anacin
Ascripton
Aspirin
Bufferin
Ecotrin
Empirin

Excedrin
Nebs
Pepto Bismol
Percogesic
Tylenol

COUGH/COLD MEDICINE

Cepacol Lozenges
Chloroseptic Mouthwash
Congesprin
Coricidin
Hills Cough Tablets
Pertussin

Robitussin
Smith Bros. Cough Drops
Terpin Hydrate Elixir
Vick's 44 Lozenges
4 Way Cold Tablets
666 Cold Preparation

ANTACIDS

Alterna Gel
Amitone
Basaljel
Bisodol Gel
Camalox
Creamalin
Gelusil, Gelusil II
Maalox, Maalox Plus

Mylanta, Mylanta II
Mylicon
Riopan
Sodium-free Rolaids
Titralac Tablets
Tums
Wingel

LAXATIVES, STOOL SOFTENERS

Cascara
Colace
Dialose
Ducolax
Haley's MO
Metamucil

Milk of Magnesia
Perdiem
Pericolace Syrup
Sal Hepatica
Senokot
Surfak

SALT IN THE KITCHEN

You don't need to add salt to the water used for boiling vegetables and pasta, even though package directions usually call for it. Many people add salt to cooking water because they believe it lowers the boiling point. Salt, in the amounts usually added in cooking, has no effect on the boiling temperature of water. When salt is added to cooking water, most is usually lost when the food is drained.

You can cut salt in many recipes by using only one-quarter of the amount called for. Start slowly, reducing salt by one-fourth each time you prepare the recipe. Continue reducing the salt until the food is just salty enough.

When a recipe calls for a salty ingredient, substitute a less salty one.

INSTEAD OF	SUBSTITUTE
catsup	salt-free salsa
garlic salt	garlic powder
canned vegetables	fresh vegetables
salt	herbs and spices, pepper
soy or worcestershire sauce	low-salt soy sauce, lemon, vinegar

KEEPING BLOOD VESSELS YOUNG

Blood vessels must dilate and contract normally for blood pressure to be normal. Excess salt can change the way blood vessels respond. In a recent study two groups of people ranging in age from 20 to 72 were given a high-salt diet; then their blood vessels were tested to see if they could dilate and contract normally. It was found that in the older people blood vessels dilated only half as much as in the younger. When the older subjects were given a low-salt diet, their blood vessels dilated as much as the younger ones. A low-salt diet can keep blood vessels youthful.

DID YOU KNOW?

High blood pressure is the most common medical problem in the United States and most other industrialized countries.

•

Blood pressure in a giraffe is about double that of an adult human. This extra pressure is necessary to get blood up the giraffe's long neck.

•

When you eat less salt, you will probably need less blood pressure medication.

•

When your intake of potassium is low, you increase your risk for high blood pressure.

•

People who consume less calcium are more likely to have high blood pressure.

•

Blood pressure goes down 20 percent during sleep.

•

Experts say that a very-low sodium intake (less than 1,500 mg daily) can lower blood pressure as much as taking one blood pressure medication.

•

For every two pounds lost, systolic blood pressure goes down 1 mm Hg (millimeter of mercury, unit used in measuring blood pressure).

•

Researchers believe that if people on high blood pressure medication ate more potassium-rich foods, one-third would be able to discontinue their medication.

•

Population studies show that increasing your potassium intake by eating more fruits, vegetables and whole grains protects against stroke.

•

Men eat more salt than women do because they usually eat more calories.

•

DID YOU KNOW?

After you have taken antihypertensive medication for several years, your doctor may suggest discontinuing it for a trial period. People who reduce their salt intake are more successful in keeping their blood pressure down without medication.

•

Drinking more than 1 ounce of alcohol (2 ounces of 100 proof whiskey, 8 ounces of wine, 24 ounces of beer) regularly can cause high blood pressure. Smokers can get high blood pressure from even less alcohol.

•

Reducing dietary salt and alcohol intake, losing weight, increasing potassium intake, and exercising regularly may have an even greater potential for preventing hypertension than for lowering high blood pressure once it has become established.

•

May is National High Blood Pressure month; use that observance as a reminder to check your blood pressure.

•

Even small increases in blood pressure are not good. Studies show that one-third of all cardiovascular disease caused by hypertension occurs in people who have high normal levels of blood pressure (diastolic pressure of 85 to 89 mm Hg). The good news about this finding is that high normal levels of blood pressure can be successfully treated, often without medication, simply by losing weight, eating less salt, and exercising.

•

People often think of high blood pressure as a stress disease resulting from tension. While stress may be a factor, no one is sure just what causes high blood pressure.

•

One bagel has more sodium (580 mg) than ten saltines (360 mg).

•

One-half cup of instant chocolate pudding has more sodium (450 mg) than 1 teaspoon soy sauce (313 mg).

•

Six ounces of tomato juice has more sodium (658 mg) than 1 ounce of potato chips (150 mg).

•

DID YOU KNOW?

Sex raises your blood pressure, as much as 25 to 120 mm Hg systolic and 24 to 48 mm Hg diastolic.

•

Researchers have recently found in animal studies that a substance in celery (3-n-butyl phthalide) lowers blood pressure. Even though celery contains more sodium than most vegetables, eating a few stalks won't hurt and may even help.

•

Dr. Claude J. Lenfant, who heads the National Heart, Lung and Blood Institute, a federal agency in Bethesda, Md., has said that gains made in detecting and treating high blood pressure were ''a major factor in the declining death rate for coronary heart disease and stroke.''

IF YOUR NUMBERS ARE UP

High blood pressure, or hypertension, is the reason for most visits to the doctor. The National Center for Health Statistics reports that in a year there are almost 58 million visits to the doctor for high blood pressure. But this doesn't tell the whole story. The National High Blood Pressure Education Program, which the federal government established twenty years ago to combat high blood pressure, estimates that 50 million Americans have hypertension. That adds up to one in four of all adults! Some are under a doctor's care, while others do not even know they have the condition.

High blood pressure can cause damage for fifteen to twenty years before there are any symptoms. Some warning signs are headache, chest pains, shortness of breath, and palpitations, but there may not be any of these. All too often, the first sign may be a heart attack or stroke. And that can be fatal. According to Dr. Edward J. Roccella, the coordinator of the National High Blood Pressure Education Program, treatment of the condition probably prevented about 180,000 fatal strokes among Americans from 1970 to 1990.

Medical experts believe that if all cases of high blood pressure were controlled, there would be a 20 percent drop in deaths among white men and women, a 30 percent decrease in deaths in black men, and 45 percent fewer deaths in black women. That is because high blood pressure increases the risk for heart attack, stroke, kidney failure and other diseases.

It's important that everyone—adults and children—have blood pressure checked regularly. The American Academy of Pediatrics recommends that all children over the age of 2 have their blood pressure checked. Adults should be checked regularly, too.

Both men and women are at risk for high blood pressure. Men have a greater chance of hypertension when they are younger. By age 55, the risk is equal for both sexes, and after age 65 women are more likely than men to develop high blood pressure.

If your parents or other close relatives have high blood pressure, there is a good chance you will, too. More black people than white, especially women, have hypertension. Other risk factors are a diet high in salt, being overweight, aging, and heavy alcohol use.

A percentage of the population—one-fifth to one-third—is salt sensitive. For these people, eating a lot of salt may be a factor in their high blood pressure. Intersalt, an international epidemiologic study of more than 10,000 people in 32 countries, found no high blood pressure in places where the sodium intake was 1,403 mg or less a day. The Intersalt study positively correlated hypertension with sodium intake. As people ate more salt, their blood pressure readings were higher.

• My doctor told me not to worry, my blood pressure was 125 over 80. Is that normal?

Yes, your blood pressure is fine. Blood pressure is the force of blood against the blood vessel walls. It is reported as two numbers written like this: 125/80. The upper figure, in your case 125, is the systolic pressure—the maximum pressure when the heart contracts and forces the blood through the arteries. The lower figure, in your case 80, is the diastolic pressure—the minimum pressure when the heart relaxes between beats. Both of these numbers are given as millimeters of mercury, or mm Hg, because a column of mercury is used to measure blood pressure. Repeated blood pressure readings of 140/90 or over indicate high blood pressure, or hypertension.

• I have high blood pressure. Do I really have to give up salty foods?

Yes. Eating less salt can help control your blood pressure. That doesn't mean that you have to give up all salty foods. Even a modest reduction in sodium can help. Not all people are sensitive to salt. Those who are older, black, or overweight are more likely to be salt sensitive. Even so, studies show that as many as 60 percent of people with hypertension can lower their blood pressure when they eat less salt.

Reducing salt can have long-term health benefits. Experts estimate that if everybody ate less than 2,000 mg of sodium a day, blood pressure would not increase as people grow older. Risk of death would be reduced:

> 16 percent for coronary heart disease
> 23 percent for stroke
> 13 percent for all other causes

• Does carrying around an extra 30 pounds affect my blood pressure?

Yes. If you are 15 to 20 percent over your desirable weight, you increase your risk of developing high blood pressure. A long-term study in Framingham, Mass., found that people who were 20 percent or more over their desirable weight were eight times more likely to become hypertensive.

In the last few years researchers have found the risk of obesity may really depend on where the excess weight is located. If it is in the midsection—abdomen and chest—it is more of a risk than when it's on the lower body—hips and thighs. Excess body weight in the trunk increases risk for high blood pressure, breast cancer, diabetes, coronary heart disease, and unhealthy levels of blood fats.

> Apple shape = too much weight in the midsection
> Pear shape = too much weight from the waist down

To find out which type you are, simply measure your waist where it is smallest and your hips where they are widest. Divide your waist measurement by your hip measurement.

Women with measurements below 0.75 are pears; above 0.85, apples.

Men with measurements below 0.80 are pears; above 0.95, apples.

Apples indicate greater risk, but you can lower your hip-to-waist ratio and your risk when you lose weight.

We don't know exactly how excess weight causes high blood pressure but we do know that even a small weight loss causes a drop in blood pressure. Losing 10 to 20 pounds can cause a 10 mm Hg drop in blood pressure. The effect of weight loss varies but it averages about 1 mm Hg for each 1 percent of weight lost.

• My husband and I have a drink every night before dinner. Will that raise my blood pressure?

Drinking a lot of alcohol can cause hypertension, but moderate alcohol intake may lower it. Alcohol is believed to be the most common cause of reversible hypertension in Western countries. But studies show that when people drink two or fewer drinks a day they have lower blood pressure than nondrinkers. Increasing alcohol consumption has been shown to raise blood pressure, regardless of age or weight.

It is clear that having five or six drinks a day causes high blood pressure, but the effect of lower intake of alcohol is not so certain. Most experts agree that one to two drinks a day will not increase blood pressure. And some believe that having one or two drinks a day may even be helpful in lowering blood pressure. Those who drink small amounts can enjoy it with the knowledge that it carries no proven harmful effects and may even be beneficial.

• **I have heard that potassium is good for high blood pressure. Should I take a potassium supplement?**

While potassium supplements can lower blood pressure, you can get all the potassium you need by eating lots of potassium-rich fruits, vegetables and grains.

Researchers have found that in areas where people eat a lot of potassium, both average blood pressure and prevalence of hypertension are low. Vegetarians who eat potassium-rich plant foods have lower blood pressure than meat eaters.

The Intersalt study found a negative correlation between potassium and blood pressure—as intake of potassium goes down, blood pressure goes up. Other studies show that people who have a lot of potassium in their diet reduce their risk of stroke. There is a relationship between the level of sodium and the level of potassium in the body. A low potassium intake is a factor in the development of high blood pressure, especially when sodium intake is high. A high potassium intake may be beneficial because it helps the body get rid of excess sodium. Because of this, some experts suggest a potassium intake of 4,000 milligrams or more a day.

POTASSIUM IN FOODS

FOOD	CALORIES	POTASSIUM (mg)
amaranth, cooked, ½ cup	59	423
apricots, dried, 10 halves	83	482
artichoke, 1	60	425
avocado, ½	162	602
baked beans, ½ cup	190	452
banana, 1	105	451
beefsteak, broiled, 6 oz	473	631
beet greens, cooked, ½ cup	20	654
black bean soup, canned, 1 cup	218	739
blackeye peas, canned, ½ cup	199	427
burritos, beef, 2	523	739
cantaloupe, cubed, 1 cup	57	494

FOOD	CALORIES	POTASSIUM (mg)
carrot juice, canned, 6 oz	73	538
cheeseburger, 1 large	608	644
chestnuts, roasted, ½ cup	350	846
chicken, roasted, ½	715	667
chickpeas, canned, 1 cup	285	413
clams, cooked, 3 oz	126	534
clams, raw, 9 large	133	565
cod, baked, 3 oz	95	465
dates, dried, 10	228	541
enchilada, cheese and beef, 1	324	574
figs, dried, 5	238	666
grapefruit juice, canned, 1 cup	116	405
great northern beans, canned, ½ cup	150	458
halibut, cooked, 3 oz	119	490
honeydew, cubed, 1 cup	60	461
ice milk, soft, 1 cup	223	412
kidney beans, canned, 1 cup	216	658
lima beans, canned, 1 cup	191	531
lima beans, cooked, ½ cup	104	485
mackerel, cooked, 3 oz	134	471
milk, chocolate, 1 cup	208	417
milk, lowfat, fortified, 1 cup	119	444
milk, skim, 1 cup	86	406
molasses, 2 tbsp	85	1171
orange juice, canned, 1 cup	104	436
orange juice, chilled, 1 cup	110	473
orange juice, fresh, 1 cup	111	496
orange juice, frozen, 1 cup	112	474
oysters, canned, 1 cup	170	568
peaches, dried, 5 halves	155	647
peanut butter, ¼ cup	379	465
pears, dried, 5 halves	229	466
pinto beans, canned, 1 cup	186	723
pompano, cooked, 3 oz	179	541
pork tenderloin, roasted, 3 oz	141	457
potato, baked, 1	220	844
potato, baked w/ cheese sauce	475	1167
potatoes, french fried, med size	235	541
prune juice, 1 cup	181	706
prunes, dried, 10	201	626
sablefish, smoked, 3 oz	218	401
salmon, baked, 3 oz	155	534
snapper, cooked, 3 oz	109	404

FOOD	CALORIES	POTASSIUM (mg)
soybeans, dry roasted, ½ cup	387	1173
soybeans, roasted, 1 oz	129	417
spaghetti sauce, marinara, 1 cup	171	1061
spinach, cooked, ½ cup	21	419
split peas, cooked, 1 cup	231	710
squash, acorn, baked, ½ cup	57	446
swiss chard, cooked, ½ cup	18	483
tomato paste, canned, ¼ cup	27	307
tomato sauce, ½ cup	37	452
tomato soup, canned, prep w/ milk, 1 cup	160	450
tomato, sun-dried in oil, ½ cup	118	860
trout, rainbow, cooked, 3 oz	129	539
tuna, baked, 3 oz	112	444
turkey, roasted, 1 cup	238	418
yam, cooked, cubed, ½ cup	79	455
yogurt, lowfat, coffee, 8 oz	194	498
yogurt, lowfat, fruit, 8 oz	225	402
yogurt, lowfat, plain, 8 oz	144	531
yogurt, lowfat, vanilla, 8 oz	194	498

• I have a pressure-cooker job as a production manager, and I work nights. Could this affect my blood pressure?

Yes, chronic stress may be a factor in causing high blood pressure. Reducing stress helps prevent and control high blood pressure. Relaxation, meditation and biofeedback techniques have been studied with varying results. Some people benefit more than others.

Exercise is another approach. Long-term physical exercise results in lower blood pressure even if no weight is lost. Endurance exercise is more efficient than strength training. Experts suggest moderate exercise for 30 minutes three times a week. Everybody is advised to see his or her doctor before starting any type of exercise program.

Nutrients Under Study

Population studies suggest a health-protecting effect of hard water. Hard water contains the minerals calcium and magnesium. Both of these minerals have been studied for their effect on blood pressure.

It was found that older women who consume less than 800 mg of calcium a day had higher systolic blood pressure than others who had more than 800 mg. A recent study of boys and girls 3 to 6 showed the same effect of calcium on blood pressure. Children who ate more calcium had lower systolic blood pressure. Some studies found that calcium supplements reduced blood pressure. A high calcium intake helps the body get rid of excess sodium.

Increasing calcium intake may not be the most important issue in reducing blood pressure, but since more than one-

---

WHITE COAT HYPERTENSION

The anxiety of a visit to the doctor's office may falsely elevate blood pressure. This effect, called "white coat hypertension" has been studied.

The presence of a doctor can raise systolic blood pressure as much as 27 mm Hg, and diastolic, 15 mm Hg. This could result in a person with normal blood pressure being treated for hypertension. More than 25 percent of those people found to have borderline high blood pressure when tested by a physician turned out to have normal readings when their blood pressure was taken automatically several times during the day.

White coat hypertension persists in some, but most people get used to having their blood pressure measured, so that the readings tend to go down over the course of several visits to the doctor. Also, when nurses instead of doctors measure blood pressure, the results are usually lower. Taking your own blood pressure a number of times has been shown to make it go down six points.

third of all women eat too little calcium, increasing calcium intake is worthwhile for all women, whether they have high blood pressure or not.

Other studies have shown a strong relationship between magnesium in the diet and blood pressure. When more magnesium-rich foods were eaten, blood pressure went down. Magnesium supplements, however, do not reduce blood presure in most people. A few studies connect vitamin C intake and blood pressure. Those with higher intakes of vitamin C tend to have lower blood pressure. More research is needed to see exactly what role, if any, there is for these nutrients in the treatment of hypertension.

BLOOD PRESSURE UPPERS AND DOWNERS

UPPER	DOWNER
winter	summer
noise	quiet
alcohol use	garlic
combining caffeine/smoking/alcohol	vegetarian diet
using too much salt	vitamin C
aging	eating less salt
headache	potassium
chronic pain	losing weight
overweight	sleep
public speaking	laughing
stress	caring for a pet
sex	exercise
	meditation

COUNT UP YOUR SODIUM

Your blood pressure depends on your weight and your salt intake. Eating less salt both prevents and helps treat high blood pressure. Losing weight makes high blood pressure go down. Recent research sponsored by the National Institutes of Health showed that weight loss worked best at lowering blood pressure. It didn't have to be dramatic. The average participant lost only 8.6 pounds during the one-and-a-half-year study. Second best was cutting down modestly on sodium. The average intake dropped from about 3,600 milligrams to 2,600 milligrams a day. No other nondrug treatment was effective in reducing blood pressure significantly.

We often eat on the run and pick foods high in sodium. By the end of the day, we've eaten too much salt. You know you shouldn't be eating so much salt, and you want to cut back. *The Sodium Counter* will help you do it. For the first time, it's simple to find out the amount of sodium in all the foods you are eating.

Let's look at a typical day. Are the food choices familiar? Let's see how much sodium this sample day has in it.

SODIUM COUNTING
A SAMPLE DAY

Breakfast	SODIUM (MG)	CALORIES
tomato juice (½ cup)	428	21
cornflakes (1 oz)	351	110
lowfat milk (½ cup)	62	51
bran muffin	189	125
coffee	4	4
w/ half & half (2 tbsp)	12	40
Lunch		
tomato soup (1 cup)	932	160
ham & cheese sandwich		
ham, sliced (1 oz)	405	37
swiss cheese (1 oz)	74	107
rye bread (2 slices)	350	130
coleslaw (½ cup)	14	42
mineral water	tr	0
Snack		
doughnut	192	210
coffee	4	4
w/ half & half (2 tbsp)	12	40
Dinner		
chicken teriyaki (¾ cup)	2,190	399
peas, (canned, ½ cup)	186	59
tossed salad	27	16
french dressing (2 tbsp)	184	176
pound cake (1 slice)	96	120
tea	0	0
w/ sugar (1 tsp)	tr	25
TV Snack		
vanilla ice cream sandwich	220	140
TOTAL	5,932	2,016

This is too much sodium for one day—5,932 milligrams.
Now you can see how easy it is to eat too much.

SODIUM COUNTING
A SAMPLE DAY OF LOWER SODIUM FOOD CHOICES

Breakfast	SODIUM (MG)	CALORIES
orange juice (½ cup)	1	56
bran flakes (1 oz)	264	90
lowfat milk (½ cup)	62	51
toast (1 slice)	106	65
butter (1 tsp)	41	36
coffee	4	4
w/ half & half (2 tbsp)	12	40
Lunch		
hamburger w/ bun	387	275
catsup (1 tbsp)	178	16
french fries (10)	15	111
cola	14	151
Snack		
lowfat fruit yogurt (8 oz)	121	225
sugar cookie	66	58
Dinner		
roasted chicken breast, w/o skin		
(½ breast)	6	142
baked potato	tr	145
w/ sour cream (2 tbsp)	10	60
carrots (½ cup)	52	35
tossed salad	0	10
w/ oil & vinegar dressing (2		
tbsp)	tr	144
dinner roll	155	85
butter (1 tsp)	41	36
fruit cocktail, juice pack (½ cup)	4	56
tea	0	0
w/ sugar (1 tsp)	tr	25
TV Snack		
vanilla ice milk (½ cup)	53	92
TOTAL	1,592	2,008

Wise food choices! A much healthier intake of sodium for the day.

Aim for between 2,400 and 3,000 milligrams of sodium a day.

Now, it's *your* turn to count your salt. Note everything you eat today, then look up the sodium in each food you have eaten to see how much sodium you ate today. While you're at it, jot down the calories, too!

SODIUM COUNTING:
A SAMPLE WORKSHEET

FOOD	SODIUM (MG)	CALORIES
Breakfast		
Lunch		
Snack		
Dinner		
Snack		
	Total ____	Total ____

Aim for between 2,400 and 3,000 milligrams of sodium a day.

Did you eat more than 3,000 milligrams of sodium today? If you did, you're eating too much. Start right now to make lower sodium food choices.

USING YOUR SODIUM COUNTER

This book lists the salt and calorie content of more than 9,000 foods. For the first time, information about sodium values is at your fingertips. Now, you will find it easy to follow a low salt diet.

Before *The Sodium Counter*, it was impossible to compare so many foods at one time. When you want to pick a frozen dinner with less sodium, look up the dinner category, page 149. Fresh foods like meat, chicken, fish and cheese do not usually have labels. The same goes for take-out items like potato salad, coleslaw and ice cream, or foods bought at the bakery. How can you tell how much sodium there is in a burger or taco that you enjoy at the local fast food restaurant? *The Sodium Counter* lists them all!

The Sodium Counter is divided into two main sections. Part I, "Brand-Name and Generic Foods," lists foods alphabetically. For each group, you will find brand-name foods listed first in alphabetical order, followed by an alphabetical listing of generic foods. Large categories are divided into subcategories—canned, fresh, frozen, ready-to-use—to make it easier to find what you are looking for.

If you want to know how much sodium is in the hamburger you are having for lunch: look under HAMBURGER where you will find all kinds of hamburgers listed, or if you are making a hamburger at home, look under ROLL where you will find the hamburger roll listed alphabetically and under BEEF where you will find a cooked chopped-beef patty. For foods like FRENCH TOAST, BACON, or SALAD DRESSING, simply look for the specific food alphabetically in the complete listing. For example, FRENCH TOAST is on pages 173–74, listed alphabetically between FRENCH FRIES and FROSTING. Two slices have 514 milligrams of sodium.

If you are eating at home, simply look up the individual foods you are eating and total the sodium for the meal. For example, your dinner may consist of:

	SODIUM (mg)
rib lamb chop, broiled	64
Green Giant Broccoli Cuts	15
Ore Ida Cheddar Browns	330
Sealtest Free Vanilla Frozen Yogurt	45
Pepperidge Farm Chocolate Chip Cookie	60
glass of white wine	5
TOTAL SODIUM FOR THE MEAL =	519

If you are eating out, you'll find most food categories have a take-out subcategory. Items in the take-out subcategory will help you estimate the sodium and calories in similar restaurant or take-out menu items. For example, if you order spaghetti and meatballs, look under PASTA DINNERS on page 264.

Most foods are listed alphabetically. But, in some cases, foods are grouped by category. For example, all pasta dishes—like spaghetti and meat balls, lasagna, and manicotti—are under the category PASTA DINNERS.

Other group categories include:

DINNER   page 149
    includes all frozen dinners by brand name

ICE CREAM AND FROZEN DESSERT   page 198
    includes all dairy and nondairy ice cream
    and frozen novelties

Part II, Restaurant, Take-Out and Fast-Food Chains, contains an alphabetical listing of 31 popular chains. Fast foods like those of BURGER KING, DOMINO'S PIZZA, TACO BELL and WENDY'S are listed alphabetically under the chain's name. For example, McDONALD'S begins on page 444, between MACHEEZO MOUSE and NATHANS.

We have tried to include all foods for which sodium values are known. There will be some foods, however, that are not listed in *The Sodium Counter* because the sodium values are not available for those particular foods.

When you can't locate your favorite brand, look at other similar foods. You will probably find a brand-name food, a generic product, or a home recipe that is like your favorite food. For example: You find that your favorite brand of cinnamon bread is not listed. Look at the different cinnamon breads listed under BREAD, ready-to-eat, on page 29. From these entries you can quickly determine that one slice of cinnamon bread has from 100 to 120 milligrams of sodium. You can then assume that your favorite brand of cinnamon bread has a comparable amount.

With *The Sodium Counter* as your guide, you will never again wonder how much sodium is in a given food. You will always be able to tell if a food is high in sodium, moderate in sodium, or low in sodium. Your goal is to pick low-sodium foods each time you eat.

DEFINITIONS

as prep (as prepared): refers to food that has been prepared according to package directions

cooked: refers to food cooked without the addition of fat (oil, butter, margarine, etc.); steaming, poaching, broiling and dry roasting are examples of this type of preparation

generic: describes a food without a brand name

home recipe: describes homemade dishes; those included can be used as a guide to the sodium and calorie values of similar products you may prepare or take-out food you buy ready to eat

lean and fat: describes meat with some fat on its edges that is not cut away before cooking, or poultry prepared with skin and fat as purchased

lean only: describes a lean portion, trimmed of all visible fat

shelf stable or **shelf ready:** refers to prepared products found on the supermarket shelf that are ready to be heated and do not require refrigeration

take-out: describes prepared dishes that you purchase ready to eat; those included serve as a guide to the sodium and calorie values of similar products you may purchase

tr (trace): value used when a food contains less than one calorie or less than one mg of sodium

ABBREVIATIONS

avg	=	average
diam	=	diameter
frzn	=	frozen
g	=	gram
lb	=	pound
lg	=	large
med	=	medium
mg	=	milligram
oz	=	ounce
pkg	=	package
prep	=	prepared
pt	=	pint
qt	=	quart
reg	=	regular
sm	=	small
sq	=	square
tbsp	=	tablespoon
tr	=	trace
tsp	=	teaspoon
w/	=	with
w/o	=	without
"	=	inch
<	=	less than

EQUIVALENT MEASURES

1 tablespoon	=	3 teaspoons
4 tablespoons	=	¼ cup
8 tablespoons	=	½ cup
12 tablespoons	=	¾ cup
16 tablespoons	=	1 cup
1000 milligrams	=	1 gram
28 grams	=	1 ounce

LIQUID MEASUREMENTS

2 tablespoons	=	1 ounce
¼ cup	=	2 ounces
½ cup	=	4 ounces
¾ cup	=	6 ounces
1 cup	=	8 ounces
2 cups	=	1 pint
4 cups	=	1 quart

DRY MEASUREMENTS

16 ounces	=	1 pound
12 ounces	=	¾ pound
8 ounces	=	½ pound
4 ounces	=	¼ pound

ALL SODIUM VALUES OF FOODS ARE GIVEN IN MILLIGRAMS (MG).

Discrepancies in figures are due to rounding, product reformulation and reevaluation.

FOOD	PORTION	CALORIES	SODIUM

ABALONE

FRESH
| fried | 3 oz | 161 | 502 |
| raw | 3 oz | 89 | 255 |

ACEROLA

| acerola | 1 | 2 | 0 |

JUICE
| juice | 1 cup | 51 | 7 |

ADZUKI BEANS

CANNED
| sweetened | 1 cup | 702 | 646 |

DRIED
| Arrowhead | 2 oz | 190 | 3 |
| cooked | 1 cup | 294 | 18 |

READY-TO-USE
| yokan, sliced | 3¼" slice | 112 | 36 |

ALE
(see BEER AND ALE and MALT)

ALFALFA

Seeds (Arrowhead)	1 cup	40	tr
sprouts	1 cup	40	2
sprouts	1 tbsp	1	0

ALLSPICE

| ground | 1 tsp | 5 | 1 |

FOOD	PORTION	CALORIES	SODIUM

ALMONDS

FOOD	PORTION	CALORIES	SODIUM
Almond Butter (Erewhon)	1 tbsp	90	18
Almonds (Planters)	1 oz	170	0
Blanched Slivered (Dole)	1 oz	170	4
Blanched Whole (Dole)	1 oz	170	4
Chopped Natural (Dole)	1 oz	170	4
Honey Roasted (Planters)	1 oz	170	180
Sliced (Planters)	1 oz	170	0
Sliced Natural (Dole)	1 oz	170	4
Slivered (Planters)	1 oz	170	0
Whole Natural (Dole)	1 oz	170	4
almond butter honey & cinnamon	1 tbsp	96	2
w/ salt	1 tbsp	101	75
w/o salt	1 tbsp	101	2
almond meal	1 oz	116	2
almond paste	1 oz	127	3
dried, blanched	1 oz	166	3
dried, unblanched	1 oz	167	3
dry roasted, unblanched	1 oz	167	3
dry roasted, unblanched, salted	1 oz	167	260
oil roasted, blanched	1 oz	174	3
oil roasted, blanched, salted	1 oz	174	3
oil roasted, unblanched	1 oz	176	3
toasted, unblanched	1 oz	167	3

AMARANTH
(*see also* COOKIES)

FOOD	PORTION	CALORIES	SODIUM
Amaranth Cereal with Bananas (Health Valley)	½ cup	110	5

FOOD	PORTION	CALORIES	SODIUM
Amaranth Crunch with Raisins (Health Valley)	¼ cup	110	10
Amaranth Flakes 100% Organic (Health Valley)	½ cup	90	5
Fast Menu Amaranth with Garden Vegetables (Health Valley)	7½ oz	140	140
Seeds (Arrowhead)	2 oz	200	tr
cooked	½ cup	59	14
uncooked	½ cup	366	21

ANASAZI BEANS

DRIED Arrowhead	2 oz	200	4

ANCHOVY

CANNED in oil	1 can (1.6 oz)	95	1651
in oil	5	42	734
FRESH raw	3 oz	62	88

ANGLERFISH

raw	3½ oz	72	109

ANISE

seed	1 tsp	7	tr

ANTELOPE

roasted	3 oz	127	46

FOOD	PORTION	CALORIES	SODIUM

APPLE

CANNED
Apple Sauce

FOOD	PORTION	CALORIES	SODIUM
Natural Packed w/ Apple Juice (White House)	4 oz	60	5
Regular or Chunky (White House)	4 oz	80	5
Unsweetened (White House)	4 oz	50	0
100% Gravenstein, Sweetened (S&W)	½ cup	90	10
100% Gravenstein Unsweetened (S&W)	½ cup	55	5

Applesauce

FOOD	PORTION	CALORIES	SODIUM
Cinnamon (Tree Top)	½ cup	80	0
Diet (S&W)	½ cup	55	10
Natural (Tree Top)	½ cup	60	0
Original (Tree Top)	½ cup	80	0
Sweetened (S&W)	½ cup	55	10
Unsweetened (S&W)	½ cup	25	5
Cinnamon Applesauce (White House)	4 oz	100	5
Escalloped Apples (White House)	4 oz	120	10
Sliced (White House)	4 oz	55	10
Spiced Apple Rings (White House)	1 ring	25	0
sliced, sweetened	1 cup	136	7

applesauce

FOOD	PORTION	CALORIES	SODIUM
sweetened	½ cup	97	4
unsweetened	½ cup	53	2

DRIED
cooked

FOOD	PORTION	CALORIES	SODIUM
w/ sugar	½ cup	116	27
w/o sugar	½ cup	172	26

FOOD	PORTION	CALORIES	SODIUM
rings	10	155	56
FRESH			
Dole	1	80	0
apple	1	81	1
w/o skin			
sliced	1 cup	62	0
sliced & cooked	1 cup	91	1
sliced & microwaved	1 cup	96	1
FROZEN			
Apple Fritters (Mrs. Paul's)	2	270	500
sliced, w/o sugar	½ cup	41	3
JUICE			
Juice & More	8 oz	120	10
Kern's Cinnamon Nectar	6 oz	110	0
Libby's Nectar	6 oz	100	25
Ocean Spray	6 oz	90	10
S&W 100% Unsweetened	6 oz	85	5
Tree Top	6 oz	90	10
Cider	6 oz	90	10
Cider frzn, as prep	6 oz	90	10
frzn, as prep	6 oz	90	10
Unfiltered	6 oz	90	10
Unfiltered frzn, as prep	6 oz	90	10
w/ Vitamin C	6 oz	90	10
White House	6 oz	90	0
apple	1 cup	116	7
frzn, as prep	1 cup	111	17
frzn, not prep	6 oz	349	54

FOOD	PORTION	CALORIES	SODIUM

APRICOTS

CANNED
Halves

FOOD	PORTION	CALORIES	SODIUM
Diet (S&W)	½ cup	35	5
Unpeeled in Heavy Syrup (S&W)	½ cup	110	15
Unsweetened (S&W)	½ cup	35	5

Whole

FOOD	PORTION	CALORIES	SODIUM
Peeled, Diet (S&W)	½ cup	28	5
Peeled in Heavy Syrup (S&W)	½ cup	100	15
heavy syrup w/ skin	3 halves	70	3
juice pack w/ skin	3 halves	40	3
light syrup w/ skin	3 halves	54	3
water pack w/ skin	3 halves	22	2
w/o skin	4 halves	20	10

DRIED

FOOD	PORTION	CALORIES	SODIUM
halves	10	83	3
halves, cooked w/o sugar	½ cup	106	4

FRESH

FOOD	PORTION	CALORIES	SODIUM
apricots	3	51	1

FROZEN

FOOD	PORTION	CALORIES	SODIUM
sweetened	½ cup	119	5

JUICE

FOOD	PORTION	CALORIES	SODIUM
Kern's Nectar	6 oz	100	10
Libby's Nectar	6 oz	110	0
S&W Nectar	6 oz	35	20
nectar	1 cup	141	9

ARROWHEAD

FOOD	PORTION	CALORIES	SODIUM
fresh, boiled	1 med (⅓ oz)	9	2

FOOD	PORTION	CALORIES	SODIUM

ARROWROOT

| flour | 1 cup | 457 | 2 |

ARTICHOKE

CANNED
| Hearts Marinated (S&W) | ½ cup | 225 | 15 |

FRESH
Dole	1 lg	23	65
boiled	1 med (4 oz)	60	114
hearts, cooked	½ cup	42	80

FROZEN
| cooked | 1 pkg (9 oz) | 108 | 127 |

ARUGULA

| raw | ½ cup | 2 | 3 |

ASPARAGUS

CANNED
| Points Water Pack (S&W) | ½ cup | 17 | 10 |

Spears
| Colossal Fancy (S&W) | ½ cup | 20 | 320 |
| Fancy (S&W) | ½ cup | 18 | 320 |

FRESH
Dole	5 spears	18	0
cooked	½ cup	22	10
cooked	4 spears	14	7
raw	½ cup	16	2
raw	4 spears	14	1

FROZEN
| Harvest Fresh Cuts (Green Giant) | ½ cup | 25 | 60 |

FOOD	PORTION	CALORIES	SODIUM
cooked	1 pkg (10 oz)	82	12
cooked	4 spears	17	2

AVOCADO

FRESH

avocado	1	324	21
puree	1 cup	370	24

BACON

(*see also* BACON SUBSTITUTES)

Nathan's Beef Bacon, cooked	3 slices	100	310
breakfast strips, beef, cooked	3 strips (34 g)	153	766
cooked	3 strips	109	303
grilled	2 slices (1.7 oz)	86	719

BACON SUBSTITUTES

Bac-Os	2 tsp	25	90
bacon substitute	1 strip	25	117

BAGEL

FRESH

egg	1 (3½" diam)	200	245
plain	1 (3½" diam)	200	245

FROZEN

Bagel Sandwich Ham & Cheese (Weight Watchers)	1 (3 oz)	210	469
Cinnamon & Raisin (Sara Lee)	1 (3 oz)	240	280
Cinnamon Raisin (Sara Lee)	1 (2.5 oz)	200	230
Cinnamon'N Raisin (Lender's)	1	200	310
Egg (Lender's)	1	150	360

FOOD	PORTION	CALORIES	SODIUM
(Sara Lee)	1 (2.5 oz)	200	360
(Sara Lee)	1 (3 oz)	250	450
Ham & Cheese On A Bagel (Great Starts)	3 oz	240	600
Oat Bran			
(Sara Lee)	1 (2.5 oz)	180	360
(Sara Lee)	1 (3 oz)	220	450
Onion			
(Lender's)	1	160	290
(Sara Lee)	1 (2.5 oz)	190	450
(Sara Lee)	1 (3 oz)	230	560
Plain			
(Lender's)	1	150	320
(Sara Lee)	1 (2.5 oz)	190	460
(Sara Lee)	1 (3 oz)	230	580
Poppy Seed			
(Sara Lee)	1 (2.5 oz)	190	450
(Sara Lee)	1 (3 oz)	230	560
Sesame Seed			
(Sara Lee)	1 (2.5 oz)	190	440
(Sara Lee)	1 (3 oz)	240	550

BAKING POWDER

FOOD	PORTION	CALORIES	SODIUM
Clabber Girl	1 tsp	0	435
Davis	1 tsp	6	450
baking powder	1 tsp	5	329
low sodium	1 tsp	5	tr

BAKING SODA

FOOD	PORTION	CALORIES	SODIUM
Arm & Hammer	1 tsp	0	1368

FOOD	PORTION	CALORIES	SODIUM

BALSAM PEAR

leafy tips

cooked	½ cup	10	4
raw	½ cup	7	3
pods, cooked	½ cup	12	4

BAMBOO SHOOTS

CANNED

Empress Sliced	2 oz	14	10
La Choy	¼ cup	6	2
sliced	1 cup	25	9

FRESH

cooked	½ cup	15	5
raw	½ cup	21	3

BANANA

DRIED

powder	1 tbsp	21	0

FRESH

Dole	1	120	0
banana	1	105	1
mashed	1 cup	207	2

JUICE

Libby's Nectar	6 oz	110	15

BARLEY

Arrowhead	2 oz	200	tr
Arrowhead Barley Flakes	2 oz	200	1
Quaker			
Medium Pearled	¼ cup	172	0
Quick Pearled	¼ cup	172	0

FOOD	PORTION	CALORIES	SODIUM
Scotch			
Medium Pearled	¼ cup	172	0
Quick Pearled	¼ cup	172	0
Pearled			
cooked	½ cup	97	2
uncooked	½ cup	352	9

BASIL

FRESH			
chopped	2 tbsp	1	0
ground	1 tsp	4	tr
leaves	5	1	0

BASS

FRESH			
freshwater, raw	3 oz	97	59
sea			
cooked	3 oz	105	74
raw	3 oz	82	58
striped, baked	3 oz	105	75

BAY LEAF

crumbled	1 tsp	2	tr

BEAN SPROUTS
(see also individual bean names)

CANNED			
La Choy	⅔ cup	8	20

BEANS
(see also individual bean names)

Baked Beans			
(Brick Oven)	½ cup	160	560
(Van Camp's)	1 cup	260	1020

FOOD	PORTION	CALORIES	SODIUM
Barbecue Beans (Campbell)	½ can (7⅞ oz)	210	900
Texas Style (S&W)	½ cup	135	550
Beanee Weenee (Van Camp's)	1 cup	326	990
Big John's Beans 'n Fixin's (Hunt's)	4 oz	170	490
Boston Baked (Health Valley)	7½ oz	190	300
No Salt Added (Health Valley)	7½ oz	190	20
Brown Sugar Beans (Van Camp's)	1 cup	290	640
Chili (Gebhardt)	4 oz	115	580
Deluxe Baked Beans (Van Camp's)	1 cup	320	970
Fast Menu Honey Baked Organic Beans With Tofu Weiner (Health Valley)	7½ oz	150	140
Home Style Beans (Campbell)	½ can (8 oz)	220	820
Hot Chili Beans (Campbell)	½ can (7¾ oz)	180	870
Maple Sugar Beans (S&W)	½ cup	150	586
Mexican Style Chili Beans (Van Camp's)	1 cup	210	730
Mixed Bean Salad Marinated (S&W)	½ cup	90	730
Old Fashioned Beans in Molasses & Brown Sugar Sauce (Campbell)	½ can (8 oz)	230	730
Pork And Beans (Hunt's)	4 oz	135	430
(Van Camp's)	1 cup	216	1000
in Tomato Sauce (Campbell)	½ can (8 oz)	200	770
in Tomato Sauce (Green Giant)	½ cup	90	420
Pork 'N Beans (S&W)	½ cup	130	135
Refried (Gebhardt)	4 oz	100	490

FOOD	PORTION	CALORIES	SODIUM
(Rosarita)	4 oz	100	480
Jalapeno (Gebhardt)	4 oz	115	270
Spicy (Rosarita)	4 oz	100	500
Vegetarian (Rosarita)	4 oz	100	480
With Bacon (Rosarita)	4 oz	110	560
w/ Green Chilies (Rosarita)	4 oz	90	460
w/ Nacho Cheese (Rosarita)	4 oz	110	490
w/ Onions (Rosarita)	4 oz	110	490
Smokey Ranch Beans (S&W)	½ cup	130	569
Three Bean Salad (Green Giant)	½ cup	70	470
Vegetarian Beans (Campbell)	½ can (7¾ oz)	170	780
With Miso (Health Valley)	7½ oz	180	60
Vegetarian Style (Van Camp's)	1 cup	206	950
baked beans plain	½ cup	118	504
vegetarian	½ cup	118	504
w/ beef	½ cup	161	632
w/ franks	½ cup	182	551
w/ pork	½ cup	133	522
w/ pork & sweet sauce	½ cup	140	423
w/ pork & tomato sauce	½ cup	123	554
refried beans	½ cup	134	534
TAKE-OUT baked beans	½ cup	190	532
barbecue beans	3.5 oz	120	460
four bean salad	3.5 oz	100	280
refried beans	½ cup	43	104
three bean salad	¾ cup	230	500

FOOD	PORTION	CALORIES	SODIUM

BEAVER

roasted	3 oz	140	50
simmered	3 oz	141	39

BEEF

(*see also* BEEF DISHES, VEAL)

Beef is graded according to its marbling, the little flecks of fat in the muscle. Beef graded "Prime" has the highest percentage of fat, followed by "Choice" with less fat and "Select" with the least fat.

FRESH

Note that the values for cooked beef may differ slightly from the values for raw beef. When meat is cooked, some moisture and fat are lost, changing the nutrition value slightly. As a rule of thumb, it can be assumed that a 4-oz raw portion will equal a 3-oz cooked portion of meat.

Filet (Double J)	3.5 oz	130	54
NY Strip (Double J)	3.5 oz	133	57
Rib Eye (Double J)	3.5 oz	134	55
Top Butt (Double J)	3.5 oz	136	55
bottom round, lean & fat			
trim 0", braised	3 oz	193	43
trim 0" Choice, roasted	3 oz	172	56
trim 0" Select, braised	3 oz	171	43
trim 0" Select, roasted	3 oz	150	56
trim ¼" Choice, braised	3 oz	241	42
trim ¼" Choice, roasted	3 oz	221	53
trim ¼" Select, braised	3 oz	220	42
trim ¼" Select, roasted	3 oz	199	54
brisket flat half, lean & fat			
trim 0", braised	3 oz	183	53
trim ¼", braised	3 oz	309	48

FOOD	PORTION	CALORIES	SODIUM
brisket point half, lean & fat			
trim 0", braised	3 oz	304	57
trim ¼", braised	3 oz	343	55
brisket whole, lean & fat			
trim 0", braised	3 oz	247	55
trim ¼", braised	3 oz	327	52
chuck arm pot roast, lean & fat			
trim 0", braised	3 oz	238	53
trim ¼", braised	3 oz	282	51
chuck blade roast, lean & fat			
trim 0", braised	3 oz	284	56
trim ¼", braised	3 oz	293	55
corned beef brisket, cooked	3 oz	213	964
eye of round, lean & fat			
trim 0" Choice, roasted	3 oz	153	53
trim 0" Select, roasted	3 oz	137	53
trim ¼" Choice, roasted	3 oz	205	50
trim ¼" Select, roasted	3 oz	184	51
flank, lean & fat			
trim 0", braised	3 oz	224	60
trim 0", broiled	3 oz	192	69
ground			
extra lean, broiled medium	3 oz	217	59
extra lean, broiled well done	3 oz	225	70
extra lean, fried medium	3 oz	216	59
extra lean, fried well done	3 oz	224	69
extra lean, raw	4 oz	265	75
ground lean, broiled medium	3 oz	231	65
ground lean, broiled well done	3 oz	238	76
ground low-fat w/ carrageenan, raw	4 oz	160	70
ground regular, broiled medium	3 oz	246	70
ground regular, broiled well done	3 oz	248	79

FOOD	PORTION	CALORIES	SODIUM
porterhouse steak			
lean & fat, trim ¼" Choice, broiled	3 oz	260	52
lean only, trim ¼" Choice, broiled	3 oz	185	56
rib eye small end, lean & fat, trim 0" Choice, broiled	3 oz	261	54
rib large end, lean & fat			
trim 0", roasted	3 oz	300	55
trim ¼", broiled	3 oz	295	54
trim ¼", roasted	3 oz	310	54
rib small end, lean & fat			
trim 0", broiled	3 oz	252	54
trim ¼", broiled	3 oz	285	53
trim ¼", roasted	3 oz	295	53
rib whole, lean & fat			
trim ¼" Choice, broiled	3 oz	306	53
trim ¼" Choice, roasted	3 oz	320	53
trim ¼" Prime, roasted	3 oz	348	54
trim ¼" Select, broiled	3 oz	274	54
trim ¼" Select, roasted	3 oz	286	54
shank crosscut, lean & fat, trim ¼" Choice, simmered	3 oz	224	52
short loin top loin, lean & fat			
trim 0" Choice, broiled	1 steak (5.4 oz)	353	104
trim 0" Choice, broiled	3 oz	193	57
trim 0" Select, broiled	1 steak (5.4 oz)	309	104
trim ¼" Choice, broiled	1 steak (6.3 oz)	536	114
trim ¼" Choice, broiled	3 oz	253	54
trim ¼" Prime, broiled	1 steak (6.3 oz)	582	114
trim ¼" Select, broiled	1 steak (6.3 oz)	473	114
short loin top loin, lean only			
trim 0" Choice, broiled	1 steak (5.2 oz)	311	101

FOOD	PORTION	CALORIES	SODIUM
trim ¼" Choice, broiled	1 steak (5.2 oz)	314	100
shortribs, lean & fat, Choice, braised	3 oz	400	43
t-bone steak			
lean & fat, trim ¼" Choice, broiled	3 oz	253	52
lean only, trim ¼" Choice, broiled	3 oz	182	56
tenderloin, lean & fat			
trim 0" Choice, broiled	3 oz	208	52
trim 0" Select, broiled	3 oz	194	52
trim ¼" Choice, broiled	3 oz	259	50
trim ¼" Choice, roasted	3 oz	288	55
trim ¼" Prime, broiled	3 oz	270	50
trim ¼" Select, roasted	3 oz	275	48
tenderloin, lean only			
trim 0" Select, broiled	3 oz	170	54
trim ¼" Choice, broiled	3 oz	188	54
trim ¼" Select, broiled	3 oz	169	54
tip round, lean & fat			
trim 0" Choice, roasted	3 oz	170	54
trim 0" Select, roasted	3 oz	158	55
trim ¼" Choice, roasted	3 oz	210	53
trim ¼" Prime, roasted	3 oz	233	53
trim ¼" Select, roasted	3 oz	191	53
top round, lean & fat			
trim 0" Choice, braised	3 oz	184	38
trim 0" Select, braised	3 oz	170	38
trim ¼" Choice, braised	3 oz	221	38
trim ¼" Choice, broiled	3 oz	190	51
trim ¼" Choice, fried	3 oz	235	58
trim ¼" Prime, broiled	3 oz	195	51

FOOD	PORTION	CALORIES	SODIUM
top round, lean & fat *(cont.)*			
trim ¼" Select, braised	3 oz	199	38
trim ¼" Select, broiled	3 oz	175	51
top sirloin, lean & fat			
trim 0" Choice, broiled	3 oz	194	55
trim 0" Select, broiled	3 oz	166	55
trim ¼" Choice, broiled	3 oz	228	53
trim ¼" Choice, fried	3 oz	277	59
trim ¼" Select, broiled	3 oz	208	54
tripe raw	4 oz	111	52
FROZEN			
patties, broiled medium	3 oz	240	66
READY-TO-USE			
Weight Watchers Deli Thin Oven Roasted Cured	5 slices (⅓ oz)	10	85

BEEF DISHES

CANNED			
Beef Stew			
(Healthy Choice)	½ can (7.5 oz)	140	540
(Wolf Brand)	1 cup	179	1043
Manwich Mexican, as prep	1 sandwich	310	690
Sloppy Joe, as prep (Manwich)	1 sandwich	310	620
FROZEN			
Banquet Entree			
Beef Patties And Mushroom Gravy	7 oz	350	1190
Meatloaf w/ Tomato Sauce	7 oz	330	1330
Salisbury Steak And Gravy	7 oz	300	1310
Ovenstuffs Beef/Cheddar Deli Melt	1 (4.75 oz)	390	820

FOOD	PORTION	CALORIES	SODIUM
MIX			
Hamburger Helper			
Beef Noodle, as prep	1 cup	330	920
Beef Romanoff, as prep	1 cup	350	1070
Beef Taco, as prep	1 cup	330	970
Cheddar 'n Bacon, as prep	1 cup	380	970
Cheeseburger Macaroni, as prep	1 cup	370	1030
Cheesy Italian, as prep	1 cup	370	1040
Chili Macaroni, as prep	1 cup	330	960
Hamburger Hash, as prep	1 cup	320	1020
Hamburger Pizza Dish, as prep	1 cup	360	1010
Hamburger Stew, as prep	1 cup	300	1010
Lasagne, as prep	1 cup	340	910
Meat Loaf, as prep	5 oz	360	710
Nacho Cheese, as prep	1 cup	360	1050
Pizzabake, as prep	⅙ pkg (4.5 oz)	320	840
Potatoes Au Gratin, as prep	1 cup	350	900
Potatoes Stroganoff, as prep	1 cup	330	990
Rice Oriental, as prep	1 cup	340	1120
Sloppy Joe Bake, as prep	5 oz	340	1100
Spaghetti, as prep	1 cup	340	1100
Stroganoff, as prep	1 cup	390	870
Tacobake, as prep	⅙ pkg (5.75 oz)	320	940
Zesty Italian, as prep	1 cup	340	980
Lipton Microeasy			
Hearty Beef Stew	¼ pkg	71	729
Homestyle Meatloaf	¼ pkg	87	630
Manwich Seasoning Mix, as prep	1 sandwich	320	590

FOOD	PORTION	CALORIES	SODIUM
SHELF STABLE			
Beef Stew (Healthy Choice)	7.5 oz cup	140	540
TAKE-OUT			
roast beef			
sandwich plain	1	346	792
sandwich w/ cheese	1	402	1634
submarine sandwich w/ tomato, lettuce & mayonnaise	1	411	845
steak sandwich w/ tomato, lettuce, salt & mayonnaise	1	459	798
stew w/ vegetables	1 cup	220	292
stroganoff	¾ cup	260	503
swiss steak	4.6 oz	214	139

BEEFALO

FOOD	PORTION	CALORIES	SODIUM
roasted	3 oz	160	70

BEER AND ALE
(*see also* MALT)

FOOD	PORTION	CALORIES	SODIUM
Coors	12 oz	132	10
Extra Gold	12 oz	147	10
Light	12 oz	101	10
Killian's	12 oz	212	10
Old Milwaukee	12 oz	145	25
Light	12 oz	122	18
Schaefer	12 oz	138	23
Light	12 oz	111	16
Schlitz	12 oz	145	23
Light	12 oz	99	9
Signature	12 oz	150	21
Stroh	12 oz	142	23
Light	12 oz	115	11

FOOD	PORTION	CALORIES	SODIUM
Winterfest	12 oz	167	11
beer			
light	12 oz can	100	10
regular	12 oz can	146	19

BEETS

CANNED			
Diced Tender (S&W)	½ cup	40	270
Julienne, French Style (S&W)	½ cup	40	270
Pickled Whole, Extra Small (S&W)	½ cup	70	215
Pickled w/ Red Wine Vinegar, Sliced (S&W)	½ cup	70	215
Sliced, Small Premium (S&W)	½ cup	40	270
Sliced, Water Pack (S&W)	½ cup	35	40
Whole Small (S&W)	½ cup	40	270
harvard	½ cup	89	199
pickled	½ cup	75	301
FRESH			
beet greens			
cooked	½ cup	20	173
raw	½ cup	4	38
raw, chopped	½ cup	4	38
cooked	½ cup	26	42
raw, sliced	½ cup	30	49
JUICE			
beet juice	3½ oz	36	200

BEVERAGES

(*see* BEER AND ALE, COCOA, COFFEE, DRINK MIXERS, FRUIT DRINKS, LIQUOR/LIQUEUR, MALT, MILK DRINKS, MINERAL WATER/BOTTLED WATER, SODA, TEA/HERBAL TEA, WINE, WINE COOLER)

FOOD	PORTION	CALORIES	SODIUM
BISCUIT			
biscuit	1 (1 oz)	100	195
FROZEN			
Egg, Canadian Bacon & Cheese (Great Starts)	5.2 oz	420	1845
Sausage (Great Starts)	4.7 oz	410	1180
Sausage Biscuit (Weight Watchers)	3 oz	220	560
MIX			
Biscuit Mix (Arrowhead)	2 oz	100	116
Bisquick (General Mills)	½ cup	240	700
Buttermilk Biscuit Mix, not prep (Health Valley)	1 oz	100	170
biscuit	1 (1 oz)	95	262
REFRIGERATED			
1869 Brand			
Baking Powder	1	100	310
Butter Tastin'	1	100	300
Buttermilk	1	100	310
Ballard			
Ovenready	1	50	180
Ovenready Buttermilk	1	50	180
Big Country Southern Style	1	100	320
Hungry Jack			
Butter Tastin', Flaky	1	90	280
Buttermilk, Flaky	1	90	300
Buttermilk, Fluffy	1	90	280
Extra Rich, Buttermilk	1	50	180
Flaky	1	80	300
Honey Tastin', Flaky	1	90	290
Pillsbury			
Big Country Butter Tastin'	1	100	320

FOOD	PORTION	CALORIES	SODIUM
Big Country Buttermilk	1	100	320
Butter	1	50	180
Buttermilk	1	50	180
Country	1	50	180
Deluxe Heat N' Eat Buttermilk	2	170	530
Good N' Buttery, Fluffy	1	90	270
Hearty Grains Multi-Grain	1	80	230
Hearty Grains Oatmeal Raisin	1	90	210
Heat N' Eat Big Premium	2	280	610
Tender Layer Buttermilk	1	50	170
biscuit	1 (¾ oz)	65	249
TAKE-OUT			
plain	1	276	tr
w/ egg	1	315	655
w/ egg & bacon	1	457	999
w/ egg & sausage	1	582	1142
w/ egg & steak	1	474	888
w/ egg, cheese & bacon	1	477	1261
w/ ham	1	387	1433
w/ sausage	1	485	1071
w/ steak	1	456	795

BISON

roasted	3 oz	122	48

BLACK BEANS

CANNED			
Health Valley Fast Menu			
Organic Black Beans With Tofu Weiners	7½ oz	150	170
Western Black Beans With Garden Vegetable	7½ oz	160	250

FOOD	PORTION	CALORIES	SODIUM
DRIED			
Arrowhead Turtle	2 oz	190	10
cooked	1 cup	227	1

BLACKBERRIES

CANNED			
in heavy syrup	½ cup	118	3
FRESH			
blackberries	½ cup	37	0
FROZEN			
unsweetened	1 cup	97	2

BLACKEYE PEAS

CANNED			
Trappey's	½ cup	90	410
Jalapeno	½ cup	90	480
w/ pork	½ cup	199	840
DRIED			
cooked	1 cup	198	6

BLINTZE

TAKE-OUT			
cheese	2	186	268

BLUEBERRIES

CANNED			
in heavy syrup	1 cup	225	9
FRESH			
blueberries	1 cup	82	9
FROZEN			
unsweetened	1 cup	78	1

FOOD	PORTION	CALORIES	SODIUM

BLUEFIN

fillet, baked	4.1 oz	186	90

BLUEFISH

FRESH			
baked	3 oz	135	65

BOK CHOY

Dole shredded	½ cup	5	23

BORAGE

FRESH			
cooked, chopped	3½ oz	25	88
raw, chopped	½ cup	9	35

BOYSENBERRIES

CANNED			
in heavy syrup	1 cup	226	9
FROZEN			
unsweetened	1 cup	66	2
JUICE			
Smucker's	8 oz	120	10
Juice Sparkler	10 oz	130	5

BRAINS

beef			
pan-fried	3 oz	167	134
simmered	3 oz	136	102
lamb			
braised	3 oz	124	114
fried	3 oz	232	133

FOOD	PORTION	CALORIES	SODIUM
pork, braised	3 oz	117	77
veal			
braised	3 oz	115	133
fried	3 oz	181	150

BRAN

FOOD	PORTION	CALORIES	SODIUM
Fast Menu Oat Bran Pilaf With Garden Vegetables (Health Valley)	7½ oz	210	330
Oat Bran			
(Arrowhead)	1 oz	110	1
(Mother's)	⅓ cup	92	1
Quaker Unprocessed Bran	2 tbsp	8	0
Super Bran (H-O)	⅓ cup	110	0
Toasted Wheat Bran (Kretschmer)	⅓ cup	57	2
Wheat Bran (Arrowhead)	2 oz	50	3
corn	⅓ cup	56	2
oat, cooked	½ cup	44	1
oat, dry	½ cup	116	1
rice, dry	⅓ cup	88	1
wheat, dry	½ cup	65	1

BRAZIL NUTS

FOOD	PORTION	CALORIES	SODIUM
DRIED			
unblanched	1 oz	186	0

BREAD

(see also BAGEL, BISCUIT, BREADSTICKS, CROISSANT, ENGLISH MUFFIN, MUFFIN, ROLL, SCONE)

FOOD	PORTION	CALORIES	SODIUM
CANNED			
Brown Bread New England Recipe (S&W)	2 slices	76	172
boston brown	1 slice	95	113

FOOD	PORTION	CALORIES	SODIUM
HOME RECIPE			
datenut	1, ½" slice	92	63
hush puppies	5 (2.7 oz)	256	965
MIX			
Corn Bread			
(Ballard)	⅛ of bread	140	570
(Dromedary)	1 piece (2" × 2")	130	480
Easy Mix (Aunt Jemima)	⅙ cake	210	690
READY-TO-EAT			
7 Grain Hearty Slice (Pepperidge Farm)	2 slices	180	340
9 Grain & Nut (Matthew's)	1 slice	80	100
Crunchy Oat 1½ lb Loaf (Pepperidge Farm)	2 slices	190	290
Cinnamon			
(Matthew's)	1 slice	70	100
(Pepperidge Farm)	1 slice	90	110
Cinnamon Raisin (Weight Watchers)	1 slice	60	120
Cracked Wheat (Pepperidge Farm)	1 slice	70	140
Date Walnut (Pepperidge Farm)	1 slice	90	110
French			
Fully Baked (Pepperidge Farm)	2 oz	150	320
Twin (Pepperidge Farm)	1 oz	80	160
Golden (Matthew's)	1 slice	70	125
Hi-Fibre (Monks' Bread)	1 slice	50	110
Honey Bran (Pepperidge Farm)	1 slice	90	160
Italian			
Brown & Serve (Pepperidge Farm)	1 oz	80	150
Light (Wonder)	1 slice	40	115
Sliced (Pepperidge Farm)	1 slice	70	125

FOOD	PORTION	CALORIES	SODIUM
Malsovit	1 slice	66	146
Multi-Grain (Weight Watchers)	1 slice	40	100
Oat Bran			
(Matthew's)	1 slice	65	110
(Weight Watcher's)	1 slice	40	100
Oatmeal			
(Pepperidge Farm)	1 slice	70	160
1½ lb Loaf (Pepperidge Farm)	1 slice	90	200
Light (Pepperidge Farm)	1 slice	45	95
Very Thin Sliced (Pepperidge Farm)	1 slice	40	80
Pita, Whole Wheat (Matthew's)	1	210	390
Pumpernickel			
Family (Pepperidge Farm)	1 slice	80	230
Party (Pepperidge Farm)	4 slices	60	160
Raisin			
(Malsovit)	1 slice	77	146
(Monks' Bread)	1 slice	70	85
With Cinnamon (Pepperidge Farm)	1 slice	90	100
Rye			
(Weight Watchers)	1 slice	40	100
Dijon (Pepperidge Farm)	1 slice	50	180
Dijon Thick Sliced (Pepperidge Farm)	1 slice	70	260
Family (Pepperidge Farm)	3 oz	80	220
Party (Pepperidge Farm)	4 slices	60	250
Seedless Family (Pepperidge Farm)	1 slice	80	210
Soft (Pepperidge Farm)	1 slice	70	120
Sesame Wheat (Pepperidge Farm)	2 slices	190	340
Sodium Free (Matthew's)	1 slice	7	<5

FOOD	PORTION	CALORIES	SODIUM
Sourdough Light (Wonder)	1 slice	40	115
Sprouted Wheat (Pepperidge Farm)	1 slice	70	100
Sunflower & Bran (Monks' Bread)	1 slice	70	80
Vienna			
Light (Pepperidge Farm)	1 slice	45	100
Thick Sliced (Pepperidge Farm)	1 slice	70	125
1½ lb Loaf (Pepperidge Farm)	1 slice	90	190
Family (Pepperidge Farm)	1 slice	70	130
Wheat			
(Weight Watchers)	1 slice	40	100
Family (Wonder)	1 slice	70	150
Light (Pepperidge Farm)	1 slice	45	90
Light (Wonder)	1 slice	40	115
Very Thin Sliced (Pepperidge Farm)	1 slice	35	75
White			
(Monks' Bread)	1 slice	60	95
(Weight Watchers)	1 slice	40	100
(Wonder)	1 slice	70	150
White Country (Pepperidge Farm)	2 slices	190	340
White Large Family Thin Slice (Pepperidge Farm)	1 slice	70	150
White Light (Wonder)	1 slice	40	115
White Sandwich (Pepperidge Farm)	2 slices	130	260
White Thin Slice (Pepperidge Farm)	1 slice	80	130
White Toasting (Pepperidge Farm)	1 slice	90	200
White Very Thin Sliced (Pepperidge Farm)	1 slice	40	80
White Whole Special Recipe (Stroehmann)	1 slice	70	160

FOOD	PORTION	CALORIES	SODIUM
White Whole Special Recipe, Kids (Stroehmann)	1 slice	60	150
Whole Wheat (Matthew's)	1 slice	70	130
Whole Wheat Thin Slice (Pepperidge Farm)	1 slice	60	110
Whole Wheat 100% Stone Ground (Monks' Bread)	1 slice	70	110
Whole Wheat 100% Stoneground (Wonder)	1 slice	80	160
cracked wheat	1 slice	65	106
cracked wheat, toasted	1 slice	65	106
french	1 loaf (1 lb)	454	2633
french	1 slice (1.2 oz)	100	203
italian	1 loaf (1 lb)	454	2656
italian	1 slice (1 oz)	85	176
oatmeal	1 slice	65	124
pita	1 (2 oz)	165	339
pumpernickel	1 slice	80	177
raisin	1 slice	65	92
rye	1 slice	65	175
vienna	1 slice (.9 oz)	70	145
wheat	1 slice	65	138
white	1 slice	65	129
white, cubed	1 cup	80	154
whole wheat	1 slice	70	180
REFRIGERATED Pillsbury			
Crusty French Loaf	1" slice	60	120
Hearty Grains Country Oatmeal Twists	1	80	120
Hearty Grains Cracked Wheat Twists	1	80	120

FOOD	PORTION	CALORIES	SODIUM
Pipin' Hot Wheat Loaf	1" slice	70	170
Pipin' Hot White Loaf	1" slice	70	170
TAKE-OUT			
cornbread	2" × 2" piece (1.4 oz)	107	276
cornstick	1 (1.3 oz)	101	195

BREAD COATING

Golden Dipt			
Breading Frying Mix	1 oz	90	630
Chicken Frying Mix	1 oz	90	1430
Onion Ring Mix	1 oz	100	570
Mrs. Dash Crispy Coating Mix	½ oz	63	3

BREADCRUMBS

Jaclyn's			
Organic Whole Wheat Italian Style	½ oz	28	5
Organic Whole Wheat Plain	½ oz	28	5
dry	1 cup	390	736
fresh	1 cup	120	231

BREADFRUIT

fresh	¼ small	99	2

BREADSTICKS

Cheese (Angonoa)	1 oz	110	210
Garlic			
(Angonoa)	1 oz	120	160
(Keebler)	2	30	20
Italian (Angonoa)	1 oz	120	240
Low Sodium (Angonoa)	1 oz	120	15

FOOD	PORTION	CALORIES	SODIUM
Mini Cheese (Angonoa)	1 oz	110	160
Mini Pizza (Angonoa)	1 oz	120	220
Mini Sesame (Angonoa)	1 oz	120	200
Mini Whole Wheat (Angonoa)	1 oz	120	170
Onion (Angonoa)	1 oz	120	150
Onion (Keebler)	2	30	25
Plain (Keebler)	2	30	30
Sesame (Keebler)	2	30	30
Sesame Royale (Angonoa)	1 oz	120	200
Soft Bread Sticks (Pillsbury)	1	100	230
onion poppyseed (home recipe)	1	64	69

BREAKFAST BAR
(*see also* BREAKFAST DRINKS, NUTRITIONAL SUPPLEMENTS)

Apple (Nutri-Grain)	1 (1.3 oz)	150	65
Blueberry (Nutri-Grain)	1 (1.3 oz)	150	65
Raspberry (Nutri-Grain)	1 (1.3 oz)	150	65
Strawberry (Nutri-Grain)	1 (1.3 oz)	150	65

BREAKFAST DRINKS
(*see also* BREAKFAST BAR, NUTRITIONAL SUPPLEMENTS)

Instant Breakfast			
Chocolate, as prep w/ whole milk (Pillsbury)	1 serving	290	310
Chocolate Malt, as prep w/ whole milk (Pillsbury)	1 serving	290	310
Strawberry, as prep w/ whole milk (Pillsbury)	1 serving	290	300
Vanilla, as prep w/ whole milk (Pillsbury)	1 serving	300	330
orange drink			
powder	3 rounded tsp	93	4
powder, as prep w/ water	6 oz	86	9

FOOD	PORTION	CALORIES	SODIUM
BROAD BEANS			
CANNED			
broad beans	1 cup	183	1161
DRIED			
cooked	1 cup	186	8
FRESH			
cooked	3½ oz	56	41
BROCCOLI			
FRESH			
Dole	1 med spear	40	75
chopped, cooked	½ cup	22	20
chopped, raw	½ cup	12	12
FROZEN			
Broccoli With Cheese In Pastry (Pepperidge Farm)	1	230	380
Cuts (Green Giant)	½ cup	12	15
Harvest Fresh			
Cut (Green Giant)	½ cup	16	95
Spears (Green Giant)	½ cup	20	115
In Butter Sauce (Green Giant)	½ cup	40	350
In Cheese Sauce (Green Giant)	½ cup	60	530
Mini Spears (Green Giant Select)	4–5 spears	18	25
One Serve			
Cuts, In Butter Sauce (Green Giant)	1 pkg	45	10
Cuts, In Cheese Sauce (Green Giant)	1 pkg	70	660
Valley Combinations Broccoli Fanfare (Green Giant)	½ cup	80	340
chopped, cooked	½ cup	25	22
spears, cooked	½ cup	25	22
spears, cooked	10 oz pkg	69	60

FOOD	PORTION	CALORIES	SODIUM
BROWNIE			
FROZEN			
Brownie a la Mode (Weight Watchers)	1	180	150
Chocolate Brownie (Weight Watchers)	1 (1.25 oz)	100	150
Mint Frosted (Weight Watchers)	1 (1.23 oz)	100	130
Monterey Hot Fudge Chocolate Chunk Brownie (Pepperidge Farm)	1	480	200
Newport Hot Fudge Brownie (Pepperidge Farm)	1	400	160
HOME RECIPE			
w/ nuts	1 (.8 oz)	95	51
MIX			
Brownie With Hot Fudge MicroRave Single (Betty Crocker)	1	350	260
Deluxe Family Size Fudge Brownie (Pillsbury)	2″ sq	150	95
Deluxe Fudge Brownie (Pillsbury)	2″ sq	150	100
With Walnuts (Pillsbury)	2″ sq	150	90
Estee Brownie Mix	1 (2″ × 2″)	50	5
Frosted MicroRave (Betty Crocker)	1	180	120
Fudge			
Family Size (Betty Crocker)	1	150	100
Light (Betty Crocker)	1	100	90
MicroRave (Betty Crocker)	1	150	110
Microwave (Pillsbury)	1	190	105
Regular Size (Betty Crocker)	1	150	105
Supreme			
Caramel (Betty Crocker)	1	120	115

FOOD	PORTION	CALORIES	SODIUM
Chocolate Chip (Betty Crocker)	1	120	75
Frosted (Betty Crocker)	1	160	120
German Chocolate (Betty Crocker)	1	160	110
Original (Betty Crocker)	1	140	80
Party (Betty Crocker)	1	160	110
Walnut (Betty Crocker)	1	140	80
The Ultimate			
Caramel Fudge Chunk Brownie (Pillsbury)	2″ sq	170	105
Chunky Triple Fudge Brownie (Pillsbury)	2″ sq	170	105
Double Fudge Brownie (Pillsbury)	2″ sq	160	105
Rockey Road Fudge Brownie (Pillsbury)	2″ sq	170	95
Walnut MicroRave (Betty Crocker)	1	160	95
READY-TO-EAT			
Charlotte Fudgey Brownie (Pepperidge Farm)	1	220	105
Little Debbie	1 pkg (2 oz)	230	120
Tahoe Milk Chocolate Pecan (Pepperidge Farm)	1	210	100
Westport Fudgey Brownies w/ Walnuts (Pepperidge Farm)	1	220	105
w/ nuts	1 (1 oz)	100	59
w/o nuts	1 (2 oz)	243	153

BRUSSELS SPROUTS

FRESH			
Dole	½ cup	19	11
cooked	½ cup	30	17

FOOD	PORTION	CALORIES	SODIUM
cooked	1 sprout	8	4
raw	½ cup	19	11
raw	1 sprout	8	5
FROZEN			
Green Giant	½ cup	7	10
In Butter Sauce (Green Giant)	½ cup	40	280
cooked	½ cup	33	18

BUCKWHEAT

FOOD	PORTION	CALORIES	SODIUM
Buckwheat Groats			
Brown (Arrowhead)	2 oz	190	tr
White (Arrowhead)	2 oz	190	tr
groats, roasted			
cooked	½ cup	91	4
uncooked	½ cup	283	9

BUFFALO

FOOD	PORTION	CALORIES	SODIUM
water, roasted	3 oz	111	48

BULGUR

FOOD	PORTION	CALORIES	SODIUM
cooked	½ cup	76	5
uncooked	½ cup	239	12

BURBOT (FISH)

FOOD	PORTION	CALORIES	SODIUM
FRESH			
baked	3 oz	98	106

BURDOCK ROOT

FOOD	PORTION	CALORIES	SODIUM
cooked	1 cup	110	5
raw	1 cup	85	6

FOOD	PORTION	CALORIES	SODIUM

BUTTER
(*see also* BUTTER BLENDS, BUTTER SUBSTITUTES, MARGARINE)

REGULAR			
Cabot	1 tsp	35	41
Cabot Unsalted	1 tsp	35	0
Land O'Lakes	1 tsp	350	40
Land O'Lakes Unsalted	1 tsp	35	0
butter	1 pat	36	41
butter	1 stick (4 oz)	813	937
WHIPPED			
Land O'Lakes	1 tsp	25	25
Land O'Lakes Unsalted	1 tsp	24	0
butter	4 oz	542	625
butter	1 pat	27	31

BUTTER BEANS

CANNED			
S&W Tender Cooked	½ cup	100	440
Trappey's Large White	½ cup	80	410
Van Camp's	1 cup	162	710

BUTTER BLENDS
(*see also* BUTTER, BUTTER SUBSTITUTES, MARGARINE)

REGULAR			
Blue Bonnet			
Better Blend	1 tbsp	90	95
Better Blend Unsalted	1 tbsp	90	0
Country Morning			
Blend	1 tsp	35	35
Blend Unsalted	1 tsp	35	0
butter blend	1 stick	811	1013

FOOD	PORTION	CALORIES	SODIUM
SOFT			
Blue Bonnet Better Blend	1 tbsp	90	95
Country Morning			
Blend	1 tsp	30	25
Blend Light Tub	1 tsp	20	30
Blend Unsalted	1 tsp	30	0
Downey's			
Cinnamon Honey-Butter	1 tbsp	52	5
Original Honey-Butter	1 tbsp	52	5
Le Slim Cow	1 tbsp	40	15
Touch of Butter			
Stick	1 tbsp	90	110
Tub	1 tbsp	50	110

BUTTER SUBSTITUTES
(*see also* BUTTER BLENDS, MARGARINE)

FOOD	PORTION	CALORIES	SODIUM
Molly McButter	½ tsp	3	90
w/ Bacon	½ tsp	4	62
w/ Cheese	½ tsp	4	55
w/ Sour Cream	½ tsp	4	69

BUTTERBUR

FOOD	PORTION	CALORIES	SODIUM
CANNED			
fuki, chopped	1 cup	3	5
FRESH			
fuki, raw	1 cup	13	7

BUTTERFISH

FOOD	PORTION	CALORIES	SODIUM
baked	3 oz	159	97
fillet, baked	1 oz	47	29

FOOD	PORTION	CALORIES	SODIUM
BUTTERNUTS			
dried	1 oz	174	0
BUTTERSCOTCH			
(*see also* CANDY)			
Nestle Butterscotch Morsels	1 oz	150	25
CABBAGE			
FRESH			
Dole	1/12 med head	18	30
Dole Napa, shredded	½ cup	6	3
chinese pak-choi, raw, shredded	½ cup	5	23
chinese pak-choi, shredded, cooked	½ cup	10	29
chinese pe-tsai, raw, shredded	1 cup	12	7
chinese pe-tsai, shredded, cooked	1 cup	16	11
green, raw, shredded	½ cup	8	6
green, raw, shredded	1 head (2 lbs)	215	164
green, shredded, cooked	½ cup	16	14
red, raw, shredded	½ cup	10	4
red, shredded, cooked	½ cup	16	6
savoy, raw, shredded	½ cup	10	10
savoy, shredded, cooked	½ cup	18	17
HOME RECIPE			
coleslaw w/ dressing	¾ cup	147	267
TAKE-OUT			
coleslaw w/ dressing	½ cup	42	14
stuffed cabbage	1 (6 oz)	373	1007
vinegar & oil coleslaw	3.5 oz	150	480

FOOD	PORTION	CALORIES	SODIUM

CAKE

(*see also* BROWNIE, COOKIES, DANISH PASTRY, DOUGHNUTS, PIE)

FOOD	PORTION	CALORIES	SODIUM
FROSTING/ICING			
Butter Pecan Ready-to-Spread (Betty Crocker)	½12 tub	170	50
Cake & Cookie Decorator			
all colors except chocolate (Pillsbury)	1 tbsp	70	0
chocolate (Pillsbury)	1 tbsp	60	0
Cherry Ready-to-Spread (Betty Crocker)	½12 tub	160	50
Chocolate Chip Ready-to-Spread (Betty Crocker)	½12 tub	170	30
Chocolate Fudge (Pillsbury)	for ⅛ cake	110	65
Chocolate Fudge, as prep (Betty Crocker)	½12 mix	180	70
Chocolate Light Ready-to-Spread (Betty Crocker)	½12 tub	130	60
Chocolate Ready-to-Spread (Betty Crocker)	½12 tub	160	60
Chocolate With Candy Coated Chocolate Chips Ready-to-Spread (Betty Crocker)	½12 tub	160	60
Chocolate With Dinosaurs Ready-to-Spread (Betty Crocker)	½12 tub	160	60
Chocolate With Turbo Racers Ready-to-Spread (Betty Crocker)	½12 tub	160	60
Coconut Almond Frosting Mix (Pillsbury)	for ½12 cake	160	85
Coconut Pecan			
as prep (Betty Crocker)	½12 mix	180	50
Frosting Mix (Pillsbury)	for ½12 cake	150	105
Ready-to-Spread (Betty Crocker)	½12 tub	160	80

FOOD	PORTION	CALORIES	SODIUM
Cream Cheese Ready-to-Spread (Betty Crocker)	¹⁄₁₂ tub	170	70
Creamy Milk Chocolate, as prep (Betty Crocker)	¹⁄₁₂ mix	170	40
Creamy Vanilla, as prep (Betty Crocker)	¹⁄₁₂ mix	170	50
Dark Dutch Fudge Ready-to-Spread (Betty Crocker)	¹⁄₁₂ tub	160	70
Fluffy White Frosting Mix (Pillsbury)	for ¹⁄₁₂ cake	60	65
Frost It Hot Chocolate (Pillsbury)	for ⅛ cake	50	50
Frost It Hot Fluffy White (Pillsbury)	for ⅛ cake	50	50
Frosting Mix, as prep (Estee)	1½ tsp	50	0
Frosting Supreme (Pillsbury)			
Caramel Pecan	for ¹⁄₁₂ cake	160	70
Chocolate Chip	for ¹⁄₁₂ cake	150	70
Chocolate Fudge	for ¹⁄₁₂ cake	150	80
Chocolate Mint	for ¹⁄₁₂ cake	150	80
Coconut Almond	for ¹⁄₁₂ cake	150	60
Coconut Pecan	for ¹⁄₁₂ cake	160	60
Cream Cheese	for ¹⁄₁₂ cake	160	115
Double Dutch	for ¹⁄₁₂ cake	140	45
Lemon	for ¹⁄₁₂ cake	160	80
Milk Chocolate	for ¹⁄₁₂ cake	150	60
Mocha	for ¹⁄₁₂ cake	150	60
Sour Cream Vanilla	for ¹⁄₁₂ cake	160	80
Strawberry	for ¹⁄₁₂ cake	160	75
Vanilla	for ¹⁄₁₂ cake	160	75
Funfetti (Pillsbury)			
Chocolate Fudge	¹⁄₁₂ can	140	80
Vanilla Pink	¹⁄₁₂ can	150	70
Vanilla White	¹⁄₁₂ can	150	70

FOOD	PORTION	CALORIES	SODIUM
Lemon, Ready-to-Spread (Betty Crocker)	1/12 tub	170	70
Milk Chocolate			
Light, Ready-to-Spread (Betty Crocker)	1/12 tub	140	50
Ready-to-Spread (Betty Crocker)	1/12 tub	160	55
Rainbow Chip Ready-to-Spread (Betty Crocker)	1/12 tub	170	30
Sour Cream			
Chocolate, Ready-to-Spread (Betty Crocker)	1/12 tub	160	100
White, Ready-to-Spread (Betty Crocker)	1/12 tub	160	50
Vanilla			
(Pillsbury)	for 1/8 cake	120	60
Ready-to-Spread (Betty Crocker)	1/12 tub	160	30
Light, Ready-to-Spread (Betty Crocker)	1/12 tub	140	30
With Teddy Bears, Ready-to-Spread (Betty Crocker)	1/12 tub	160	25
White Fluffy, as prep (Betty Crocker)	1/12 mix	70	40
FROZEN			
Amhurst Apple Crumb Coffee Cake (Pepperidge Farm)	1	220	150
Apple 'N Spice Bake Dessert Lights (Pepperidge Farm)	1 piece (4 1/4 oz)	170	105
Apple Crisp			
(Weight Watchers)	1 (3.5 oz)	190	190
Light (Sara Lee)	1 (3 oz)	150	130
Apple Turnover (Pepperidge Farm)	1	300	210
Banana Single Layer, Iced (Sara Lee)	1 slice (1.7 oz)	170	160

FOOD	PORTION	CALORIES	SODIUM
Berkshire Apple Crisp (Pepperidge Farm)	1	250	130
Black Forest			
Light (Sara Lee)	1 (3.6 oz)	170	85
Two Layer (Sara Lee)	1 slice (2.5 oz)	190	100
Blueberry Turnovers (Pepperidge Farm)	1	310	230
Boston Cream Supreme (Pepperidge Farm)	1 piece (2⅞ oz)	290	190
Brownie Cheesecake (Weight Watchers)	1 (3.5 oz)	200	260
Butter Pound (Pepperidge Farm)	1 slice (1 oz)	130	150
Carrot			
Classic (Pepperidge Farm)	1 cake	260	280
Light (Sara Lee)	1 (2.5 oz)	170	75
Single Layer Iced (Sara Lee)	1 slice (2.4 oz)	250	240
w/ Cream Cheese Icing (Pepperidge Farm)	1 slice (1½ oz)	150	160
Charleston Peach Melba Shortcake (Pepperidge Farm)	1	220	170
Cheesecake (Sara Lee)			
Original Cherry	1 slice (3.2 oz)	243	184
Original Plain	1 slice (2.8 oz)	230	153
Original Strawberry	1 slice (3.2 oz)	222	171
Cherries And Cream Cake (Weight Watchers)	1 (3 oz)	150	200
Cherries Supreme Dessert Lights (Pepperidge Farm)	1 piece (3¼ oz)	170	35
Cherry Turnover (Pepperidge Farm)	1	310	280
Chocolate Cake (Weight Watchers)	1 (2.5 oz)	180	250
Chocolate Eclair (Weight Watchers)	1 (2.1 oz)	120	110

FOOD	PORTION	CALORIES	SODIUM
Chocolate Free & Light (Sara Lee)	1 slice (1.7 oz)	110	140
Chocolate Fudge Large Layer (Pepperidge Farm)	1 slice (1⅝ oz)	180	140
Chocolate Fudge Strip, Large Layer (Pepperidge Farm)	1 piece (1⅝ oz)	170	140
Chocolate Mousse Cake Dessert Lights (Pepperidge Farm)	1 piece (2½ oz)	190	260
Chocolate Supreme (Pepperidge Farm)	1 piece (2⅞ oz)	300	140
Cholesterol Free Pound (Pepperidge Farm)	1 slice (1 oz)	110	85
Coconut			
Classic (Pepperidge Farm)	1 cake	230	160
Large Layer (Pepperidge Farm)	1 slice (1⅝ oz)	180	120
Coffee Cake			
All Butter Butter Streusel (Sara Lee)	1 slice (1.4 oz)	160	160
All Butter Cheese (Sara Lee)	1 slice (2 oz)	210	220
All Butter Pecan (Sara Lee)	1 slice (1.4 oz)	160	180
Devil's Food Large Layer (Pepperidge Farm)	1 slice (1⅝ oz)	180	135
Double Chocolate			
Classic (Pepperidge Farm)	1 cake	250	180
Light (Sara Lee)	1 (2.5 oz)	150	85
Three Layer (Sara Lee)	1 slice (2.2 oz)	220	130
Double Fudge (Weight Watchers)	1 piece (2.75 oz)	190	150
Elfin Loaves			
Apple Cinnamon	1	180	260
Banana	1	190	260
Blueberry	1	170	220
Carrot	1	210	170
French Cheesecake Light (Sara Lee)	1 (3.2 oz)	150	90

FOOD	PORTION	CALORIES	SODIUM
French Cheese (Sara Lee)	1 slice (2.9 oz)	250	120
Fruit Squares (Pepperidge Farm)			
Apple	1	220	170
Cherry	1	230	180
Fudge Golden Classic (Pepperidge Farm)	1 cake	260	160
German Chocolate			
Classic (Pepperidge Farm)	1 cake	250	230
Large Layer (Pepperidge Farm)	1 slice (1⅝ oz)	180	170
Golden Large Layer (Pepperidge Farm)	1 slice (1⅝ oz)	180	110
Lemon Cake Supreme Dessert Lights (Pepperidge Farm)	1 piece (2¾ oz)	170	100
Lemon Coconut Supreme (Pepperidge Farm)	1 piece (3 oz)	280	220
Lemon Cream			
Light (Sara Lee)	1 (3.2 oz)	180	60
Supreme (Pepperidge Farm)	1 piece (1⅝ oz)	170	120
Manhattan Strawberry Cheesecake (Pepperidge Farm)	1	300	250
Peach Parfait Dessert Lights (Pepperidge Farm)	1 piece (4¼ oz)	150	70
Peach Melba Supreme (Pepperidge Farm)	1 (3⅛ oz)	270	135
Peach Turnover (Pepperidge Farm)	1	310	260
Pineapple Cream Supreme (Pepperidge Farm)	1 piece (2 oz)	190	130
Pound (Sara Lee)			
All Butter Family Size	1 slice (1 oz)	130	85
All Butter Original	1 slice (1 oz)	130	85
Free & Light	1 slice (1 oz)	70	105
Raspberry			
Turnovers (Pepperidge Farm)	1	310	260

FOOD	PORTION	CALORIES	SODIUM
Raspberry Vanilla Swirl, Dessert Lights (Pepperidge Farm)	1 piece (3¼ oz)	160	140
Strawberry Cheesecake (Weight Watchers)	1 piece (3.9 oz)	180	210
Strawberry Cream Supreme (Pepperidge Farm)	1 piece (2 oz)	190	120
Strawberry French Cheesecake Light (Sara Lee)	1 (3.5 oz)	150	65
Strawberry Shortcake, Dessert Lights (Pepperidge Farm)	1 piece (3 oz)	170	50
Strawberry Shortcake Two Layer (Sara Lee)	1 slice (2.5 oz)	190	90
Strawberry Strip Large Layer (Pepperidge Farm)	1 piece (1½ oz)	160	120
Strawberry Yogurt Dessert Free & Light (Sara Lee)	1 slice (2.2 oz)	120	90
Vanilla Large Layer (Pepperidge Farm)	1 slice (1⅝ oz)	190	120
Vanilla Fudge Swirl Classic (Pepperidge Farm)	1 cake	250	160
HOME RECIPE			
carrot w/ cream cheese icing	1 cake 10″ diam	6175	4470
carrot w/ cream cheese icing	¹⁄₁₆ of cake	385	279
fruitcake, dark	1 cake 7½″ × 2¼″	5185	2123
fruitcake, dark	⅔″ slice	165	67
pound cake	1 loaf 8½″ × 3½″	1935	1645
pound cake	1 slice (1 oz)	120	96
sheet cake			
w/ white frosting	1 cake 9″ sq	4020	2488
w/ white frosting	⅑ of cake	445	275
w/o frosting	1 cake 9″ sq	2830	2331

FOOD	PORTION	CALORIES	SODIUM
w/o frosting	⅑ of cake	315	258
MIX			
Angel Food (Betty Crocker)			
Confetti	¹⁄₁₂ cake	150	300
Lemon Custard	¹⁄₁₂ cake	150	300
Traditional	¹⁄₁₂ cake	130	170
White	¹⁄₁₂ cake	150	300
Apple Cinnamon Coffee Cake (Pillsbury)	⅛ cake	240	150
Apple Streusel			
MicroRave (Betty Crocker)	⅙ cake	240	190
No Cholesterol Recipe (Betty Crocker)	⅙ cake	210	200
Banana Quick Bread (Pillsbury)	¹⁄₁₂ loaf	170	200
Blueberry Nut Quick Bread (Pillsbury)	¹⁄₁₂ loaf	150	150
Butter Chocolate (Betty Crocker)	¹⁄₁₂ cake	280	400
Butter Pecan			
No Cholesterol Recipe (Betty Crocker)	¹⁄₁₂ cake	220	320
SuperMoist (Betty Crocker)	¹⁄₁₂ cake	250	320
Butter Recipe (Pillsbury Plus)	¹⁄₁₂ cake	260	370
Butter Yellow (Betty Crocker)	¹⁄₁₂ cake	260	340
Carrot			
(Betty Crocker)	¹⁄₁₂ cake	250	300
(Dromedary)	¹⁄₁₂ cake	232	292
(Estee)	¹⁄₁₀ cake	100	65
No Cholesterol Recipe (Betty Crocker)	¹⁄₁₂ cake	210	300
Cheese Cake (Royal)			
Lite No-Bake	⅛ pie	130	230
Real No-Bake	⅛ pie	160	250
Cherry Chip (Betty Crocker)	¹⁄₁₂ cake	190	270

FOOD	PORTION	CALORIES	SODIUM
Cherry Nut Quick Bread (Pillsbury)	1/12 loaf	180	150
Chocolate (Estee)	1/10 cake	100	100
Chocolate Chocolate Chip (Betty Crocker)	1/12 cake	260	400
Chocolate Microwave (Pillsbury)	1/8 cake	210	260
Chocolate Pudding Classic Dessert (Betty Crocker)	1/6 cake	230	250
Chocolate With Chocolate Frosting (Pillsbury)	1/8 cake	300	310
Chocolate With Vanilla Frosting (Pillsbury)	1/8 cake	300	300
Chocolate Chip			
(Betty Crocker)	1/12 cake	290	300
(Pillsbury Plus)	1/12 cake	270	290
No Cholesterol Recipe (Betty Crocker)	1/12 cake	220	300
Chocolate Fudge (Betty Crocker)	1/12 cake	260	450
Cinnamon Pecan Streusel			
Microwave (Betty Crocker)	1/6 cake	280	220
No Cholesterol (Betty Crocker)	1/6 cake	230	220
Cobbler (Dromedary)			
Apple Crumb	1/8 of cake	237	490
Cherry Crumb	1/8 of cake	231	160
Coffee Cake Easy Mix (Aunt Jemima)	1/8 cake	160	290
Cranberry Quick Bread (Pillsbury)	1/12 loaf	160	200
Date Quick Bread (Pillsbury)	1/12 loaf	160	150
Date Nut (Dromedary)	1/12 of cake	183	248
Date Nut Roll (Dromedary)	1/2" slice	80	160
Devil's Food (Betty Crocker)	1/12 cake	260	430
Devil's Food (Pillsbury Plus)	1/12 cake	270	370
Devil's Food Chocolate Frosting MicroRave (Betty Crocker)	1/6 cake	310	250

FOOD	PORTION	CALORIES	SODIUM
Devil's Food No Cholesterol Recipe (Betty Crocker)	1/12 cake	220	430
Devil's Food SuperMoist Light (Betty Crocker)	1/12 cake	200	340
Devil's Food SuperMoist Light No Cholesterol Recipe (Betty Crocker)	1/12 cake	180	370
Devil's Food With Chocolate Frosting MicroRave Single (Betty Crocker)	1	440	480
Double Chocolate Supreme Microwave (Pillsbury)	1/8 cake	330	340
Double Lemon Supreme Microwave (Pillsbury)	1/8 cake	300	210
Fudge Marble (Pillsbury Plus)	1/12 cake	270	300
German Chocolate (Betty Crocker)	1/12 cake	260	420
No Cholesterol Recipe (Betty Crocker)	1/12 cake	220	420
Chocolate Frosting MicroRave (Betty Crocker)	1/8 cake	320	250
Gingerbread (Dromedary)	1 piece 2" × 2"	100	190
(Pillsbury)	3" sq	190	310
Classic Dessert (Betty Crocker)	1/8 cake	22	330
Classic Dessert No Cholesterol Recipe (Betty Crocker)	1/8 cake	21	330
Golden Pound Classic Dessert (Betty Crocker)	1/12 cake	200	170
Golden Vanilla (Betty Crocker)	1/12 cake	280	270
No Cholesterol Recipe (Betty Crocker)	1/12 cake	220	270
Rainbow Chip Frosting MicroRave (Betty Crocker)	1/8 cake	320	230

FOOD	PORTION	CALORIES	SODIUM
Lemon			
(Betty Crocker)	1/12 cake	260	280
(Estee)	1/10 cake	100	67
(Pillsbury Plus)	1/12 cake	250	290
Microwave (Pillsbury)	1/8 cake	220	180
No Cholesterol Recipe (Betty Crocker)	1/12 cake	220	280
Lemon Pudding Classic Dessert (Betty Crocker)	1/6 cake	230	270
Lemon Cake With Lemon Frosting (Pillsbury)	1/8 cake	300	220
Lemon Chiffon Classic Dessert (Betty Crocker)	1/12 cake	200	200
Marble			
(Betty Crocker)	1/12 cake	260	290
No Cholesterol Recipe (Betty Crocker)	1/12 cake	220	290
Milk Chocolate			
(Betty Crocker)	1/12 cake	260	340
No Cholesterol Recipe (Betty Crocker)	1/12 cake	210	340
Nut Quick Bread (Pillsbury)	1/12 loaf	170	190
Pineapple Upsidedown Classic Dessert (Betty Crocker)	1/9 cake	250	210
Pound			
(Dromedary)	1/2" slice	150	160
(Estee)	1/10 cake	100	77
Rainbow Chip (Betty Crocker)	1/12 cake	250	320
Sour Cream			
Chocolate (Betty Crocker)	1/12 cake	260	430
Chocolate No Cholesterol Recipe (Betty Crocker)	1/12 cake	220	430
White (Betty Crocker)	1/12 cake	180	290
Spice			
(Betty Crocker)	1/12 cake	260	320

FOOD	PORTION	CALORIES	SODIUM
No Cholesterol Recipe (Betty Crocker)	1/12 cake	220	320
Streusel Swirl			
Cinnamon (Pillsbury)	1/16 cake	260	200
Cinnamon Microwave (Pillsbury)	1/8 cake	240	180
Lemon (Pillsbury)	1/16 cake	270	340
Tunnel of Fudge Bundt Microwave (Pillsbury)	1/8 cake	290	320
White			
(Betty Crocker)	1/12 cake	240	270
(Estee)	1/10 cake	100	67
(Pillsbury Plus)	1/12 cake	240	290
No Cholesterol Recipe (Betty Crocker)	1/12 cake	220	270
SuperMoist Light (Betty Crocker)	1/12 cake	180	330
Yellow			
(Betty Crocker)	1/12 cake	260	300
(Pillsbury Plus)	1/12 cake	260	300
Chocolate Frosting MicroRave (Betty Crocker)	1/6 cake	300	220
Microwave (Pillsbury)	1/8 cake	220	170
No Cholesterol Recipe (Betty Crocker)	1/12 cake	220	300
SuperMoist Light (Betty Crocker)	1/12 cake	200	310
SuperMoist Light No Cholesterol Recipe (Betty Crocker)	1/12 cake	190	330
With Chocolate Frosting (Pillsbury)	1/8 cake	300	220
With Chocolate Frosting MicroRave, Single (Betty Crocker)	1	440	500

FOOD	PORTION	CALORIES	SODIUM
angelfood	1 cake 9¾" diam	1510	3226
angelfood	¹⁄₁₂ of cake	125	269
crumb coffeecake	1 cake 7¾" × 5⅝"	1385	1853
crumb coffeecake	⅙ of cake	230	310
devil's food w/ chocolate frosting	1 cake 9" diam	3755	2900
devil's food w/ chocolate frosting	¹⁄₁₆ of cake	235	181
gingerbread	1 cake 8" sq	1575	1733
gingerbread	⅑ cake	175	192
yellow w/ chocolate frosting	1 cake 9" diam	3735	2515
yellow w/ chocolate frosting	¹⁄₁₆ of cake	235	157
READY-TO-USE			
cheesecake	1 cake 9" diam	3350	2464
cheesecake	¹⁄₁₂ of cake	280	204
pound cake	1 cake 8½ × 3½ × 3	1935	1857
pound cake	1 slice (1 oz)	110	108
white w/ white frosting	1 cake 9" diam	4170	2827
white w/ white frosting	¹⁄₁₆ cake	260	176
yellow w/ chocolate frosting	1 cake 9" diam	3895	3080
yellow w/ chocolate frosting	¹⁄₁₆ cake	245	192
REFRIGERATED			
Apple Turnovers (Pillsbury)	1	170	330
Cheesecake (Baby Watson)	1 pkg (4 oz)	420	480
Cherry Turnovers (Pillsbury)	1	170	320

FOOD	PORTION	CALORIES	SODIUM
Coffee Cake (Pillsbury)			
Cinnamon Swirl	⅛ of cake	180	170
Pecan Streusel	⅛ of cake	180	170
Pastry Pockets	1	240	520
SNACK			
All Butter Pound (Sara Lee)	1	200	190
Apple Delights (Little Debbie)	1 pkg (1.25 oz)	160	105
Apple Light & Fruity (Drake)	1 (1.2 oz)	90	110
Apple Spice (Little Debbie)	1 pkg (2.2 oz)	300	200
Banana Slices (Little Debbie)	1 pkg (3 oz)	380	240
Banana Twins (Little Debbie)	1 pkg (2.2 oz)	280	170
Be My Valentine (Little Debbie)	1 pkg (2.2 oz)	290	120
Blueberry Light & Fruity (Drake)	1 (1.2 oz)	90	95
Cherry Cordials (Little Debbie)	1 pkg (1.3 oz)	180	85
Choc-O-Jel (Little Debbie)	1 pkg (1.16 oz)	170	100
Choco-Cakes (Little Debbie)	1 pkg (2.17 oz)	270	220
Chocolate Chip (Little Debbie)	1 pkg (2.4 oz)	310	180
Chocolate Fudge Cake (Sara Lee)	1	190	125
Chocolate Slices (Little Debbie)	1 pkg (3 oz)	360	310
Chocolate Twins (Little Debbie)	1 pkg (2.2 oz)	260	220
Christmas Tree Cakes (Little Debbie)	1 pkg (1.5 oz)	200	95
Cinnamon Raisin Light & Fruity (Drake)	1 (1.2 oz)	90	105
Classic Cheesecake (Sara Lee)	1	200	150
Coconut (Little Debbie)	1 pkg (2.17 oz)	310	130
Coconut Crunch (Little Debbie)	1 pkg (2 oz)	340	50
Coconut Rounds (Little Debbie)	1 pkg (1.13 oz)	160	85
Coffee Cake			
(Drake's)	1 (1.1 oz)	140	90
(Little Debbie)	1 pkg (2 oz)	220	210

FOOD	PORTION	CALORIES	SODIUM
Coffee Cake *(cont.)*			
Apple Cinnamon (Sara Lee)	1	290	270
Butter Streusel (Sara Lee)	1	230	270
Chocolate Crumb (Drake's)	1 (2.5 oz)	245	206
Cinnamon Crumb (Drake's)	¹⁄₁₂ cake (1.3 oz)	150	110
Pecan (Sara Lee)	1	280	270
Small (Drake's)	1 (2 oz)	220	160
Deluxe Carrot Cake (Sara Lee)	1	180	200
Devil Cremes (Little Debbie)	1 pkg (1.3 oz)	170	170
Devil Dog (Drake's)	1 (1.5 oz)	160	135
Devil Squares (Little Debbie)	1 pkg (2.2 oz)	300	135
Easter Bunny Cakes (Little Debbie)	1 pkg (2.5 oz)	320	140
Easter Puffs (Little Debbie)	1 pkg (1.25 oz)	150	60
Fancy Cakes (Little Debbie)	1 pkg (2.4 oz)	310	135
Figaroos (Little Debbie)	1 pkg (1.5 oz)	160	105
Fudge Crispy (Little Debbie)	1 pkg (2.08 oz)	330	55
Fudge Rounds (Little Debbie)	1 pkg (1.19 oz)	150	75
Funny Bones (Drake's)	1 (1.25 oz)	150	110
Golden Cremes (Little Debbie)	1 pkg (1.47 oz)	160	150
Holiday Cakes			
Chocolate (Little Debbie)	1 pkg (2.4 oz)	330	135
Vanilla (Little Debbie)	1 pkg (2.5 oz)	350	160
Jelly Rolls (Little Debbie)	1 pkg (2.17 oz)	240	140
Lemon Stix (Little Debbie)	1 pkg (1.5 oz)	220	60
Marshmallow Supremes (Little Debbie)	1 pkg (1.25 oz)	150	65
Mint Sprints (Little Debbie)	1 pkg (1.5 oz)	240	45
Nutty Bar (Little Debbie)	1 pkg (2 oz)	320	80
Pecan Twins (Little Debbie)	1 pkg (2 oz)	220	170

FOOD	PORTION	CALORIES	SODIUM
Pop-Tarts			
Apple Cinnamon	1	210	170
Blueberry	1	210	210
Brown Sugar Cinnamon	1	210	200
Cherry	1	210	220
Chocolate Graham	1	210	220
Frosted Brown Sugar Cinnamon	1	210	190
Frosted Cherry	1	210	220
Frosted Chocolate Vanilla Creme	1	200	230
Frosted Chocolate Fudge	1	200	220
Frosted Grape	1	200	200
Frosted Raspberry	1	200	210
Frosted Strawberry	1	200	190
Strawberry	1	210	200
Pound Cake (Drake's)	1/10 cake	110	70
Pumpkin Delights (Little Debbie)	1 pkg (1.13 oz)	140	110
Ring Ding (Drake's)	1 (1.5 oz)	180	115
Ring Ding Mint (Drake's)	1 (1.5 oz)	190	115
Snack Cake			
Chocolate (Little Debbie)	1 pkg (2.5 oz)	340	140
Vanilla (Little Debbie)	1 pkg (2.6 oz)	360	160
Star Crunch (Little Debbie)	1 pkg (1.08 oz)	150	75
Sunny Doodle (Drake's)	1 (1 oz)	100	100
Swiss Cake Roll (Little Debbie)	1 pkg (2.17 oz)	270	130
Toaster Tart (Pepperidge Farm)			
Apple Cinnamon	1	170	120
Cheese	1	190	180
Strawberry	1	190	120

FOOD	PORTION	CALORIES	SODIUM
Toastettes (Nabisco)			
Apple	1	190	170
Blueberry	1	190	200
Cherry	1	190	200
Frosted Apple	1	190	170
Frosted Blueberry	1	190	200
Frosted Brown Sugar Cinnamon	1	190	180
Frosted Cherry	1	190	200
Frosted Fruit Punch	1	190	200
Frosted Fudge	1	200	280
Frosted Strawberry	1	190	200
Strawberry	1	190	200
Vanilla Cremes (Little Debbie)	1 pkg (1.3 oz)	160	140
Yankee Doodle (Drake's)	1 (1 oz)	100	110
Yodel's (Drake's)	1 (1 oz)	150	65
devil's food cupcake w/ chocolate frosting	1	120	92
devil's food w/ creme filling	1 (1 oz)	105	105
sponge w/ creme filling	1 (1.5 oz)	155	155
toaster pastries	1 (1.9 oz)	210	248
TAKE-OUT			
baklava	1 oz	126	78
strudel	1 piece (4.1 oz)	272	142

CANADIAN BACON

unheated	2 slices (1.9 oz)	89	799

CANDY
(see also MARSHMALLOW)

5th Avenue	1 (2.1 oz)	290	140

FOOD	PORTION	CALORIES	SODIUM
After Eight Dark Chocolate Wafer Thin Mints (Rowntree)	1	35	0
Almond Joy	1 (1.76 oz)	250	70
Alpine White Bar w/ Almonds (Nestle)	1.25 oz	200	30
Baby Ruth	2.2 oz	300	130
Bar None	1.5 oz	240	50
Bit-O-Honey	1.7 oz	200	125
Breath Savers Sugar Free Cinnamon	1 candy	2	0
Peppermint	1 candy	2	0
Spearmint	1 candy	2	0
Wintergreen	1 candy	2	0
Butter Mints (Kraft)	1	8	0
Butterfinger	2.1 oz	280	105
Caramel Nip (Pearson)	1 oz	120	70
Caramello	1 (1.6 oz)	220	60
Caramels (Kraft)	1	30	25
Chocolate (Estee)	1	30	15
Vanilla (Estee)	1	30	15
Chocolate Bar Almond (Estee)	2 sq	60	10
Coconut (Estee)	2 sq	60	10
Fruit & Nut (Estee)	2 sq	60	10
Peanut (Estee)	2 sq	60	10
Chocolate Coated Raisins (Estee)	10 pieces	30	10
Chocolate Fudgies (Kraft)	1	35	25
Chocolate Parfait (Pearson)	1 oz	120	70
Chunky	1.4 oz	210	20
Coffee Nip (Pearson)	1 oz	120	70

FOOD	PORTION	CALORIES	SODIUM
Coffico Mocha Parfait (Pearson)	1 oz	120	70
Crunch Chocolate Bar (Estee)	2 sq	45	20
Dark Chocolate Bar (Estee)	2 sq	60	0
Dark Chocolate Mint Bar (Estee)	2 sq	60	0
Estee-ets (Estee)	5 pieces	35	10
Fruit and Nut Mix (Estee)	4 pieces	35	10
Golden Almond	½ bar	260	35
Golden III	½ bar	250	40
Goobers	1⅜ oz	220	15
Gum Drops (Estee)	4 pieces	25	0
Gummy Bears (Estee)	3 pieces	20	0
Hard Candy (Estee)	2	25	0
Hershey Bar	1 (1.55 oz)	240	40
Hershey Bar With Almonds	1 (1.45 oz)	230	55
Hershey's Kisses	9 pieces	220	35
Kit Kat Wafer	1 (1.625 oz)	250	60
Krackel	1 (1.55 oz)	230	80
Laffy Taffy (Beich's)			
Apple Chews	1 oz	110	55
Banana Chews	1 oz	110	55
Grape Chews	1 oz	110	60
Passion Punch Chews	1 oz	110	50
Strawberry Chews	1 oz	110	55
Sweet & Sour Cherry Chews	1 oz	110	55
Watermelon Chews	1 oz	110	55
Licorice Nip (Pearson)	1 oz	120	70
Lifesaver Holes			
Sunshine Fruits	1 candy	2	0
Tangerine	1 candy	2	0

FOOD	PORTION	CALORIES	SODIUM
Lifesavers			
Christmas Lollipops	1	40	0
Easter Pops	1	40	0
Fancy Fruits	1 candy	8	0
Fruit Juicers Citrus Fruits	1 candy	8	0
Fruit Juicers Easter Egg-Sortments	1 candy	10	0
Fruit Juicers Fruit Punch	1 candy	8	0
Fruit Juicers Grape	1 candy	8	0
Fruit Juicers Lollipops	1	40	0
Fruit Juicers Mixed Berries	1 candy	8	0
Fruit Juicers Strawberry	1 candy	8	0
Gummi Savers Grape	1 candy	12	0
Gummi Savers Mixed Berry	1 candy	12	0
Sunshine Fruits	1 candy	8	0
Tropical Fruits	1 candy	8	0
Valentine Pops	1	40	0
Wild Cherry	1 candy	8	0
Lollipops (Estee)	1	25	0
Milk Chocolate Bar (Estee)	2 sq	60	10
Milky Way II	1 bar (2 oz)	193	154
Mounds	1 (1.9 oz)	260	85
Mr. Goodbar	1 (1.75 oz)	290	20
Nestle			
Crunch	1.4 oz	210	35
Milk Chocolate	1.45 oz	220	25
Milk Chocolate With Almonds	1.45 oz	230	25
Oh Henry!	2 oz	280	85
Party Mints (Kraft)	1	8	0
Peanut Brittle (Estee)	¼ oz	35	30

FOOD	PORTION	CALORIES	SODIUM
Peanut Brittle (cont.)			
(Kraft)	1 oz	130	135
Peanut Butter Cups (Estee)	1	40	20
Raisinets	1⅜ oz	180	10
Reese's Peanut Butter Cups	1.8 oz	280	180
Reese's Pieces	1.85 oz	260	90
Rolo Carmels in Milk Chocolate	8 pieces	270	110
Skor Toffee Bar	1 (1.4 oz)	220	125
Sno-Caps Nonpareils	1 oz	140	0
Solitaires With Almonds	½ bag	260	25
Special Dark Sweet Chocolate Bar (Hershey)	1 (1.45 oz)	220	5
Symphony			
Almond/Butterchips	1 (1.4 oz)	220	40
Milk Chocolate	1 (1.4 oz)	220	35
Turtles Pecan Caramel Candy (Demet's)	1 (.6 oz)	90	15
Whatchamacallit	1 (1.8 oz)	260	130
Y&S Bites Cherry	1 oz	100	85
Y&S Nibs Cherry	1 oz	180	80
Y&S Twizzlers Strawberry	1 oz	100	95
York Peppermint Patty	1 (1.5 oz)	180	20
candied citron	1 oz	89	82
candied lemon peel	1 oz	90	14
candied orange peel	1 oz	90	14
candy corn	1 oz	105	57
caramels, chocolate	1 oz	115	64
caramels, plain	1 oz	115	64
chocolate	1 oz	145	23
chocolate crisp	1 oz	140	46
chocolate w/ almonds	1 oz	150	23

FOOD	PORTION	CALORIES	SODIUM
chocolate w/ peanuts	1 oz	155	19
dark chocolate	1 oz	150	5
fudge, chocolate	1 oz	115	54
fudge, vanilla	1 oz	115	54
gum drops	1 oz	100	10
hard candy	1 oz	110	7
jelly beans	1 oz	105	7
marzipan	3½ oz	497	5
mint fondant	1 oz	105	57

CANTALOUPE

Dole	¼	50	35
cubed	1 cup	57	14
half	½	94	23

CARAMBOLA

fresh	1	42	2

CARAWAY

seed	1 tsp	7	tr

CARDAMON

ground	1 tsp	6	tr

CARDOON

fresh, cooked	3½ oz	22	176
raw, shredded	½ cup	36	151

CARIBOU

roasted	3 oz	142	51

FOOD	PORTION	CALORIES	SODIUM

CARISSA

| fresh | 1 | 12 | 1 |

CAROB

carob mix	3 tsp	45	12
carob mix, as prep w/ whole milk	9 oz	195	132
flour	1 cup	185	36
flour	1 tbsp	14	3

CARP

FRESH			
cooked	1 fillet (6 oz)	276	107
cooked	3 oz	138	54
raw	3 oz	108	42

CARROTS

CANNED			
Diced Fancy (S&W)	½ cup	30	240
Julienne French Style Fancy (S&W)	½ cup	30	240
Sliced Fancy (S&W)	½ cup	30	240
Sliced Water Pack (S&W)	½ cup	30	50
Whole Tiny Fancy (S&W)	½ cup	30	240
slices	½ cup	17	176
slices, low sodium	½ cup	17	31
FRESH			
Dole	1 med	40	40
baby, raw	1 (½ oz)	6	5
raw	1 (2.5 oz)	31	25
raw, shredded	½ cup	24	19
slices, cooked	½ cup	35	52

FOOD	PORTION	CALORIES	SODIUM
FROZEN			
Harvest Fresh Baby (Green Giant)	½ cup	18	75
slices, cooked	½ cup	26	43
JUICE			
canned	6 oz	73	54
CASABA			
cubed	1 cup	45	20
fresh	¹⁄₁₀	43	20
CASHEWS			
Fancy (Planters)	1 oz	170	110
Honey Roasted (Planters)	1 oz	170	140
Unsalted Halves (Planters)	1 oz	170	0
cashew butter w/o salt	1 tbsp	94	2
dry roasted	1 oz	163	4
dry roasted, salted	1 oz	163	213
oil roasted	1 oz	163	5
oil roasted, salted	1 oz	163	209
CASSAVA			
raw	3½ oz	120	8
CATFISH			
FRESH			
channel, breaded & fried	3 oz	194	238
channel, raw	3 oz	99	54
CATSUP			
Estee	1 tbsp	6	20
Heinz	1 tbsp	16	200

FOOD	PORTION	CALORIES	SODIUM
Heinz Hot	1 tbsp	14	185
Heinz Lite	1 tbsp	8	115
Hunt's	1 tbsp	15	160
Hunt's No Salt Added	1 tbsp	20	0
Smucker's	1 tsp	8	0
Weight Watchers	2 tsp	8	110
catsup	1 pkg (.2 oz)	6	71
catsup	1 tbsp	16	178
low sodium	1 tbsp	16	3

CAULIFLOWER

FRESH			
Dole	⅛ med head	18	45
cooked	½ cup	15	4
raw	½ cup	12	7
FROZEN			
Cuts (Green Giant)	½ cup	12	25
In Cheese Sauce (Green Giant)	½ cup	60	500
One Serve In Cheese Sauce (Green Giant)	1 pkg	80	690
With Cheddar Cheese Sauce (Budget Gourmet)	1 pkg	130	410
cooked	½ cup	17	16
JARRED			
Hot & Spicy (Vlasic)	1 oz	4	435
Sweet (Vlasic)	1 oz	35	225

CAVIAR

black granular	1 oz	71	420
black granular	1 tbsp	40	240

FOOD	PORTION	CALORIES	SODIUM
red granular	1 oz	71	420
red granular	1 tbsp	40	240

CELERIAC

fresh, cooked	3½ oz	25	61
raw	½ cup	31	78

CELERY

DRIED			
seed	1 tsp	8	3
FRESH			
Dole	2 med stalks	20	140
diced, cooked	½ cup	13	68
raw	1 stalk (1.3 oz)	6	35
raw, diced	½ cup	10	52

CELTUCE

raw	3½ oz	22	11

CEREAL

COOKED			
5-Bran Kashi (Kashi)	2½ oz	281	13
Barley Plus (Erewhon)	1 oz	110	0
Bear Mush (Arrowhead)	1 oz	100	tr
Brown Rice Cream (Erewhon)	1 oz	110	20
Bulgar Wheat (Arrowhead)	2 oz	200	0
Coco Wheat (Little Crow)	3 tbsp	130	12
Cracked Wheat Cereal (Arrowhead)	2 oz	180	1
Cream of Rice (Nabisco)	1 oz	100	0

FOOD	PORTION	CALORIES	SODIUM
Cream of Wheat			
Instant (Nabisco)	1 oz	100	0
Quick (Nabisco)	1 oz	100	80
Regular (Nabisco)	1 oz	100	0
Enriched White Hominy Grits			
Quick (Quaker)	3 tbsp	101	1
Regular (Aunt Jemima)	3 tbsp	101	1
Enriched Yellow Hominy Quick Grits (Quaker)	3 tbsp	101	1
Farina			
(H-O)	3 tbsp	120	0
as prep (Pillsbury)	⅔ cup	80	170
Instant (H-O)	1 pkg	110	235
Four Grain Cereal (Arrowhead)	2 oz	94	tr
High Fiber Hot Cereal, as prep (Ralston)	⅓ cup	90	5
Instant Grits			
White Hominy (Quaker)	1 pkg	79	440
With Imitation Bacon Bits (Quaker)	1 pkg	101	590
With Imitation Ham Bits (Quaker)	1 pkg	99	800
With Real Cheddar Cheese (Quaker)	1 pkg	104	497
Kashi (Kashi)	2 oz	177	5
Mix'n Eat Cream of Wheat			
Apple and Cinnamon (Nabisco)	1 pkg (1¼ oz)	130	250
Brown Sugar Cinnamon (Nabisco)	1 pkg (1¼ oz)	130	230
Maple Brown Sugar (Nabisco)	1 pkg (1¼ oz)	130	180
Our Original (Nabisco)	1 pkg (1¼ oz)	100	170
Oat Bran			
(Quaker)	⅓ cup	92	1

FOOD	PORTION	CALORIES	SODIUM
Natural Apples & Cinnamon (Health Valley)	¼ cup	100	10
Natural Raisins & Spice (Health Valley)	¼ cup	100	10
w/ Toasted Wheat Germ (Erewhon)	1 oz	115	15
Oat Groats (Arrowhead)	2 oz	220	tr
Oat Steel Cut (Arrowhead)	2 oz	220	tr
Oatmeal Instant			
(H-O)	1 pkg	110	230
(H-O)	½ cup	130	<5
Apple Cinnamon (Erewhon)	1.25 oz	145	100
Apple Cinnamon (H-O)	1 pkg	130	220
Apple Date & Almond (Arrowhead)	1 oz	130	3
Apple Raisin (Erewhon)	1.3 oz	150	100
Apple Spice (Arrowhead)	1 oz	130	2
Apples & Cinnamon, cooked (Quaker)	1 pkg	118	128
Cinnamon & Spice, cooked (Quaker)	1 pkg	164	322
Cinnamon Raisin & Almond (Arrowhead)	1 oz	140	3
Dates & Walnuts (Erewhon)	1.2 oz	130	60
Extra Fortified Apples & Spice, cooked (Quaker)	1 pkg	133	191
Extra Fortified Raisins & Cinnamon, cooked (Quaker)	1 pkg	129	119
Extra Fortified Regular, cooked (Quaker)	1 pkg	95	219
Maple & Brown Sugar, cooked (Quaker)	1 pkg	152	320
Maple Brown Sugar (H-O)	1 pkg	160	285

FOOD	PORTION	CALORIES	SODIUM
Oatmeal Instant *(cont.)*			
Maple Spice (Erewhon)	1.2 oz	140	100
Peaches & Cream Flavors, cooked (Quaker)	1 pkg	129	179
Raisin & Spice (H-O)	1 pkg	150	140
Raisin & Spice, cooked (Quaker)	1 pkg	149	266
Raisin, Dates & Walnuts, cooked (Quaker)	1 pkg	141	216
Regular (Arrowhead)	1 oz	100	0
Regular, cooked (Quaker)	1 pkg	94	270
Strawberries & Cream Flavors, cooked (Quaker)	1 pkg	129	204
Sweet 'n Mellow (H-O)	1 pkg	150	270
With Added Oat Bran (Erewhon)	1.25 oz	125	0
Oats Gourmet (H-O)	⅓ cup	100	0
Oats 'n Fiber			
(H-O)	1 pkg	110	140
(H-O)	⅓ cup	100	5
Apple & Bran (H-O)	1 pkg	130	140
Raisin & Bran (H-O)	1 pkg	150	140
Oats Old Fashion, cooked (Quaker)	⅔ cup	99	1
Oats Quick			
(H-O)	½ cup	130	<5
cooked (Quaker)	⅔ cup	99	1
Rice & Shine (Arrowhead)	¼ oz	160	tr
Seven Grain (Arrowhead)	1 oz	100	tr
White Corn Grits (Arrowhead)	2 oz	200	tr
Whole Wheat Hot Natural Cereal, cooked (Quaker)	⅔ cup	92	1
Yellow Corn Grits (Arrowhead)	2 oz	200	tr

FOOD	PORTION	CALORIES	SODIUM
corn grits			
instant, as prep	1 pkg (.8 oz)	82	344
quick	1 cup	579	1
quick	1 tbsp	36	0
quick, cooked	1 cup	146	0
regular	1 cup	579	1
regular, cooked	1 cup	146	0
farina			
cooked	¾ cup	87	1
dry	1 tbsp	40	0
oatmeal			
cooked	1 cup	145	1
dry	1 cup	311	3
instant, cooked w/o salt	1 cup	145	2
quick, cooked w/o salt	1 cup	145	2
regular, cooked w/o salt	1 cup	145	2
READY-TO-EAT			
100% Bran (Nabisco)	⅓ cup	70	130
100% Natural Bran With Apples & Cinnamon (Health Valley)	¼ cup	100	10
All-Bran			
(Kellogg's)	⅓ cup (1 oz)	70	260
With Extra Fiber (Kellogg's)	½ cup (1 oz)	50	140
Almond Delight (Ralston)	¾ cup	110	200
Apple Cinnamon Squares (Kellogg's)	½ cup (1 oz)	90	5
Apple Corns (Arrowhead)	1 oz	100	23
Apple Jacks (Kellogg's)	1 cup (1 oz)	110	125
Apple Raisin Crisp (Kellogg's)	⅔ cup (1 oz)	130	230
Arrowhead Crunch (Arrowhead)	1 oz	120	13
Aztec (Erewhon)	1 oz	100	85
Basic 4 (General Mills)	¾ cup	130	290

FOOD	PORTION	CALORIES	SODIUM
Batman (Ralston)	1 cup	110	140
Blue Corn Flakes 100% Organic (Health Valley)	½ cup	90	10
Blueberry Squares (Kellogg's)	½ cup (1 oz)	90	5
Body Buddies Natural Fruit (General Mills)	1 cup (1 oz)	110	280
Booberry (General Mills)	1 cup (1 oz)	110	210
Bran Buds (Kellogg's)	⅓ cup (1 oz)	70	200
Bran Cereal With			
Dates 100% Organic (Health Valley)	¼ cup	100	5
Raisins 100% Organic (Health Valley)	¼ cup	100	5
Bran Flakes			
(Arrowhead)	1 oz	100	1
(Kellogg's)	⅔ cup (1 oz)	90	220
Bran News (Ralston)	¾ cup	100	160
Breakfast With Barbie (Ralston)	1 cup	110	70
Cap'n Crunch (Quaker)	¾ cup	113	241
Cap'n Crunch's (Quaker)			
Crunchberries	¾ cup	113	247
Peanut Butter Crunch	¾ cup	119	281
Cheerios (General Mills)	1¼ cup (1 oz)	110	290
Apple Cinnamon	¾ cup (1 oz)	110	180
Honey Nut	¾ cup (1 oz)	110	250
Cheerios-To-Go (General Mills)	¾ oz pkg	80	220
Apple Cinnamon	1 oz pkg	110	180
Honey Nut	1 oz pkg	110	250
Chex (Ralston)			
Corn	1 cup	110	310
Double	⅔ cup	100	190
Honey Graham	⅔ cup	110	180
Honey Nut Oat	½ cup	100	220

FOOD	PORTION	CALORIES	SODIUM
Multi-Bran	⅔ cup	90	200
Rice	1⅛ cup	110	280
Wheat	⅔ cup	100	130
Cinnamon Mini Buns (Kellogg's)	¾ cup (1 oz)	110	220
Cinnamon Toast Crunch (General Mills)	¾ cup (1 oz)	120	210
Clusters (General Mills)	½ cup (1 oz)	110	140
Cocoa Krispies (Kellogg's)	¾ cup (1 oz)	110	190
Cocoa Puffs (General Mills)	1 cup (1 oz)	110	180
Common Sense Oat Bran (Kellogg's)	¾ cup (1 oz)	100	250
Oat Bran With Raisins (Kellogg's)	¾ cup (1 oz)	130	250
Cookie-Crisp Chocolate Chip (Ralston)	1 cup	110	190
Vanilla Wafer (Ralston)	1 cup	110	220
Corn Flakes (Arrowhead)	1 oz	110	5
(Kellogg's)	1 cup (1 oz)	100	290
Corn Pops (Kellogg's)	1 cup (1 oz)	110	90
Count Chocula (General Mills)	1 cup (1 oz)	110	210
Country Corn Flakes (General Mills)	1 cup (1 oz)	110	260
Cracklin' Oat Bran (Kellogg's)	½ cup (1 oz)	110	140
Crispix (Kellogg's)	1 cup (1 oz)	110	220
Crispy Brown Rice (Erewhon)	1 oz	110	185
Crispy Brown Rice Cereal Low Sodium (Erewhon)	1 oz	110	5
Crispy Wheats 'N Raisins (General Mills)	¾ cup (1 oz)	100	140
Crunchy Bran (Quaker)	⅔ cup	89	316
Crunchy Not Oh!s (Quaker)	1 cup	127	164

FOOD	PORTION	CALORIES	SODIUM
Dinersaurs (Ralston)	1 cup	110	70
Double Dip Crunch (Kellogg's)	⅔ cup (1 oz)	120	160
Fiber 7 Flakes			
100% Organic (Health Valley)	½ cup	90	0
With Raisins 100% Organic (Health Valley)	½ cup	90	0
Fiber One (General Mills)	½ cup (1 oz)	60	140
Fiberwise (Kellogg's)	⅔ cup (1 oz)	90	140
Frankenberry (General Mills)	1 cup (1 oz)	110	210
Froot Loops (Kellogg's)	1 cup (1 oz)	110	125
Frosted Bran (Kellogg's)	1½ oz	150	290
Frosted Flakes (Kellogg's)	¾ cup (1 oz)	110	200
Frosted Krispies (Kellogg's)	¾ cup (1 oz)	110	220
Frosted Mini-Wheats (Kellogg's)	4 biscuits (1 oz)	100	0
Frosted Mini-Wheats Bite Size (Kellogg's)	½ cup	100	0
Fruit & Fitness (Health Valley)	1 cup	220	5
Fruit 'n Wheat (Erewhon)	1 oz	100	75
Fruit Lites (Health Valley)			
Corn	½ cup	45	2
Rice	½ cup	45	2
Wheat	½ cup	45	2
Fruit Muesli (Ralston)			
Raisins, Apples And Almonds	½ cup	150	140
Raisins, Dates And Almonds	½ cup	140	95
Raisins, Peaches And Pecans	½ cup	150	95
Raisins, Walnuts And Cranberries	½ cup	150	95
Fruit Wheats, Apple (Nabisco)	1 oz	90	15
Fruitful Bran (Kellogg's)	⅔ cup (1.4 oz)	120	220
Fruity Marshmallow Krispies (Kellogg's)	1¼ cups (1.3 oz)	140	210

FOOD	PORTION	CALORIES	SODIUM
Fruity Yummy Mummy (General Mills)	1 cup (1 oz)	110	160
Golden Grahams (General Mills)	¾ cup (1 oz)	110	280
Healthy Crunch (Health Valley) Almond Date	¼ cup	110	5
Apple Cinnamon	¼ cup	110	10
Healthy O's, 100% Organic (Health Valley)	¾ cup	90	1
Honey Graham Oh!s (Quaker)	1 cup	122	217
Hot Wheels (Ralston)	1 cup	110	160
Just Right (Kellogg's) With Fiber Nuggets	⅔ cup (1 oz)	100	200
With Raisins, Dates & Nuts	¾ cup (1.3 oz)	140	190
Kaboom (General Mills)	1 cup (1 oz)	110	270
Kashi Brittles Sesame/Maple (Kashi)	3½ oz	473	85
Kashi Puffed (Kashi)	¾ oz	74	2
Kenmei (Kellogg's)	¾ cup (1 oz)	110	230
King Vitaman (Quaker)	1½ cup	110	280
Kix (General Mills)	1½ cup (1 oz)	110	260
Life (Quaker)	⅔ cup	101	186
Life Cinnamon (Quaker)	⅔ cup	101	182
Lites Puffed Corn (Health Valley)	½ cup	50	0
Rice (Health Valley)	½ cup	50	0
Wheat (Health Valley)	½ cup	50	0
Lucky Charms (General Mills)	1 cup (1 oz)	110	240
Maple Corns (Arrowhead)	1 oz	100	25
Morning Funnies (Ralston)	1 cup	110	70
Mueslix (Kellogg's) Crispy Blend	⅔ cup (1.5 oz)	150	150
Golden Crunch	½ cup (1.2 oz)	120	170

FOOD	PORTION	CALORIES	SODIUM
Nature O's (Arrowhead)	1 oz	110	5
Nintendo Cereal System (Ralston)	1 cup	110	70
Nut & Honey Crunch (Kellogg's)	⅔ cup (1 oz)	110	200
Nut & Honey Crunch O's (Kellogg's)	⅔ cup (1 oz)	110	190
Nutri-Grain (Kellogg's)			
Almond Raisin	⅔ cup (1.4 oz)	140	220
Raisin Bran	1 cup (1.4 oz)	130	200
Wheat	⅔ cup (1 oz)	90	170
Oat Bran Flakes			
(Arrowhead)	1 oz	110	10
100% Organic (Health Valley)	½ cup	100	0
Almonds/Dates 100% Organic (Health Valley)	½ cup	100	0
With Raisins 100% Organic (Health Valley)	½ cup	100	0
Oat Bran O's (Health Valley)			
100% Organic	½ cup	110	0
Fruit & Nuts	½ cup	110	0
Oat Brand Options (Ralston)	¾ cup	130	150
Oat Squares (Quaker)	½ cup	105	159
Oatbake (Kellogg's)			
Honey Bran	⅓ cup (1 oz)	110	190
Raisin Nut	⅓ cup (1 oz)	110	200
Oatmeal			
Crisp (Kellogg's)	½ cup (1 oz)	110	180
Raisin Crisp (General Mills)	½ cup (1.2 oz)	130	170
Orangeola (Health Valley)			
Almonds & Dates	¼ cup	110	5
Bananas & Hawaiian Fruit	¼ cup	120	10
Popeye Sweet Crunch (Quaker)	1 cup	113	254
Poppets (US Mills)	1 oz	110	10

FOOD	PORTION	CALORIES	SODIUM
Product 19 (Kellogg's)	1 cup (1 oz)	100	320
Puffed Corn (Arrowhead)	½ oz	50	tr
Puffed Millet (Arrowhead)	½ oz	50	tr
Puffed Rice			
(Arrowhead)	½ oz	50	tr
(Quaker)	1 cup	54	1
Puffed Wheat			
(Arrowhead)	½ oz	50	tr
(Quaker)	1 cup	50	1
Quaker 100% Natural	¼ cup	127	14
Apples & Cinnamon	¼ cup	126	13
Raisins & Date	¼ cup	123	14
Raisin Bran			
(Erewhon)	1 oz	100	80
(Kellogg's)	¾ cup (1.4 oz)	120	210
Flakes 100% Organic (Health Valley)	½ cup	100	5
Raisin Nut Bran (General Mills)	½ cup (1 oz)	110	140
Raisin Squares (Kellogg's)	½ cup (1 oz)	90	0
Real Oat Bran (Health Valley)			
Almond Crunch	¼ cup	110	2
Hawaiian Fruit	¼ cup	130	2
Raisin Nut	¼ cup	130	2
Rice Bran O's (Health Valley)	½ cup	110	5
Rice Bran With Almonds & Dates (Health Valley)	½ cup	110	2
Rice Brand Options (Ralston)	⅔ cup	120	120
Rice Krispies (Kellogg's)	1 cup (1 oz)	110	290
S'Mores Grahams (General Mills)	¾ cup (1 oz)	120	250
Shredded Wheat			
(Quaker)	2 biscuits	132	1
(Sunshine)	1 biscuit	90	0

FOOD	PORTION	CALORIES	SODIUM
Shredded Wheat *(cont.)*			
Bite Size (Sunshine)	⅔ cup	110	0
'n Bran (Nabisco)	⅔ cup	90	0
Spoon Size (Nabisco)	⅔ cup	90	0
With Oat Bran (Nabisco)	⅔ cup	100	0
Slimer! And The Real Ghostbusters (Ralston)	1 cup	110	115
Special K (Kellogg's)	1 cup (1 oz)	100	230
Sprouts 7 (Health Valley) Bananas & Hawaiian Fruit	¼ cup	90	5
Raisin	¼ cup	90	5
Strawberry Squares (Kellogg's)	½ cup (1 oz)	90	5
Sunflakes Multi-Grain (Ralston)	1 cup	100	240
Super-O's (Erewhon)	1 oz	110	5
Swiss Breakfast (Health Valley) Raisin Nut	¼ cup	100	10
Tropical Fruit	¼ cup	100	10
Team (Nabisco)	1 cup	110	180
Teenage Mutant Ninja Turtles (Ralston)	1 cup	110	190
Total (General Mills)	1 cup (1 oz)	100	200
Total Corn Flakes (General Mills)	1 cup (1 oz)	110	200
Total Raisin Bran (General Mills)	1 cup (1.5 oz)	140	190
Triples (General Mills)	¾ cup (1 oz)	110	250
Trix (General Mills)	1 cup (1 oz)	110	140
Uncle Sam Cereal (US Mills)	1 oz	110	65
Wheat Flakes (Arrowhead)	1 oz	110	5
(Erewhon)	1 oz	100	75
Wheaties (General Mills)	1 cup (1 oz)	100	200
Whole Grain Shredded Wheat (Kellogg's)	½ cup (1 oz)	90	0

FOOD	PORTION	CALORIES	SODIUM
all bran	½ cup (1 oz)	76	196
bran flakes	¾ cup (1 oz)	90	264
corn flakes	1¼ cup (1 oz)	110	351
corn flakes, low sodium	1 cup	100	3
crispy rice	1 cup	111	205
fortified oat flakes	1 cup	177	429
granola	¼ cup	138	3
puffed rice	1 cup	57	0
puffed wheat	1 cup	44	0
shredded wheat	1 biscuit	83	0
sugar-coated corn flakes	¾ cup (1 oz)	110	230

CHAYOTE

fresh, cooked	1 cup	38	1
raw	1 (7 oz)	49	8
raw, cut up	1 cup	32	198

CHEESE
(*see also* CHEESE DISHES, CHEESE SUBSTITUTES, COTTAGE CHEESE, CREAM CHEESE)

NATURAL			
Asiago (Frigo)	1 oz	110	400
Baby Swiss (Cracker Barrel)	1 oz	110	65
Blue			
(Frigo)	1 oz	100	400
(Kraft)	1 oz	100	330
(Sargento)	1 oz	100	396
Brick			
(Kraft)	1 oz	110	180
(Land O'Lakes)	1 oz	110	160
Brie (Sargento)	1 oz	95	178

FOOD	PORTION	CALORIES	SODIUM
Burger Cheese (Sargento)	1 oz	106	406
Cajun (Sargento)	1 oz	110	164
Camembert (Sargento)	1 oz	85	239
Ched-R-Lo (Alpine Lace)	1 oz	80	95
Cheda-Jack Reduced Fat Low Sodium (Dorman)	1 oz	80	140
Chedarella (Land O'Lakes)	1 oz	100	180
Cheddar			
(Cabot)	1 oz	110	175
(Dorman)	1 oz	110	200
(Frigo)	1 oz	110	200
(Kraft)	1 oz	110	180
(Land O'Lakes)	1 oz	110	180
(Sargento)	1 oz	114	176
Reduced Fat Low Sodium (Dorman)	1 oz	80	140
Cheddar Light			
(Bristol Gold)	1 oz	70	150
w/ Simplesse (White Clover)	1 oz	80	160
Cheddar Lite (Frigo)	1 oz	80	190
Cheddar Mild			
Low Sodium White (Weight Watchers)	1 oz	80	70
Low Sodium Yellow (Weight Watchers)	1 oz	80	70
MooTown Snackers Light (Sargento)	1 stick	70	140
Preferred Light (Sargento)	1 oz	90	180
Reduced Fat (Kraft Light)	1 oz	80	220
Shredded (Weight Watchers)	1 oz	80	150
Shredded Preferred Light (Sargento)	1 oz	90	180

FOOD	PORTION	CALORIES	SODIUM
White (Weight Watchers)	1 oz	80	150
Yellow (Weight Watchers)	1 oz	80	150
Cheddar New York (Sargento)	1 oz	114	176
Cheddar Sharp			
Nut Log (Sargento)	1 oz	97	252
Reduced Fat (Kraft Light)	1 oz	80	220
Reduced Fat White (Cracker Barrel Light)	1 oz	80	220
White (Weight Watchers)	1 oz	80	150
Yellow (Weight Watchers)	1 oz	80	150
Cherve (Brier Run)	1 oz	61	70
Colbi-Lo (Alpine Lace)	1 oz	80	85
Colby			
(Dorman)	1 oz	110	190
(Kraft)	1 oz	110	180
(Land O'Lakes)	1 oz	110	170
(Sargento)	1 oz	112	171
(Weight Watchers)	1 oz	80	150
And Monterey Jack, Reduced Fat Shredded (Kraft Light)	1 oz	80	220
Light With Simplesse (White Clover)	1 oz	80	180
Reduced Fat (Kraft Light)	1 oz	80	220
Colby-Jack (Sargento)	1 oz	109	162
Edam			
(Dorman)	1 oz	100	200
(Kraft)	1 oz	90	310
(Land O'Lakes)	1 oz	110	270
(Sargento)	1 oz	101	274
Farmer's			
Cheese (Sargento)	1 oz	102	129

FOOD	PORTION	CALORIES	SODIUM
Farmer's *(cont.)*			
MooTown Snackers Light (Sargento)	1 stick	70	140
Preferred Light (Sargento)	1 oz	80	180
Shredded Preferred Light (Sargento)	1 oz	80	180
Feta (Frigo)	1 oz	100	400
Feta (Sargento)	1 oz	75	316
Finland Swiss (Sargento)	1 oz	107	74
French Onion Light (Bristol Gold)	1 oz	70	150
Fruit Moos (Dannon)			
Apricot	3.5 oz	150	40
Banana	3.5 oz	150	40
Raspberry	3.5 oz	150	40
Strawberry	3.5 oz	150	40
Garlic & Herb Light (Bristol Gold)	1 oz	70	150
Gjetost (Sargento)	1 oz	132	170
Gouda			
(Dorman)	1 oz	100	210
(Kraft)	1 oz	110	200
(Land O'Lakes)	1 oz	110	230
(Sargento)	1 oz	101	232
Gourmet Parm (Sargento)	1 tbsp	20	95
Havarti			
(Casino)	1 oz	120	140
(Sargento)	1 oz	118	200
Horseradish Light (Bristol Gold)	1 oz	70	150
Impastata (Frigo)	1 oz	60	50
Italian Style Grated Cheeses (Sargento)	1 oz	108	106
Jarlsberg (Sargento)	1 oz	100	130

FOOD	PORTION	CALORIES	SODIUM
Limburger			
(Sargento)	1 oz	93	227
Little Gem Size (Mohawk Valley)	1 oz	90	250
Monterey Jack			
(Cabot)	1 oz	80	200
(Dorman)	1 oz	100	180
(Kraft)	1 oz	110	190
(Land O'Lakes)	1 oz	110	150
(Sargento)	1 oz	106	152
(Weight Watchers)	1 oz	80	150
Hot Pepper (Land O'Lakes)	1 oz	110	150
Light With Simplesse (White Clover)	1 oz	70	190
Reduced Fat (Kraft Light)	1 oz	80	220
With Caraway Seeds (Kraft)	1 oz	100	180
With Jalapeno Peppers (Kraft)	1 oz	110	190
With Peppers, Reduced Fat (Kraft Light)	1 oz)	80	220
Monterey Reduced Fat Low Sodium (Dorman)	1 oz	80	140
Monti-Jack-Lo (Alpine Lace)	1 oz	80	75
Mozzarella			
(Weight Watchers)	1 oz	70	150
Lite, Low Moisture, Whole Milk (Frigo)	1 oz	60	140
Low Moisture (Kraft)	1 oz	90	190
Low Moisture, Part Skim (Alpine Lace)	1 oz	70	75
Low Moisture, Part Skim (Frigo)	1 oz	80	190
Low Moisture, Part Skim (Kraft)	1 oz	80	200

FOOD	PORTION	CALORIES	SODIUM
Mozzarella *(cont.)*			
Low Moisture, Part Skim (Sargento)	1 oz	79	150
Low Moisture, Whole Milk (Frigo)	1 oz	90	190
Part Skim (Dorman)	1 oz	90	190
Part Skim (Land O'Lakes)	1 oz	80	150
Preferred Light (Sargento)	1 oz	60	150
Reduced Fat (Kraft Light)	1 oz	80	200
Reduced Fat, Low Sodium (Dorman)	1 oz	80	140
Shredded (Weight Watchers)	1 oz	80	150
Shredded, Preferred Light (Sargento)	1 oz	60	150
Whole Milk (Sargento)	1 oz	90	118
Muenster			
(Alpine Lace)	1 oz	100	85
(Dorman)	1 oz	110	190
(Land O'Lakes)	1 oz	100	180
Light With Simplesse (White Clover)	1 oz	70	190
Low Sodium (Dorman)	1 oz	110	95
Red Rind (Sargento)	1 oz	104	180
Reduced Fat, Low Sodium (Dorman)	1 oz	80	140
Parmazest (Frigo)	1 oz	120	410
Parmesan			
(Dorman)	1 oz	110	350
& Romano Dry Grated (Frigo)	1 oz	130	510
& Romano Grated (Frigo)	1 oz	110	350
& Romano Grated (Sargento)	1 oz	111	397
Dry Grated (Frigo)	1 oz	130	510

FOOD	PORTION	CALORIES	SODIUM
Fresh (Sargento)	1 oz	111	454
Grated (Frigo)	1 oz	110	350
Grated (Kraft)	1 oz	130	430
Grated (Sargento)	1 oz	129	528
Natural (Kraft)	1 oz	100	290
Whole (Frigo)	1 oz	110	350
Pizza Shredded (Frigo)	1 oz	65	150
Port Wine			
Cup Cheese (Weight Watchers)	1½ tbsp (1 oz)	70	190
Nut Log (Sargento)	1 oz	97	252
Provo-Lo (Alpine Lace)	1 oz	70	85
Provolone			
(Dorman)	1 oz	90	290
(Frigo)	1 oz	100	230
(Kraft)	1 oz	100	260
(Land O'Lakes)	1 oz	100	250
(Sargento)	1 oz	100	248
Lite (Frigo)	1 oz	70	205
Reduced Fat, Low Sodium (Dorman)	1 oz	80	140
Quark (Brier Run)	1 oz	34	15
Queso			
Blanco (Sargento)	1 oz	104	178
Queso			
de Papa (Sargento)	1 oz	114	176
Ricotta			
Lite (Sargento)	1 oz	24	23
Low Fat, Low Salt (Frigo)	1 oz	30	10
Part Skim (Frigo)	1 oz	40	30
Part Skim (Sargento)	1 oz	32	27
Whole Milk (Frigo)	1 oz	60	40

FOOD	PORTION	CALORIES	SODIUM
Romano			
(Dorman)	1 oz	100	350
(Sargento)	1 oz	110	340
Dry, Grated (Frigo)	1 oz	130	510
Grated (Casino)	1 oz	130	350
Grated (Frigo)	1 oz	110	350
Natural (Casino)	1 oz	100	250
Whole (Frigo)	1 oz	110	350
Sharp Cheddar Cup Cheese (Weight Watchers)	1½ tbsp (1 oz)	70	190
Sheep's Milk (Hallow Road Farms)	1 oz	45	65
Smoke Light (Bristol Gold)	1 oz	70	150
Smokestick (Sargento)	1 oz	103	388
String			
(Frigo)	1 oz	80	190
(Sargento)	1 oz	79	150
Lite (Frigo)	1 oz	60	140
MooTown Snackers Light (Sargento)	1 stick	40	125
Smoked (Sargento)	1 oz	79	150
With Jalapeno Peppers (Kraft)	1 oz	80	230
Swiss			
(Casino)	1 oz	110	35
(Dorman)	1 oz	100	80
(Frigo)	1 oz	110	80
(Kraft)	1 oz	110	40
(Land O'Lakes)	1 oz	110	75
(Sargento)	1 oz	107	74
Aged (Kraft)	1 oz	110	45
Almond Nut Log (Sargento)	1 oz	94	349
No Salt Added (Dorman)	1 oz	100	10

FOOD	PORTION	CALORIES	SODIUM
Reduced Fat (Kraft Light)	1 oz	90	70
Reduced Fat, Low Sodium (Dorman)	1 oz	90	60
Very Low (Kraft)	1 oz	110	10
Wafer Thin, Preferred Light (Sargento)	1 oz	80	75
Swiss-Lo (Alpine Lace)	1 oz	100	35
Taco (Sargento)	1 oz	109	162
Shredded (Frigo)	1 oz	110	200
Shredded (Kraft)	1 oz	110	190
Tilsiter (Sargento)	1 oz	96	213
Tybo Red Wax (Sargento)	1 oz	98	200
Vitalait (Cabot)	1 oz	70	170
Jalapeno (Cabot)	1 oz	70	170
Wine Light (Bristol Gold)	1 oz	70	150
blue	1 oz	100	396
blue, crumbled	1 cup	477	1884
brick	1 oz	105	159
brie	1 oz	95	178
camembert	1 oz	85	239
camembert	1 wedge (1⅓ oz)	114	320
caraway	1 oz	107	196
cheddar	1 oz	114	176
cheddar, shredded	1 cup	455	701
cheshire	1 oz	110	198
colby	1 oz	112	171
edam	1 oz	101	274
emmentaler	3½ oz	403	450
feta	1 oz	75	316

FOOD	PORTION	CALORIES	SODIUM
gjetost	1 oz	132	170
goat			
hard	1 oz	128	98
semisoft	1 oz	103	146
soft	1 oz	76	104
gouda	1 oz	101	232
gruyere	1 oz	117	95
limburger	1 oz	93	227
monterey	1 oz	106	152
mozzarella	1 lb	1276	1692
mozzarella	1 oz	80	106
low moisture	1 oz	90	118
low moisture, part skim	1 oz	79	150
part skim	1 oz	72	132
muenster	1 oz	104	178
parmesan			
grated	1 oz	129	528
grated	1 tbsp	23	93
hard	1 oz	111	454
port du salut	1 oz	100	151
provolone	1 oz	100	248
quark			
20% fat	3½ oz	116	35
40% fat	3½ oz	167	34
made w/ skim milk	3½ oz	78	40
ricotta	1 cup	428	207
ricotta	½ cup	216	104
part skim	1 cup	340	307
part skim	½ cup	171	155
romano	1 oz	110	340
roquefort	1 oz	105	513

FOOD	PORTION	CALORIES	SODIUM
swiss	1 oz	107	74
tilsit	1 oz	96	213
PROCESSED			
Alpine Lace			
American	1 oz	80	200
Free N'Lean American	1 oz	35	290
Free N'Lean Cheddar	1 oz	40	290
Free N'Lean Mozzarella	1 oz	40	290
Borden			
American Slices	1 oz	110	490
American, Very Sharp	1 oz	110	490
Swiss Slices	1 oz	100	380
Cheez Whiz	1 oz	80	470
Mild Mexican	1 oz	80	430
With Jalapeno Peppers	1 oz	80	430
Cracker Barrel			
Cheese Ball, Sharp Cheddar With Almonds	1 oz	100	250
Cheese Log, Port Wine With Almonds	1 oz	90	260
Cheese Log, Sharp Cheddar With Almonds	1 oz	90	250
Cheese Log, Smokey Cheddar With Almonds	1 oz	90	250
Extra Sharp Cheddar	1 oz	90	240
Port Wine Cheddar	1 oz	100	230
Sharp Cheddar	1 oz	100	230
With Bacon	1 oz	90	280
Dorman's Lo-Chol			
Cheddar	1 oz	100	140
Colby	1 oz	100	140
Mozzarella	1 oz	90	140

FOOD	PORTION	CALORIES	SODIUM
Dorman's Lo-Chol *(cont.)*			
Muenster	1 oz	100	140
Swiss	1 oz	100	140
Frigo			
Imitation Cheddar	1 oz	90	280
Imitation Mozzarella	1 oz	90	240
Harvest Moon American	1 oz	70	420
Kraft			
American Cheese Spread	1 oz	80	470
American Grated	1 oz	130	740
Cheese Food With Garlic	1 oz	90	370
Cheese Food With Jalapeno Peppers	1 oz	90	390
Cheese Spread With Bacon	1 oz	80	560
Deluxe American Cheese	1 oz	110	450
Deluxe Pimento Cheese	1 oz	100	440
Deluxe Swiss Cheese	1 oz	90	420
Jalapeno Cheese Spread	1 oz	80	470
Jalapeno Pepper Spread	1 oz	70	95
Olives & Pimento Spread	1 oz	60	160
Pimento Spread	1 oz	70	120
Pineapple Spread	1 oz	70	75
Kraft Singles			
American	1 oz	90	390
Cheez 'N Bacon	1 oz	90	400
Free	1 oz	45	420
Jalapeno	1 oz	90	450
Light	1 oz	70	410
Light American	1 oz	70	70
Light Sharp Cheddar	1 oz	70	380
Light Swiss	1 oz	70	350

FOOD	PORTION	CALORIES	SODIUM
Monterey Jack	1 oz	90	390
Pimento	1 oz	90	390
Sharp	1 oz	100	400
Swiss	1 oz	90	440
White American	1 oz	90	400
Lactaid American	3.5 oz	328	1189
Land O'Lakes			
American	1 oz	110	450
American & Swiss	1 oz	100	400
Cheddar & Bacon	1 oz	110	350
Extra Sharp Cheddar	1 oz	100	370
Golden Velvet Cheese Spread	1 oz	80	370
Italian Herb Cheese Food	1 oz	90	430
Jalapeno Cheese Food	1 oz	90	400
Jalapeno Jack	1 oz	90	430
Onion Cheese Food	1 oz	90	70
Pepperoni Cheese Food	1 oz	90	430
Salami Cheese Food	1 oz	90	410
Sharp American	1 oz	100	360
Light N' Lively Singles			
American	1 oz	70	420
American White	1 oz	70	410
Sharp Cheddar	1 oz	70	380
Swiss	1 oz	70	350
Lunch Wagon Sandwich Slices	1 oz	90	370
Mohawk Valley Limburger Cheese Spread	1 oz	70	420
Nippy Cheese Food	1 oz	90	380
Old English			
Sharp American	1 oz	110	440
Sharp Cheese Spread	1 oz	90	480

FOOD	PORTION	CALORIES	SODIUM
Roka Blue Spread	1 oz	70	270
Sargento			
American Hot Pepper	1 oz	106	406
American Sharp Spread	1 oz	106	406
American w/ Pimento	1 oz	106	405
Brick	1 oz	95	431
Imitation Cheddar	1 oz	85	350
Imitation Mozzarella	1 oz	80	310
Swiss	1 oz	95	388
Smart Beat			
American	1 slice (⅔ oz)	35	180
Low Sodium	1 slice (⅔ oz)	35	90
Sharp	1 slice (⅔ oz)	35	210
Spreadery			
Medium Cheddar	1 oz	70	250
Mild Mexican With Jalapeno Peppers	1 oz	70	260
Nacho	1 oz	70	240
Port Wine	1 oz	70	250
Sharp Cheddar	1 oz	70	240
Vermont White Cheddar	1 oz	70	230
Squeez-A-Snak			
Garlic	1 oz	80	430
Hickory Smoke	1 oz	80	440
Sharp	1 oz	80	440
With Bacon	1 oz	90	500
With Jalapeno Pepper	1 oz	80	510
Velveeta			
Cheese Spread	1 oz	80	430
Light Singles	1 oz	70	470
Mexican Hot	1 oz	80	520
Mexican Mild	1 oz	80	440

FOOD	PORTION	CALORIES	SODIUM
Pimento	1 oz	80	400
Shredded	1 oz	100	210
Shredded Hot Mexican w/ Jalapeno Peppers	1 oz	100	430
Shredded Mild Mexican w/ Jalapeno Peppers	1 oz	100	420
Slices	1 oz	90	400
Weight Watchers			
American Slices Low Sodium White	2 slices (⅔ oz)	35	80
American Slices Low Sodium Yellow	2 slices (⅔ oz)	35	80
American Slices White	2 slices (⅔ oz)	35	270
American Slices Yellow	2 slices (⅔ oz)	35	270
Sharp Cheddar Slices	2 slices (⅔ oz)	35	270
Swiss Slices	2 slices (⅔ oz)	35	270
american	1 oz	93	337
american cheese food	1 pkg (8 oz)	745	2700
american cheese spread	1 jar (5 oz)	412	1910
american cheese spread	1 oz	82	381
american cold pack	1 pkg (8 oz)	752	2193
pimento	1 oz	106	405
swiss	1 oz	92	440
swiss	1 oz	95	388
swiss cheese food	1 pkg (8 oz)	734	3523

CHEESE DISHES

FROZEN			
Mozzarella Cheese Nuggets (Banquet)	2.5 oz	230	510
TAKE-OUT			
fondue	½ cup	303	194

FOOD	PORTION	CALORIES	SODIUM
CHEESE SUBSTITUTES			
Borden Taco-Mate	1 oz	100	360
Cheese Two	1 oz	90	360
Golden Image			
American	1 oz	90	360
Colby	1 oz	110	190
Mild Cheddar	1 oz	110	190
mozzarella	1 oz	70	194
CHERRIES			
CANNED			
sour			
in heavy syrup	½ cup	232	18
in light syrup	½ cup	189	18
water packed	1 cup	87	17
sweet			
in heavy syrup	½ cup	107	3
in light syrup	½ cup	85	3
juice pack	½ cup	68	3
water pack	½ cup	57	2
DRIED			
Bing (Chukar)	2 oz	160	3
Rainer (Chukar)	2 oz	160	3
Tart (Chukar)	2 oz	170	10
Tart 'n Sweet (Chukar)	2 oz	180	10
FRESH			
Dole	1 cup	90	0
sour	1 cup	51	3
sweet	10	49	0
FROZEN			
sour, unsweetened	1 cup	72	1

FOOD	PORTION	CALORIES	SODIUM
sweet, sweetened	1 cup	232	3
JUICE			
Dole Pure & Light	6 oz	90	10
Smucker's			
Black Cherry	8 oz	130	10
Black Cherry Sparkler	10 oz	120	5
Wyler's			
Drink Mix Unsweetened Cherry	8 oz	2	15
Drink Mix Wild Cherry	8 oz	81	tr

CHERVIL

seed	1 tsp	1	tr

CHESTNUTS

chinese			
cooked	1 oz	44	1
dried	1 oz	103	2
raw	1 oz	64	1
roasted	1 oz	68	1
cooked	1 oz	37	8
dried, peeled	1 oz	105	11
japanese			
cooked	1 oz	16	1
dried	1 oz	102	10
raw	1 oz	44	4
raw, peeled	1 oz	56	1
roasted	1 cup	350	3
roasted	1 oz	70	1

CHEWING GUM

Beech-Nut			
Cinnamon	1 piece	10	0

FOOD	PORTION	CALORIES	SODIUM
Beech-Nut *(cont.)*			
Fruit	1 piece	10	0
Peppermint	1 piece	10	0
Spearmint	1 piece	10	0
Big Red	1 stick	10	0
Bubble Yum			
Fruit Juice Variety	1 piece	20	0
Luscious Lime	1 piece	25	0
Extra Sugar Free			
Cinnamon	1 piece	8	0
Spearmint & Peppermint	1 stick	8	0
Winter Fresh	1 piece	8	0
Freedent			
Cinnamon	1 stick	10	0
Peppermint	1 stick	10	0
Spearmint	1 stick	10	0
Fruit Stripe	1 piece	8	0
Bubble Gum	1 piece	8	0
Variety Pack	1 piece	8	0
Hubba Bubba			
Bubble Gum Cola	1 piece	23	0
Bubble Gum Sugarfree Original	1 piece	14	0
Bubble Gum Sugarfree Grape	1 piece	13	0
Original	1 piece	23	0
Grape	1 piece	23	0
Raspberry	1 piece	23	0
Strawberry	1 piece	23	0
Juicy Fruit	1 stick	10	0
Wrigley's			
Doublemint	1 piece	10	0
Spearmint	1 stick	10	0

FOOD	PORTION	CALORIES	SODIUM

CHICKEN
(*see also* CHICKEN DISHES, CHICKEN SUBSTITUTES, DINNER, HOT DOG)

CANNED			
Chunk Style Mixin' Chicken (Swanson)	2½ oz	130	230
White (Swanson)	2½ oz	100	235
White & Dark (Swanson)	2½ oz	100	240
w/ broth	1 can (5 oz)	234	714
w/ broth	½ can (2.5 oz)	117	357
FRESH			
Breast			
Oven Stuffer Roaster w/ Skin, cooked (Perdue)	1 oz	42	11
Quarters, Fresh Young w/ Skin, cooked (Perdue)	1 oz	48	14
Skinless & Boneless Oven Stuffer Roaster, cooked (Perdue)	1 oz	31	9
Skinless Boneless, cooked (Perdue)	1 oz	30	10
Split Fresh Young w/ Skin, cooked (Perdue)	1 oz	45	12
Tender Skinless & Boneless, cooked (Perdue)	1 oz	29	14
Thin-Sliced Skinless & Boneless Oven Stuffer, cooked (Perdue)	1 oz	31	9
Whole Fresh Young w/ Skin, cooked (Perdue)	1 oz	45	12
Cornish Hen			
Dark Meat w/ Skin, cooked (Perdue)	1 oz	43	10
White Meat w/ Skin, cooked (Perdue)	1 oz	42	12

FOOD	PORTION	CALORIES	SODIUM
Drumsticks			
Fresh Young w/ Skin, cooked (Perdue)	1 oz	42	21
Oven Stuffer Roaster w/ Skin, cooked (Perdue)	1 oz	41	16
Ground Fresh Young, cooked (Perdue)	1 oz	49	14
Leg Quarters, Fresh Young w/ Skin, cooked (Perdue)	1 oz	49	15
Legs, Fresh Young w/ Skin, cooked (Perdue)	1 oz	51	16
Soup & Stew			
Baking Hen, Dark Meat w/ Skin, cooked (Perdue)	1 oz	41	9
Baking Hen, White Meat w/ Skin, cooked (Perdue)	1 oz	41	11
Thighs			
Fresh Young w/ Skin, cooked (Perdue)	1 oz	57	15
Skinless & Boneless, cooked (Perdue)	1 oz	30	10
Skinless & Boneless Oven Stuffer Roaster, cooked (Perdue)	1 oz	34	13
Whole			
Fresh Young, Dark Meat w/ Skin, cooked (Perdue)	1 oz	47	12
Fresh Young, White Meat w/ Skin, cooked (Perdue)	1 oz	43	11
Oven Stuffer Roaster, Dark Meat w/ Skin, cooked (Perdue)	1 oz	49	16
Oven Stuffer Roaster White Meat w/ Skin, cooked (Perdue)	1 oz	44	12
Wing Drumettes, Fresh Young w/ Skin, cooked (Perdue)	1 oz	50	13

FOOD	PORTION	CALORIES	SODIUM
Wingettes Oven Stuffer Roaster w/ Skin, cooked (Perdue)	1 oz	52	17
Wings, Fresh Young w/ Skin, cooked (Perdue)	1 oz	54	19
broiler/fryer			
back w/ skin, batter dipped & fried	½ back (2.5 oz)	238	228
back w/ skin, floured & fried	1.5 oz	146	40
back w/ skin, roasted	1 oz	96	28
back w/ skin, stewed	½ back (2.1 oz)	158	39
back w/o skin, fried	½ back (2 oz)	167	58
breast w/ skin, batter dipped & fried	½ breast (4.9 oz)	364	385
breast w/ skin, batter dipped & fried	2.9 oz	218	231
breast w/ skin, roasted	½ breast (3.4 oz)	193	69
breast w/ skin, roasted	2 oz	115	41
breast w/ skin, stewed	½ breast (3.9 oz)	202	68
breast w/o skin, fried	½ breast (3 oz)	161	68
breast w/o skin, roasted	½ breast (3 oz)	142	63
breast w/o skin, stewed	2 oz	86	36
dark meat w/ skin, batter dipped & fried	5.9 oz	497	493
dark meat w/ skin, floured & fried	3.9 oz	313	98
dark meat w/ skin, roasted	3.5 oz	256	88
dark meat w/ skin, stewed	3.9 oz	256	77
dark meat w/o skin, fried	1 cup (5 oz)	334	136
dark meat w/o skin, roasted	1 cup (5 oz)	286	130
dark meat w/o skin, stewed	1 cup (5 oz)	269	104
dark meat w/o skin, stewed	3 oz	165	64

FOOD	PORTION	CALORIES	SODIUM
broiler/fryer *(cont.)*			
drumstick w/ skin, batter dipped & fried	1 (2.6 oz)	193	194
drumstick w/ skin, floured & fried	1 (1.7 oz)	120	44
drumstick w/ skin, roasted	1 (1.8 oz)	112	47
drumstick w/ skin, stewed	1 (2 oz)	116	43
drumstick w/o skin, fried	1 (1.5 oz)	82	40
drumstick w/o skin, roasted	1 (1.5 oz)	76	42
drumstick w/o skin, stewed	1 (1.6 oz)	78	37
leg w/ skin, batter dipped & fried	1 (5.5 oz)	431	442
leg w/ skin, floured & fried	1 (3.9 oz)	285	99
leg w/ skin, roasted	1 (4 oz)	265	99
leg w/ skin, stewed	1 (4.4 oz)	275	92
leg w/o skin, fried	1 (3.3 oz)	195	90
leg w/o skin, roasted	1 (3.3 oz)	182	87
leg w/o skin, stewed	1 (3.5 oz)	187	78
light meat w/ skin, batter dipped & fried	4 oz	312	324
light meat w/ skin, floured & fried	2.7 oz	192	60
light meat w/ skin, roasted	2.8 oz	175	59
light meat w/ skin, stewed	3.2 oz	181	57
light meat w/o skin, fried	1 cup (5 oz)	268	114
light meat w/o skin, roasted	1 cup (5 oz)	242	108
light meat w/o skin, stewed	1 cup (5 oz)	223	91
neck w/ skin, stewed	1 (1.3 oz)	94	20
neck w/o skin, stewed	1 (.6 oz)	32	12
skin, batter dipped & fried	4 oz	449	663
skin, batter dipped & fried	½ chicken (6.7 oz)	748	1105

FOOD	PORTION	CALORIES	SODIUM
skin, floured & fried	1 oz	166	18
skin, floured & fried	½ chicken (2 oz)	281	30
skin, roasted	½ chicken (2 oz)	254	36
skin, stewed	½ chicken (2.5 oz)	261	40
thigh w/ skin, batter dipped & fried	1 (3 oz)	238	248
thigh w/ skin, floured & fried	1 (2.2 oz)	162	55
thigh w/ skin, roasted	1 (2.2 oz)	153	52
thigh w/ skin, stewed	1 (2.4 oz)	158	49
thigh w/o skin, fried	1 (1.8 oz)	113	49
thigh w/o skin, roasted	1 (1.8 oz)	109	46
thigh w/o skin, stewed	1 (1.9 oz)	107	41
w/ skin, floured & fried	½ breast (3.4 oz)	218	75
w/o skin, fried	1 cup	307	127
w/o skin, roasted	1 cup (5 oz)	266	120
w/o skin, stewed	1 cup (5 oz)	248	98
w/o skin, stewed	1 oz	54	18
wing w/ skin, batter dipped & fried	1 (1.7 oz)	159	157
wing w/ skin, floured & fried	1 (1.1 oz)	103	25
wing w/ skin, roasted	1 (1.2 oz)	99	28
wing w/ skin, stewed	1 (1.4 oz)	100	27
w/ skin, floured & fried	½ chicken (11 oz)	844	264
w/ skin, fried	½ chicken (16.4 oz)	1347	1360
w/ skin, neck & giblets, batter dipped & fried	1 chicken (2.3 lb)	2987	2921

FOOD	PORTION	CALORIES	SODIUM
broiler/fryer *(cont.)*			
w/ skin, neck & giblets, roasted	1 chicken (1.5 lb)	1598	536
w/ skin, neck & giblets, stewed	1 chicken (1.6 lb)	1625	494
w/ skin, roasted	½ chicken (10.5 oz)	715	244
w/ skin, stewed	½ chicken (11.7 oz)	730	224
capon w/ skin, neck & giblets, roasted	1 chicken (3.1 lb)	3211	704
roaster			
dark meat w/o skin, roasted	1 cup (5 oz)	250	133
light meat w/o skin, roasted	1 cup (5 oz)	214	71
w/ skin, neck & giblets, roasted	1 chicken (2.4 lb)	2363	760
w/ skin, roasted	½ chicken (1.1 lb)	1071	349
w/o skin, roasted	1 cup (5 oz)	469	105
stewing			
dark meat w/o skin, stewed	1 cup (5 oz)	361	133
w/ skin, neck & giblets, stewed	1 chicken (1.3 lb)	1636	419
w/ skin, stewed	½ chicken (9.2 oz)	744	190
w/ skin, stewed	6.2 oz	507	130
FROZEN PREPARED			
Banquet			
Fried Chicken Breast Portions	5.75 oz	220	710
Fried Chicken Thighs & Drumsticks	6.25 oz	250	790
Hot'n Spicy Chicken Nuggets	2.5 oz	240	360
Hot'n Spicy Fried Chicken	6.4 oz	330	1210
Hot'n Spicy Snack'n Chicken	3.75 oz	140	480

FOOD	PORTION	CALORIES	SODIUM
Original Fried Chicken	5.6 oz	290	1060
Southern Fried Chicken	5.6 oz	290	1060
Banquet Boneless			
Breast Tenders	2.25 oz	150	280
Chicken Nuggets	2.5 oz	200	530
Chicken Nuggets w/ Cheddar	2.5 oz	240	530
Chicken Patties	2.5 oz	190	440
Chicken Sticks	2.5 oz	210	340
Drum-Snackers	2.5 oz	210	510
Fried Breast Tenders	2.25 oz	160	340
Southern Fried Chicken Nuggets	2.5 oz	210	500
Southern Fried Chicken Patties	2.5 oz	200	590
Country Skillet			
Chicken Chunks	3 oz	260	470
Chicken Nuggets	3 oz	250	580
Chicken Patties	3 oz	230	560
Southern Fried Chicken Chunks	3 oz	270	570
Southern Fried Chicken Patties	3 oz	240	540
Healthy Balance			
Baked Boneless Breast Nuggets	2.25 oz	120	310
Baked Boneless Breast Patties	2.25 oz	120	310
Baked Boneless Breast Tenders	2.25 oz	120	310
Swanson			
Chicken Nibbles	3¼ oz	300	690
Chicken Nuggets	3 oz	230	360
Fried Chicken Breast Portion	4½ oz	360	800
Pre-fried Chicken Parts	3¼ oz	270	650
Thighs And Drumsticks	3¼ oz	290	610
Weight Watchers Chicken Nuggets	5.9 oz	220	500

FOOD	PORTION	CALORIES	SODIUM
READY-TO-USE			
Carl Buddig	1 oz	60	340
Perdue Done It!			
BBQ Breast Half	1 oz	46	150
BBQ Drumsticks	1 oz	53	106
BBQ Half Dark Meat	1 oz	57	108
BBQ Half White Meat	1 oz	40	110
BBQ Thighs	1 oz	59	98
BBQ Wings	1 oz	62	169
Breast Roasted	1 oz	45	116
Cornish Hen Roasted Dark Meat	1 oz	45	72
Cornish Hen Roasted White Meat	1 oz	39	93
Cutlets	3.5 oz	250	445
Drumsticks Roasted	1 oz	40	115
Nuggets Cheese	1 (.67 oz)	54	108
Nuggets Fun Shaped	1 (.73 oz)	54	92
Nuggets Original	1 (.67 oz)	48	85
Tenders	1 oz	62	116
Thighs Roasted	1 oz	46	114
Whole Or Half Roasted Dark Meat	1 oz	51	73
Whole Or Half Roasted White Meat	1 oz	37	85
Wings Garlic & Herb	1 oz	61	172
Wings Hot & Spicy	1 oz	60	190
Weight Watchers			
Roasted And Smoked Breast	2 slices (¾ oz)	25	220
Roasted Ham	2 slices (¾ oz)	25	210
chicken roll, light meat	1 pkg (6 oz)	271	992
chicken roll, light meat	2 oz	90	331

FOOD	PORTION	CALORIES	SODIUM
poultry salad, sandwich spread	1 oz	238	107
poultry salad, sandwich spread	1 tbsp	109	49
TAKE-OUT			
boneless, breaded & fried			
w/ barbecue sauce	6 pieces (4.6 oz)	330	830
w/ honey	6 pieces (4 oz)	339	537
w/ mustard sauce	6 pieces (4.6 oz)	323	791
w/ sweet & sour sauce	6 pieces (4.6 oz)	346	791
breast & wing, breaded & fried	2 pieces (5.7 oz)	494	975
drumstick, breaded & fried	2 pieces (5.2 oz)	430	756
thigh, breaded & fried	2 pieces (5.2 oz)	430	756

CHICKEN DISHES
(*see also* CHICKEN SUBSTITUTES, DINNER)

FOOD	PORTION	CALORIES	SODIUM
CANNED			
Chicken & Dumplings (Swanson)	7½ oz	220	980
Chicken Ala King (Swanson)	5¼ oz	190	690
Chicken Stew (Swanson)	7⅝ oz	160	990
FROZEN			
MicroMagic Chicken Sandwich	1 pkg (4.5 oz)	390	650
Ovenstuffs Chicken Turnover	1 (4.75 oz)	350	690
Weight Watchers			
Chicken & Broccoli Pita	1 (5.4 oz)	190	420
Grilled Chicken Sandwich	1 (4 oz)	210	420
HOME RECIPE			
chicken & noodles	1 cup	365	600
chicken a la king	1 cup	470	760

FOOD	PORTION	CALORIES	SODIUM
MIX			
Lipton Microeasy			
Barbecue Chicken	¼ pkg	108	981
Country Chicken	¼ pkg	78	844
Skillet Chicken Helper			
Cheesy Broccoli, as prep	⅕ pkg (7.5 oz)	270	790
Creamy Chicken, as prep	⅕ pkg (8.25 oz)	290	800
Creamy Mushroom, as prep	⅕ pkg (8 oz)	280	800
Fettucine Alfredo, as prep	⅕ pkg (7.5 oz)	270	800
Stir-Fried Chicken, as prep	⅕ pkg (7 oz)	330	940
TAKE-OUT			
chicken & dumplings	¾ cup	256	1283
chicken cacciatore	¾ cup	394	671
fillet sandwich			
plain	1	515	957
w/ cheese, lettuce, mayonnaise & tomato	1	632	1238

CHICKEN SUBSTITUTES

FOOD	PORTION	CALORIES	SODIUM
Jaclyn's			
Salsa Chicken Style Dinner	11.5 oz	325	290
Sesame Chicken Style Dinner	11.5 oz	345	635

CHICKPEAS

FOOD	PORTION	CALORIES	SODIUM
CANNED			
Goya Spanish Style	7.5 oz	150	890
Green Giant Garbanzo	½ cup	90	320
S&W Garbanzo			
Lite, 50% Less Salt	½ cup	110	295
Premium Large	½ cup	110	470
Water Pack	½ cup	105	5
chickpeas	1 cup	285	718

FOOD	PORTION	CALORIES	SODIUM
DRIED			
Arrowhead Garbonzo	2 oz	200	10
cooked	1 cup	269	11

CHICORY

FOOD	PORTION	CALORIES	SODIUM
FRESH			
greens, raw, chopped	½ cup	21	41
roots, raw, cut up	½ cup	33	23
witloof, raw	½ cup	7	3

CHILI

FOOD	PORTION	CALORIES	SODIUM
CANNED			
Gebhardt			
Hot With Beans	1 cup	470	1000
Plain	1 cup	530	990
With Beans	1 cup	495	1010
Health Valley			
Mild Vegetarian With Beans	5 oz	160	290
Mild Vegetarian With Beans, No Salt Added	5 oz	160	30
Mild Vegetarian With Lentils	5 oz	140	290
Mild Vegetarian With Lentils, No Salt Added	5 oz	140	50
Spicy Vegetarian With Beans	5 oz	160	280
Spicy Vegetarian With Beans, No Salt Added	5 oz	160	30
Spicy w/ Beans & Ground Turkey	½ can (7.5 oz)	210	530
Turkey w/ Beans	½ can (7.5 oz)	200	560
Hunt's Chili Beans	4 oz	100	490
Just Rite			
Hot With Beans	4 oz	195	495
With Beans	4 oz	200	500

FOOD	PORTION	CALORIES	SODIUM
Just Rite *(cont.)*			
Without Beans	4 oz	180	515
Manwich Chili Fixin's, as prep	8 oz	290	980
S&W			
Chili Beans	½ cup	130	520
Chili Makin's Original	½ cup	100	782
Van Camp's			
Chili Weenee	1 cup	309	1057
Chili With Beans	1 cup	352	1215
Chili Without Beans	1 cup	412	1499
Wolf Brand			
Chili-Mac	7.5 oz	317	854
Extra Spicy With Beans	7.5 oz	324	926
Extra Spicy Without Beans	7.5 oz	363	962
Plain	7.5 oz	330	1165
With Beans	7.5 oz	345	1013
Without Beans	1 cup	387	1042
chili w/ beans	1 cup	286	1330
DRIED			
Gebhardt			
Chili Powder	1 tsp	15	0
Chili Quik Seasoning	1 tsp	10	165
powder	1 tsp	8	26
FROZEN			
Swanson Homestyle Chili Con Carne	8¼ oz	270	740
TAKE-OUT			
con carne w/ beans	8.9 oz	254	1008

CHINESE CABBAGE
(*see* CABBAGE)

FOOD	PORTION	CALORIES	SODIUM

CHINESE FOOD
(*see* ORIENTAL FOOD)

CHINESE PRESERVING MELON

cooked	½ cup	11	93

CHIPS
(*see also* POPCORN, PRETZELS, SNACKS)

CORN
Arrowhead

Blue Corn Curls	1 oz	120	126
Blue Corn Curls Unsalted	1 oz	120	2
Yellow Corn Chips	¾ oz	90	96
Yellow Corn Chips With Cheese	¾ oz	90	94
Health Valley	1 oz	160	90
No Salt Added	1 oz	160	1
With Cheddar Cheese	1 oz	160	120
Weight Watchers			
Corn Snackers	½ oz	60	230
Corn Snackers Nacho Cheese	½ oz	60	270

POTATO
Health Valley

Dip Chips No Salt Added	1 oz	160	1
Natural	1 oz	160	60
Natural No Salt Added	1 oz	160	1
Country Ripple	1 oz	160	60
Country Ripple No Salt Added	1 oz	160	1
Dip Chips	1 oz	160	60
Kelly's	1 oz	150	160
Bar-B-Q	1 oz	150	230
Crunchy	1 oz	150	140
Rippled	1 oz	150	160

FOOD	PORTION	CALORIES	SODIUM
Kelly's *(cont.)*			
Sour Cream n' Onion	1 oz	150	170
Unsalted	1 oz	150	5
Old Dutch Foods	1 oz	150	160
Augratin	1 oz	150	220
BBQ	1 oz	140	360
Dill Flavored	1 oz	150	340
Onion & Garlic	1 oz	150	420
Ripple	1 oz	150	150
Sour Cream & Onion	1 oz	150	220
Weight Watchers			
Great Snackers Barbecue	½ oz	70	100
Great Snackers Cheddar Cheese	½ oz	70	130
Great Snackers Sour Cream & Onion	½ oz	70	140
potato	1 oz	148	133
potato	10 chips	105	94
sticks	1 oz pkg	148	71
sticks	½ cup	94	45

CHITTERLINGS

pork, simmered	3 oz	258	33

CHIVES

fresh, chopped	1 tbsp	1	0
fresh, chopped	1 tsp	0	0

CHOCOLATE
(*see also* CANDY, CAROB, COCOA, ICE CREAM TOPPINGS, MILK DRINKS)

BAKING			
Chocolate Semi-Sweet (Nestle)	1 oz	160	0

FOOD	PORTION	CALORIES	SODIUM
Chocolate Unsweetened (Nestle)	1 oz	180	0
Pre-Melted Unsweetened (Nestle)	1 oz	190	0
Premier White (Nestle)	½ oz	80	15
Premium Baking Bar, Unsweetened (Hershey)	1 oz	190	5
baking	1 oz	145	1
CHIPS			
Milk Chocolate			
Chips (Hershey)	1 oz	150	55
Chunks (Hershey)	1 oz	160	25
Morsels (Nestle)	1 oz	150	15
Mint-Chocolate Morsels (Nestle)	1 oz	140	0
Premier White Teasures (Nestle)	1 oz	160	25
Semi-Sweet Chocolate Chips			
Miniature (Hershey)	¼ cup	220	5
Regular (Hershey)	¼ cup	220	5
SemiSweet Chocolate Morsels (Nestle)	1 oz	140	0
Toll House			
Merry Morsels (Nestle)	1 oz	140	0
Milk Chocolate Treasures (Nestle)	1 oz	150	20
Rainbow Morsels (Nestle)	½ oz	70	0
Semi-Sweet Chocolate Morsels (Nestle)	1 oz	140	0
Semi-Sweet Chocolate Treasures (Nestle)	1 oz	150	0
MIX			
Hershey Chocolate Milk Mix	3 tbsp	90	40
powder	2-3 heaping tsp	75	45
powder, as prep w/ whole milk	9 oz	226	165

FOOD	PORTION	CALORIES	SODIUM
SYRUP			
Estee	1 tbsp	20	5
Hershey's	2 tbsp	80	20
chocolate	1 cup	653	287
chocolate	2 tbsp	82	36
chocolate, as prep w/ whole milk	9 oz	232	156

CHOCOLATE MILK
(see CHOCOLATE, COCOA, MILK DRINKS)

CHUTNEY

apple cranberry	1 tbsp	16	1

CILANTRO

fresh	¼ cup	1	1

CINNAMON

ground	1 tsp	6	1

CISCO

smoked	1 oz	50	135
smoked	3 oz	151	409
fresh, raw	3 oz	84	47

CLAMS

CANNED			
Empress Whole Baby	4 oz	60	540
Gorton's Minced & Chopped	½ can	70	640
S&W Fancy Chopped	2 oz	28	280
S&W Fancy Minced	2 oz	28	280
liquid only	1 cup	6	516
liquid only	3 oz	2	183

FOOD	PORTION	CALORIES	SODIUM
meat only	1 cup	236	179
meat only	3 oz	126	95
FRESH			
cooked	20 sm	133	100
cooked	3 oz	126	95
raw	9 lg	133	100
raw	20 sm	133	100
raw	3 oz	63	47
FROZEN			
Fried (Mrs. Paul's)	2½ oz	200	450
Microwave			
Crunchy Clam Strips (Gorton's)	3.5 oz	330	430
Fried Claims (Mrs. Paul's)	2.5 oz	260	410
HOME RECIPE			
breaded & fried	20 sm	379	684
breaded & fried	3 oz	171	309
TAKE-OUT			
breaded & fried	¾ cup	451	833

CLOVES

FOOD	PORTION	CALORIES	SODIUM
ground	1 tsp	7	5

COCOA
  (*see also* CHOCOLATE)

FOOD	PORTION	CALORIES	SODIUM
Hershey	⅓ cup	120	10
Hershey European Cocoa	1 oz	90	15
Nestle	⅓ cup (1 oz)	80	<5
Nestle Hot Cocoa Mix	1 oz	110	100
as prep w/ 2% milk	6 oz	210	190
as prep w/ skim milk	6 oz	180	200

FOOD	PORTION	CALORIES	SODIUM
Nestle Hot Cocoa Mix *(cont.)*			
as prep w/ whole milk	6 oz	230	240
With Marshmallows	1 oz	120	115
With Marshmallows, as prep w/ 2% milk	6 oz	220	190
With Marshmallows, as prep w/ skim milk	6 oz	190	200
With Marshmallows, as prep w/ whole milk	6 oz	240	240
Swiss Miss Cocoa			
Diet	4 oz	20	180
Lite, as prep	6 oz	70	160
Sugar Free, as prep	6 oz	60	125
Sugar Free With Sugar Free Marshmallows, as prep	6 oz	50	120
Swiss Miss Hot Cocoa			
Bavarian Chocolate	6 oz	110	170
Double Rich	4 oz	110	150
Milk Chocolate	6 oz	110	125
With Mini Marshmallows	4 oz	110	170
Weight Watchers	1 pkg	60	160
hot cocoa	1 cup	218	123
mix, as prep w/ water	7 oz	103	149
mix w/ nutrasweet, as prep w/ water	7 oz	48	173
powder	1 oz	102	143

COCONUT

FOOD	PORTION	CALORIES	SODIUM
coconut water	1 cup	46	252
coconut water	1 tbsp	3	16
cream, canned	1 cup	568	149
cream, canned	1 tbsp	36	10

FOOD	PORTION	CALORIES	SODIUM
dried			
sweetened, flaked	1 cup	351	189
sweetened, flaked	7 oz. pkg	944	509
sweetened, flaked, canned	1 cup	341	15
sweetened, shredded	1 cup	466	244
sweetened, shredded	7 oz pkg	997	522
toasted	1 oz	168	11
unsweetened	1 oz	187	11
fresh	1 piece (1½ oz)	159	9
fresh, shredded	1 cup	283	16
milk, canned	1 cup	445	29
milk, canned	1 tbsp	30	2
milk, frozen	1 cup	486	29
milk, frozen	1 tbsp	30	2

COD

FOOD	PORTION	CALORIES	SODIUM
CANNED			
atlantic	1 can (11 oz)	327	680
atlantic	3 oz	89	185
DRIED			
atlantic	3 oz	246	5973
FRESH			
atlantic, cooked	1 fillet (6.3 oz)	189	141
atlantic, cooked	3 oz	89	66
atlantic, raw	3 oz	70	46
pacific, baked	3 oz	95	82
FROZEN			
Fishmarket Fresh (Gorton's)	5 oz	110	90
Light Fillets (Mrs. Paul's)	1 fillet	240	430

FOOD	PORTION	CALORIES	SODIUM

COFFEE
(*see also* COFFEE BEVERAGES, COFFEE SUBSTITUTES)

INSTANT

FOOD	PORTION	CALORIES	SODIUM
cappuccino mix, as prep	7 oz	62	104
decaffeinated	1 rounded tsp	4	0
decaffeinated, as prep	6 oz	4	6
mocha mix, as prep	7 oz	51	36
regular	1 rounded tsp	4	1
regular, as prep	6 oz	4	6
regular w/ chicory	1 rounded tsp	6	5
regular w/ chicory, as prep	6 oz	6	10

REGULAR

FOOD	PORTION	CALORIES	SODIUM
brewed	6 oz	4	4

COFFEE BEVERAGES
(*see also* COFFEE, COFFEE SUBSTITUTES)

FOOD	PORTION	CALORIES	SODIUM
Chock o'ccino			
Cinnamon	8 oz	120	55
Coffee	8 oz	120	55
Mocha	8 oz	120	55

COFFEE SUBSTITUTES
(*see also* COFFEE, COFFEE SUBSTITUTES)

FOOD	PORTION	CALORIES	SODIUM
powder	1 tsp	9	2
powder, as prep	6 oz	9	7
powder, as prep w/ milk	6 oz	121	91

COFFEE WHITENERS
(*see also* MILK SUBSTITUTES)

LIQUID

FOOD	PORTION	CALORIES	SODIUM
nondairy, frzn	1 tbsp	20	12

POWDER

FOOD	PORTION	CALORIES	SODIUM
N-Rich Creamer	1 tsp	10	0

FOOD	PORTION	CALORIES	SODIUM
Weight Watchers Dairy Creamer, Instant Non-fat Dry Milk	1 pkg	10	15
nondairy	1 tsp	11	4

COLLARDS

FRESH
cooked	½ cup	17	10
raw, chopped	½ cup	6	4

FROZEN
chopped, cooked	½ cup	31	42

COOKIES
(*see also* BROWNIE, CAKE, DOUGHNUTS, PIE)

HOME RECIPE
chocolate chip	4 (1½ oz)	185	82
peanut butter	4 (1.7 oz)	245	142
shortbread	2 (1 oz)	145	125

MIX
Chocolate Chip Big Batch (Betty Crocker)	2	120	100
Chocolate Chip Cookie Mix (Estee)	1 (2")	50	40
Date Bar Classic Dessert (Betty Crocker)	1	60	35

READY-TO-EAT
7-Grain Oatmeal (Frookie)	1	45	35
Almond Crecents (Sunshine)	2	70	55
Almost Home (Nabisco)			
Oatmeal Raisin	1	70	40
Real Chocolate Chip	1	60	45
Amaranth Cookies (Health Valley)	1	70	30
Animal Crackers (Sunshine)	7	70	60

FOOD	PORTION	CALORIES	SODIUM
Animal Crackers *(cont.)*			
Barnum's	5	60	70
Animal Frackers (Frookie)	6	60	25
Apple Cinnamon Oat Bran (Frookie)	1	45	35
Apple Cinnamon Oat Bran (Frookie)	1 lg	120	100
Apple Fruitins (Frookie)	1	60	25
Apple Raisin Bar (Weight Watchers)	1	100	115
Arrowroot Biscuit, National (Nabisco)	1	20	15
Baked Apple Bar (Sunbelt)	1 pkg (1.31 oz)	130	130
Bakers Bonus Oatmeal (Nabisco)	1	80	65
Bavarian Fingers (Sunshine)	1	70	55
Beacon Hill Chocolate Chocolate Walnut (Pepperidge Farm)	1	120	65
Biscos			
Sugar Wafers (Nabisco)	4	70	20
Waffle Cremes (Nabisco)	1	40	10
Bordeaux (Pepperidge Farm)	2	70	40
Brown Edge Wafers (Nabisco)	2½	70	45
Brownie Chocolate Nut (Pepperidge Farm)	2	110	45
Brownie Nut Large Cookie (Pepperidge Farm)	1	140	65
Brussels (Pepperidge Farm)	2	110	65
Brussels Mint (Pepperidge Farm)	2	130	40
Bugs Bunny Graham Cookies (Nabisco)	5	60	70
Butter Chessman (Pepperidge Farm)	2	90	60
Butter Flavored Cookies (Sunshine)	2	60	55

FOOD	PORTION	CALORIES	SODIUM
Buttercup (Keebler)	3	70	110
Cappucino (Pepperidge Farm)	1	50	20
Capri (Pepperidge Farm)	1	80	45
Chantilly (Pepperidge Farm)	1	80	35
Chesapeake Chocolate Chunk Pecan (Pepperidge Farm)	1	120	60
Cheyenne Peanut Butter Milk, Chocolate Chunk (Pepperidge Farm)	1	110	80
Chip-A-Roos (Sunshine)	1	60	45
Chips Ahoy!			
Chewy	1	60	40
Chocolate Chocolate Chunk	1	90	65
Chocolate Chocolate Walnut	1	100	70
Chocolate Chunk Pecan	1	100	65
Chunky Chocolate Chip	1	90	90
Mini	6	70	45
Oatmeal Chocolate Chip	1	90	50
Pure Chocolate Chip	1	50	40
Sprinkled	1	60	40
Striped	1	90	45
Chocolate			
(Weight Watchers)	3	80	135
Cookiesaurus (Sunshine)	7	120	140
Sandwich (Weight Watchers)	2	90	90
Snaps (Nabisco)	4	70	75
Chocolate Chip			
(Drake's)	2 (1 oz)	140	110
(Frookie)	1	45	35
(Frookie)	1 lg	120	100
(Nutra/Balance)	1 (2 oz)	260	81
(Pepperidge Farm)	2	100	45

FOOD	PORTION	CALORIES	SODIUM
Chocolate Chip (cont.)			
(Weight Watchers)	2	90	65
Large Cookie (Pepperidge Farm)	1	130	60
Mint (Frookie)	1	45	35
Snaps (Nabisco)	3	70	50
Chocolate Chunk Pecan (Pepperidge Farm)	1	70	25
Chocolate Fudge Sandwich (Keebler)	1	80	70
Chocolate-Chocolate Chip (Drake's)	2 (1 oz)	130	85
Coconut (Drake's)	2 (1 oz)	130	95
Coconut Macaroon (Drake's)	1 (1 oz)	135	80
Commodore (Keebler)	1	60	65
Cookie Break (Nabisco)	1	50	35
Cookie Caramel Bars (Little Debbie)	1 pkg (1.17 oz)	170	85
Cookies 'N Fudge (Nabisco)			
Party Grahams	1	45	35
Striped Shortbread	1	60	50
Striped Wafers	1	70	30
Cookies Mates (Keebler)	2	50	55
Creme Filled			
Chocolate (Little Debbie)	1 pkg (1.8 oz)	250	260
Wafers, Assorted (Estee)	1	30	5
Wafers, Chocolate (Estee)	1	20	5
Wafers, Vanilla (Estee)	1	20	5
Dakota Milk Chocolate, Oatmeal (Pepperidge Farm)	1	110	70
Date Pecan (Pepperidge Farm)	2	110	40
Devil's Food Cakes (Nabisco)	1	70	40
Dinosaur Grrrahams (Mother's)	1	70	50

FOOD	PORTION	CALORIES	SODIUM
Dixi Vanilla (Sunshine)	2	130	110
Famous Chocolate Wafers (Nabisco)	2½	70	110
Fancy Fruit Chunks (Health Valley)			
Apricot Almond	2	90	45
Date Pecan	2	90	45
Raisin Oat Bran	2	70	95
Tropical Fruit	2	90	45
Fancy Peanut Chunks (Health Valley)	2	90	55
Fat Free (Health Valley)			
Apple Spice	3	75	40
Apricot Delight	3	75	40
Date Delight	3	75	40
Hawaiian Fruit	3	75	40
Raisin Oatmeal	3	75	40
Fat Free Jumbos (Health Valley)			
Apple Raisin	1	70	35
Raisin	1	70	35
Raspberry	1	70	35
Fiber Jumbos (Health Valley)			
Blueberry Nut	1	100	45
Chunky Pecan	1	100	45
Raisin Nut	1	100	45
Fig Bar (Mother's)	1 oz	100	75
Fig Bars (Sunshine)	1	50	35
Fig Fruitins (Frookie)	1	60	25
Fig Newtons (Nabisco)	1	60	60
Fortune (La Choy)	1	15	1
French Vanilla Creme (Keebler)	1	80	80
Fruit & Fitness (Health Valley)	5	200	115

FOOD	PORTION	CALORIES	SODIUM
Fruit Filled (Pepperidge Farm)			
Apricot-Raspberry	2	100	50
Strawberry	2	100	50
Fruit Filled Bar (Weight Watchers)			
Apple	1	80	35
Raspberry	1	80	45
Fruit Jumbos (Health Valley)			
Almond Date	1	70	30
Oat Bran	1	70	35
Raisin Nut	1	70	35
Tropical Fruit	1	70	35
Fudge (Estee)	1	30	0
Fudge Dipped Grahams (Sunshine)	2	80	40
Fudge Family Bears (Sunshine)			
Chocolate With Vanilla Filling	1	70	60
Peanut Butter	1	70	65
Vanilla With Fudge Filling	1	60	50
Fudge Striped Shortbread (Sunshine)	3	160	80
Geneva (Pepperidge Farm)	2	130	50
Ginger Snaps			
(Bakery Wagon)	4-5 (1 oz)	140	105
(Sunshine)	3	60	70
Old Fashioned (Nabisco)	2	60	80
Ginger Spice (Frookie)	1	45	35
Gingerman (Pepperidge Farm)	2	70	50
Golden Fruit (Sunshine)	1	70	40
Graham			
(Nabisco)	2	60	90
Amaranth (Health Valley)	7	110	110
Chocolate (Nabisco)	1	50	30

FOOD	PORTION	CALORIES	SODIUM
Honey (Health Valley)	7	100	125
Honey (Honey Maid)	2	60	90
Honey Fiber, Enriched (Keebler)	2	90	110
Kitchen Rich (Keebler)	2	60	55
Oat Bran (Health Valley)	7	120	45
Grahamy Bears (Sunshine)	4	60	55
Hazelnut (Pepperidge Farm)	2	110	75
Hermit (Drake's)	1 (2 oz)	230	280
Heyday (Nabisco)			
Caramel & Peanut	1	110	40
Fudge	1	110	40
Homeplate (Keebler)	1	60	130
Honey Jumbos (Health Valley)			
Crisp Cinnamon	1	70	35
Crisp Peanut Butter	1	70	35
Fancy Oat Bran	2	130	50
Hydrox	1	50	45
Doubles, Peanut Butter	1	60	65
Iced Gingerbread Cookies (Sunshine)	3	70	75
Ideal Bars (Nabisco)	1	90	80
Irish Oatmeal (Pepperidge Farm)	2	90	80
Jingles (Sunshine)	3	70	55
Keebies (Keebler)	1	80	80
Krisp Kreem Wafers (Keebler)	2	50	20
Lemon Coolers (Sunshine)	2	60	45
Lemon Nut Crunch (Pepperidge Farm)	2	110	50
Lido (Pepperidge Farm)	1	90	30
Linzer (Pepperidge Farm)	1	120	55

FOOD	PORTION	CALORIES	SODIUM
Lorna Doone	2	70	65
Mallomars	1	60	20
Mallopuffs (Sunshine)	1	70	35
Mandarin Chocolate Chip (Frookie)	1	45	35
Marie LU (LU)	1	50	45
Marshmallow (Nabisco)			
Puffs	1	90	40
Twirls	1	130	50
Milano (Pepperidge Farm)	2	120	45
Mini Chocolate Chip Cookies (Sunshine)	2	70	50
Mint Milano (Pepperidge Farm)	2	150	60
Molasses Crisps (Pepperidge Farm)	2	70	50
Molasses Iced (Bakery Wagon)	1	100	120
My Goodness (Nabisco)			
Banana Nut	1	90	70
Chocolate Chip And Raisin	1	90	70
Oatmeal Raisin	1	90	85
Mystic Mint	1	90	65
Nantucket Chocolate Chunk (Pepperidge Farm)	1	120	60
Nassau (Pepperidge Farm)	1	80	45
Newtons (Nabisco)			
Apple	1	70	70
Raspberry	1	70	70
Strawberry	1	70	70
Nilla Wafers (Nabisco)	3½	60	45
Nutter Butter			
Peanut Butter (Nabisco)	1	70	50
Peanut Creme (Nabisco)	2	80	45

FOOD	PORTION	CALORIES	SODIUM
Oat Bran Animal Cookies (Health Valley)	7	110	50
Oat Bran Fruit & Nut (Health Valley)	2	110	70
Oat Bran Muffin (Frookie)	1	45	35
Oat Bran Muffin (Frookie)	1 lg	120	100
Oat Bran With Nuts And Raisins (Sunshine)	1	60	55
Oatmeal			
(Drake's)	2 (1 oz)	120	50
(Little Debbie)	1 pkg (2.75 oz)	340	440
(Mother's)	1	60	80
Country Style (Sunshine)	1	70	65
Large Cookie (Pepperidge Farm)	1	120	105
Oatmeal Creme (Drake's)	1 (2 oz)	240	250
Oatmeal Date Filled (Bakery Wagon)	1	90	100
Oatmeal Raisin			
(Frookie)	1	45	35
(Frookie)	1 lg	120	100
(Nutra/Balance)	1 (2 oz)	240	50
(Pepperidge Farm)	2	110	115
(Weight Watchers)	2	90	75
Oatmeal			
Soft (Bakery Wagon)	1	100	105
Spice (Weight Watchers)	3	80	75
Old Fashion (Keebler)			
Chocolate Chip	1	80	75
Double Fudge	1	80	65
Oatmeal	1	80	110
Peanut Butter	1	80	100
Sugar	1	80	70

FOOD	PORTION	CALORIES	SODIUM
Old Fashioned Chocolate Chip (Pepperidge Farm)	2	100	45
Orange Milano (Pepperidge Farm)	2	150	60
Oreo	1	50	75
Big Stuf	1	200	220
Double Stuf	1	70	75
Fudge Covered	1	110	75
Mini	5	70	85
White Fudge Covered	1	110	75
Orleans (Pepperidge Farm)	3	90	30
Orleans Sandwich (Pepperidge Farm)	2	120	40
Pantry Molasses (Nabisco)	1	80	75
Pecan Shortbread (Nabisco)	1	80	40
Peanut Butter & Jelly Sandwiches (Little Debbie)	1 pkg (1.13 oz)	150	105
Peanut Butter Bars (Little Debbie)	1 pkg (1.83 oz)	290	180
Peanut Butter Naturals (Sunbelt)	1 pkg (1.2 oz)	170	90
Peanut Butter Wafers (Drake's)	1 (2.25 oz)	324	135
Peanut Clusters (Little Debbie)	1 pkg (1.44 oz)	210	110
Pecan Shortbread (Pepperidge Farm)	1	70	15
Pinwheels (Nabisco)	1	130	40
Pirouettes (Pepperidge Farm)			
Chocolate Laced	2	70	20
Original	2	70	35
Pitter Patter (Keebler)	1	90	115
Pure Chocolate Middles (Nabisco)	1	80	35
Raisin Bran (Pepperidge Farm)	2	110	55
Sandwich Cookies (Estee)			
Chocolate	1	50	15
Original	1	45	5

FOOD	PORTION	CALORIES	SODIUM
Peanut Butter	1	50	35
Sante Fe Oatmeal Raisin (Pepperidge Farm)	1	100	70
Sausalito Milk Chocolate Macadamia (Pepperidge Farm)	1	120	65
School House Cookies (Sunshine)	15	120	100
Sea Flappers (Sunshine)	7	140	80
Shortbread (Pepperidge Farm)	2	150	85
(Weight Watchers)	3	80	95
Snack Wafer Chocolate Coated (Estee)	1	130	10
Social Tea (Nabisco)	3	70	60
Sprinkles Rainbow Topping (Sunshine)	1	70	25
Suddenly S'Mores (Nabisco)	1	100	90
Sugar (Pepperidge Farm)	2	100	55
Sugar Wafers (Sunshine) Assorted	2	90	25
Chocolate	2	90	15
Peanut Butter	2	80	35
Vanilla	2	90	25
Taffy Creme Sandwich (Mother's)	1-2 (1 oz)	140	80
Tahiti (Pepperidge Farm)	1	90	25
Teddy Grahams (Nabisco) Chocolate Graham	11	60	90
Cinnamon Graham	11	60	80
Honey Graham	11	60	90
Vanilla Graham	11	60	75
Teddy Grahams Bearwich (Nabisco) Chocolate And Vanilla Creme	4	70	60
Cinnamon With Vanilla Creme	4	70	60
Vanilla And Chocolate Creme	4	70	65

FOOD	PORTION	CALORIES	SODIUM
The Great Tofu (Health Valley)	2	90	30
The Great Wheat Free (Health Valley)	2	80	35
Tru Blu (Sunshine)			
Chocolate	2	160	140
Lemon	1	70	65
Vanilla	1	8	65
Vanilla Wafers			
(Keebler)	4	80	60
(Sunshine)	3	70	50
Vienna Fingers (Sunshine)	12	70	60
Zurich (Pepperidge Farm)	1	60	30
animal crackers	1 box (2.4 oz)	299	274
chocolate chip	1 box (1.9 oz)	233	188
chocolate chip	4 (1½ oz)	180	140
chocolate sandwich	4 (1.4 oz)	195	189
fig bars	4 (2 oz)	210	180
graham	2 sq	60	86
oatmeal raisin	4 (1.8 oz)	245	148
shortbread	4 (1 oz)	155	123
vanilla sandwich	4 (1.4 oz)	195	189
vanilla wafers	10 (1¼ oz)	185	150
REFRIGERATED			
Chocolate Chip (Pillsbury)	1	70	55
Oatmeal Raisin (Pillsbury)	1	60	55
Peanut Butter (Pillsbury)	1	70	75
Sugar (Pillsbury)	1	70	70
chocolate chip	4 (1.7 oz)	225	173
sugar	4 (1.7 oz)	235	261

FOOD	PORTION	CALORIES	SODIUM

CORIANDER

FOOD	PORTION	CALORIES	SODIUM
leaf, dried	1 tsp	2	1
leaf, fresh	¼ cup	1	1
seed	1 tsp	5	1

CORN

(*see also* BRAN, CEREAL, CORNMEAL, FLOUR)

FOOD	PORTION	CALORIES	SODIUM
CANNED			
50% Less Salt No Sugar Added (Green Giant)	½ cup	50	140
Corn (Green Giant)	½ cup	70	350
Cream Style (Green Giant)	½ cup	100	390
Diet (S&W)	½ cup	100	0
Premium Homestyle (S&W)	½ cup	105	435
Deli Corn (Green Giant)	½ cup	80	350
Golden Kernal, 50% Less Salt (Green Giant)	½ cup	70	175
Golden Vacuum Packed (Green Giant)	½ cup	80	330
Mexi Corn (Green Giant)	½ cup	80	450
No Salt, No Sugar (Green Giant)	½ cup	80	0
Sweet 'N Natural (S&W)	½ cup	90	180
Sweet Select (Green Giant)	½ cup	60	280
White, Vacuum Packed (Green Giant)	½ cup	80	290
Whole Kernel (S&W)			
Tender Young	½ cup	90	295
Water Pack	½ cup	80	0
cream style	½ cup	93	365
w/ red & green peppers	½ cup	86	396

FOOD	PORTION	CALORIES	SODIUM
DRIED			
Blue (Arrowhead)	2 oz	210	tr
Yellow (Arrowhead)	2 oz	210	tr
FRESH			
on-the-cob w/ butter, cooked	1 ear	155	30
white, cooked	½ cup	89	14
white, raw	½ cup	66	12
yellow, cooked	1 ear (2.7 oz)	83	13
yellow, cooked	½ cup	89	14
yellow, raw	1 ear (3 oz)	77	14
yellow, raw	½ cup	66	12
FROZEN			
Cob Corn (Ore Ida)	1 ear (5.3 oz)	190	10
Cob Corn Mini-Gold (Ore Ida)	1 (2.65 oz)	90	5
Cream Style (Green Giant)	½ cup	110	370
Fritters (Mrs. Paul's)	2	240	560
Harvest Fresh (Green Giant)			
Niblets	½ cup	80	40
White Shoepeg	½ cup	90	60
In Butter Sauce (Green Giant)	½ cup	100	310
Nibblers Corn On The Cob (Green Giant)	2 ears	120	10
Niblet Ears (Green Giant)	1 ear	120	10
Niblets (Green Giant)	½ cup	90	5
One Serve (Green Giant)			
Niblets In Butter Sauce	1 pkg	120	350
On The Cob	1 pkg	120	10
Super Sweet			
Nibblers Corn On The Cob (Green Giant)	2 ears	90	10
Niblet (Green Giant Select)	½ cup	60	5
Niblet Ears (Green Giant)	1 ear	90	10

FOOD	PORTION	CALORIES	SODIUM
White			
(Green Giant Select)	½ cup	90	5
In Butter Sauce (Green Giant)	½ cup	100	280
cooked	½ cup	67	4
on-the-cob, cooked	1 ear (2.2 oz)	59	3
SHELF STABLE Golden Whole Kernel (Pantry Express)	½ cup	60	210
TAKE-OUT			
fritters	1 (1 oz)	62	126
scalloped	½ cup	258	246

CORN CHIPS
(see CHIPS)

CORNISH HENS
(see CHICKEN)

CORNMEAL

FOOD	PORTION	CALORIES	SODIUM
Arrowhead			
Blue	2 oz	210	1
Hi-Lysine	2 oz	210	tr
Yellow	2 oz	210	tr
Aunt Jemima			
White	3 tbsp	102	1
Yellow	3 tbsp	102	1
Quaker			
White	3 tbsp	102	1
Yellow	3 tbsp	102	1
corn grits, cooked	1 cup	146	0
corn grits, uncooked	1 cup	579	1
degermed	1 cup	506	5
self-rising, degermed	1 cup	489	1860
whole grain	1 cup	442	43

FOOD	PORTION	CALORIES	SODIUM
MIX			
Arrowhead Corn Bread	1 oz	100	75
Aunt Jemima			
Bolted White Mix	3 tbsp	99	337
Buttermilk, Self-Rising White Mix	3 tbsp	101	439
Self-Rising White Mix	3 tbsp	98	381
Self-Rising Yellow Mix	3 tbsp	100	490
Golden Dipt			
Corny Dog Batter Mix	1 oz	100	490
Hush Puppy Deluxe Mix	1¼ oz	120	520
Hush Puppy Jalapeno Mix	1¼ oz	120	570
Hush Puppy With Onion	1¼ oz	120	520
CORNSTARCH			
Argo	1 cup	460	tr
Argo	1 tbsp	30	0
Kingsford's	1 cup	460	tr
Kingsford's	1 tbsp	30	0
cornstarch	⅓ cup	164	4
COTTAGE CHEESE			
Breakstone			
2%	4 oz	100	510
4% Small Curd	4 oz	110	370
4% With Pineapple	4 oz	140	260
Dry Curd, No Salt Added	4 oz	90	65
Cabot	4 oz	120	455
Cabot Light	4 oz	90	360
Knudsen			
2%	4 oz	100	370
2% With Fruit Cocktail	4 oz	130	330

FOOD	PORTION	CALORIES	SODIUM
2% With Mandarin Orange	4 oz	110	320
2% With Peach	4 oz	170	270
2% With Pear	4 oz	110	320
2% With Pineapple	4 oz	170	300
2% With Spiced Apple	4 oz	180	280
2% With Strawberry	4 oz	170	320
4% Large Curd	4 oz	120	340
4% Small Curd	4 oz	120	370
Nonfat	4 oz	90	420
Lactaid 1%	4 oz	72	406
Light N' Lively			
1%	4 oz	80	370
1% Garden Salad	4 oz	80	350
1% Peach And Pineapple	4 oz	100	320
Sargento Pot Cheese	1 oz	26	1
Sealtest 2%	4 oz	100	340
Viva Nonfat	½ cup	70	430
Weight Watchers			
1%	½ cup	90	460
2%	½ cup	100	460
creamed	1 cup	217	850
creamed	4 oz	117	457
creamed w/ fruit	4 oz	140	457
dry curd	1 cup	123	19
dry curd	4 oz	96	14
lowfat 1%	1 cup	164	918
lowfat 1%	4 oz	82	459
lowfat 2%	1 cup	203	918
lowfat 2%	4 oz	101	459

FOOD	PORTION	CALORIES	SODIUM

COTTONSEED

FOOD	PORTION	CALORIES	SODIUM
kernels, roasted	1 tbsp	51	3

COUSCOUS

FOOD	PORTION	CALORIES	SODIUM
Couscous, Lemon Thyme Salad Mix, as prep (Nile Spice)	½ cup	103	146
Golden Couscous (Nile Spice)			
Lentil Curry Soup Mix, as prep	10 oz	220	590
Tomato Minestrone Soup, as prep	10 oz	200	590
Vegetable Chicken Soup, as prep	10 oz	220	400
Vegetable Parmesan Soup, as prep	10 oz	200	550
Whole Wheat, Lentil & Onion Couscous Pilaf, as prep (Nile Spice)	½ cup	153	188
cooked	½ cup	101	4
dry	½ cup	346	9

COWPEAS

FOOD	PORTION	CALORIES	SODIUM
CANNED			
common	1 cup	184	718
DRIED			
catjang, cooked	1 cup	200	32
FRESH			
leafy tips			
chopped, cooked	1 cup	12	3
raw, chopped	1 cup	10	2
FROZEN			
cooked	½ cup	112	5

FOOD	PORTION	CALORIES	SODIUM

CRAB

CANNED

Dungeness Crab (S&W)	3.25 oz	81	920
blue	1 cup	133	5
blue	3 oz	84	283

FRESH

alaska king, cooked	1 leg (4.7 oz)	129	1436
alaska king, cooked	3 oz	82	911
alaska king, raw	1 leg (6 oz)	144	1438
alaska king, raw	3 oz	71	711
blue, cooked	1 cup	138	376
blue, cooked	3 oz	87	237
blue, raw	1 crab (.7 oz)	18	62
blue, raw	3 oz	74	249
dungeness, raw	1 crab (5.7 oz)	140	481
dungeness, raw	3 oz	73	251
queen, steamed	3 oz	98	587

FROZEN

| Deviled Crab (Mrs. Paul's) | 1 cake | 180 | 480 |
| Miniatures | 3½ oz | 240 | 540 |

READY-TO-USE

| crab cakes | 1 cake (2.1 oz) | 93 | 198 |

TAKE-OUT

baked	1 (3.8 oz)	160	550
cake	1 (2 oz)	160	492
soft-shell, fried	1 (4.4 oz)	334	1118

CRACKER CRUMBS

| Corn Flake Crumbs (Kellogg's) | ¼ cup (1 oz) | 100 | 290 |

FOOD	PORTION	CALORIES	SODIUM
Cracker Meal			
(Golden Dipt)	1 oz	100	0
(Keebler)	1 cup	100	5
Graham Crumbs (Keebler)	1 cup	520	630
Zesty Meal (Keebler)	1 cup	85	100

CRACKERS
 (*see also* CRACKER CRUMBS)

FOOD	PORTION	CALORIES	SODIUM
6 Calorie Wafer (Estee)	1	6	0
American Classic (Nabisco)			
Cracked Wheat	4	70	140
Dairy Butter	4	70	140
Golden Sesame	4	70	120
Minced Onion	4	70	120
Toasted Poppy	4	70	140
Bacon Flavored Thins (Nabisco)	7	70	210
Better Cheddars (Nabisco)	10	70	130
Low Salt	10	70	65
Butter Crackers (Goya)	1	40	60
Butter Thins (Pepperidge Farm)	4	70	115
Cheddar Wedges (Nabisco)	31	70	150
Cheese Crackers (Little Debbie)			
With Peanut Butter	1 pkg (.93 oz)	140	250
With Peanut Butter	1 pkg (1.4 oz)	210	380
Cheez-It	12	70	135
Low Salt	12	70	65
Cheez 'n Crackers (Handi-Snacks)	1 pkg	120	360
Bacon	1 pkg	130	410
Chicken In A Biskit (Nabisco)	7	80	130
Club (Keebler)	2	30	75
Cracked Wheat (Pepperidge Farm)	3	100	180

FOOD	PORTION	CALORIES	SODIUM
Crispbread, Garlic (Weight Watchers)	2	30	55
Crispy Graham (Pepperidge Farm)	4	70	115
Crown Pilot (Nabisco)	1	70	70
English Water Biscuits (Pepperidge Farm)	4	70	100
Escort (Nabisco)	3	70	115
Flutters (Pepperidge Farm)			
Garden Herb	¾ oz	100	190
Golden Sesame	¾ oz	110	150
Original Butter	¾ oz	100	150
Toasted Wheat	¾ oz	110	170
Garden Vegetable (Pepperidge Farm)	5	60	125
Goldfish (Pepperidge Farm)			
Cheddar Cheese	1 oz	120	230
Cheddar Cheese	1 pkg (1½ oz)	190	340
Cheese Thins	4	50	160
Original	1 oz	130	190
Parmesan Cheese	1 oz	120	330
Pizza Flavored	1 oz	130	220
Pretzel	1 oz	110	160
Gourmet Flatbread (Adrienne's)			
Caraway & Rye	2	20	45
Classic Island	2	20	45
Slightly Onion	2	20	45
Ten Grain	2	20	45
Goya Crackers	1	30	45
Harvest Crisps (Nabisco)			
5 Grain	6	60	135
Oat	6	60	135
Rice	6	60	135

FOOD	PORTION	CALORIES	SODIUM
Hearty Wheat (Pepperidge Farm)	4	100	140
Herb Stoned Wheat (Health Valley)	13	55	80
No Salt	13	55	30
Ideal Crispbread			
Extra Thin	3	48	86
Fiber Thins	2	41	81
Oatbran Thins	2	50	80
Krispy Saltine (Sunshine)	5	60	210
Unsalted Tops	5	60	120
Meal Mates Sesame Bread Wafers (Nabisco)	3	70	160
Melba Toast (Keebler)			
Garlic	2	25	35
Long	2	30	10
Onion	2	25	35
Plain	2	25	35
Sesame	2	25	35
Multi Grain (Pepperidge Farm)	4	70	115
Nips Cheese (Nabisco)	13	70	130
Oat Bran Krisp (Ralston)	2	60	140
Oat Thins (Nabisco)	8	70	90
Oyster Crackers (Keebler)			
Large	26	80	175
Small	50	80	175
Oysterettes (Nabisco)	18	60	140
Peanut Butter 'n Cheez Crackers (Handi-Snacks)	1 pkg	190	180
Premium Plus Saltines, Whole Wheat (Nabisco)	5	60	130
Premium Saltine (Nabisco)	5	60	180
Fat Free	5	50	115

FOOD	PORTION	CALORIES	SODIUM
Low Salt	5	60	115
Unsalted Tops	5	60	135
Premium Soup And Oyster (Nabisco)	20	60	210
Rice Bran (Health Valley)	7	130	65
Ritz (Nabisco)	4	70	120
Low Salt	4	70	60
Whole Wheat	5	70	110
Ritz Bits (Nabisco)	22	70	120
Cheese	22	70	130
Cheese Sandwiches	6	80	135
Low Salt	22	70	60
Peanut Butter Sandwiches	6	80	80
Royal Lunch (Nabisco)	1	60	80
Rykrisp			
Natural	2	40	75
Seasoned	2	45	105
Seasoned Twindividuals	2	45	105
Sesame	2	50	105
Snack Crackers, Toasted Rye (Keebler)	2	30	70
Sesame (Pepperidge Farm)	4	80	140
Sesame Stoned Wheat (Health Valley)	13	55	80
No Salt Added (Health Valley)	13	55	30
Seven Grain (Health Valley)			
Vegetable Stoned Wheat	13	55	80
No Salt Added	13	55	30
Snack Crackers (Keebler)			
Toasted Sesame	2	30	65
Toasted Wheat	2	30	60
Snack Mix (Pepperidge Farm)			
Classic	1 oz	140	360

FOOD	PORTION	CALORIES	SODIUM
Snack Mix *(cont.)*			
Lightly Smoked	1 oz	150	350
Snack Sticks (Pepperidge Farm)			
Cheese	8	130	400
Pretzel	8	120	430
Pumpernickel	8	140	330
Sesame	8	140	280
Sociables (Nabisco)	6	70	135
Spicy, Lightly Smoked (Pepperidge Farm)	1 oz	140	340
Stoned Wheat (Health Valley)	13	55	80
No Salt Added	13	55	30
Swiss Cheese (Nabisco)	7	70	170
Tam Tams (Manischewitz)	10	147	171
Tams (Manischewitz)			
Garlic	10	153	165
Onion	10	150	157
Wheat	10	150	180
Tid Bits, Cheese (Nabisco)	15	70	200
Toast Peanut Butter Sandwich (Planters)	6 (1.4 oz)	200	330
Toasted Rice (Pepperidge Farm)	4	60	140
Toasted Snack (Keebler)			
Bacon	2	30	65
Onion	2	30	70
Pumpernickel	2	30	55
Toasted Wheat With Onion (Pepperidge Farm)	4	80	140
Toasty Crackers With Peanut Butter (Little Debbie)	1 pkg (.93 oz)	140	250
Town House (Keebler)	2	35	60
Triscuit (Nabisco)	3	60	75
Bits	15	60	75

FOOD	PORTION	CALORIES	SODIUM
Deli-Style Rye	3	60	80
Low Salt	3	60	35
Wheat 'n Bran	3	60	75
Twigs Sesame & Cheese Sticks (Nabisco)	5	70	140
Uneeda Biscuit, Unsalted Tops (Nabisco)	2	60	100
Unsalted (Estee)	4	60	0
Vegetable Thins (Nabisco)	7	70	140
Waldorf, Sodium Free (Keebler)	2	30	0
Wasa Crispbread			
Breakfast	1	50	70
Extra Crisp	1	25	40
Falu Rye	1	30	60
Fiber Plus	1	35	60
Golden Rye	1	30	50
Hearty Rye	1	50	75
Light Rye	1	25	40
Royal	½	26	54
Savory Sesame	1	30	45
Sesame Rye	1	30	45
Sesame Wheat	1	60	65
Toasted Wheat	1	50	70
Waverly (Nabisco)	4	70	160
Low Salt	4	70	80
Wheat Thins (Nabisco)	8	70	120
Low Salt	8	70	60
Nutty	7	70	170
Wheatsworth, Stone Ground (Nabisco)	4	70	135
Wholegrain Wheat (Keebler)	2	30	70

FOOD	PORTION	CALORIES	SODIUM
Zesta Saltine (Keebler)	2	25	75
Unsalted Top	2	25	35
Zings! (Nabisco)	15	70	115
Zwieback (Nabisco)	2	60	20
cheese	10 (⅓ oz)	50	112
crispbread	3½ oz	317	436
melba toast, plain	1	20	44
peanut butter sandwich	1 (⅓ oz)	40	90
saltines	4	50	165
zwieback	3½ oz	374	263

CRANBERRIES

FOOD	PORTION	CALORIES	SODIUM
CANNED			
CranFruit Cranberry (Ocean Spray)			
Orange Sauce	2 oz	100	10
Raspberry Sauce	2 oz	100	10
Strawberry Sauce	2 oz	100	10
Cranberry Sauce			
Jellied (Ocean Spray)	2 oz	90	10
Jellied Old Fashioned (S&W)	½ cup	90	20
Whole Berry, Old Fashioned (S&W)	½ cup	90	20
Whole Berry Sauce (Ocean Spray)	2 oz	90	10
cranberry sauce, sweetened	½ cup	209	40
FRESH			
Ocean Spray	½ cup	25	0
chopped	1 cup	54	1
JUICE			
Ocean Spray Cranberry Juice Cocktail	6 oz	100	10

FOOD	PORTION	CALORIES	SODIUM
Ocean Spray Cranberry Juice Cocktail Low Calorie	6 oz	40	10
Smucker's Juice Sparkler	10 oz	140	5
cranberry juice cocktail	1 cup	147	10
cranberry juice cocktail	6 oz	108	4
cranberry juice cocktail, low calorie	6 oz	33	6
cranberry juice cocktail, frzn	12 oz	821	13
cranberry juice cocktail, frzn, as prep	6 oz	102	6

CRANBERRY BEANS

CANNED
cranberry beans	1 cup	216	863

DRIED
cooked	1 cup	240	1

CRAYFISH

cooked	3 oz	97	58
raw	3 oz	76	45
raw	8	24	14

CREAM
(*see also* SOUR CREAM, SOUR CREAM SUBSTITUTES, WHIPPED TOPPINGS)

LIQUID
half & half	1 cup	315	98
half & half	1 tbsp	20	6
heavy whipping	1 tbsp	52	6
light coffee	1 cup	496	95
light coffee	1 tbsp	29	6
light whipping	1 tbsp	44	5

FOOD	PORTION	CALORIES	SODIUM
WHIPPED			
heavy whipping	1 cup	411	89
light whipping	1 cup	345	82

CREAM CHEESE

FOOD	PORTION	CALORIES	SODIUM
NEUFCHATEL			
Philadelphia Brand Light	1 oz	80	115
Spreadery			
With Classic Ranch	1 oz	70	190
With French Onion	1 oz	70	135
With Garden Vegetable	1 oz	70	220
With Garlic & Herb	1 oz	70	140
With Strawberries	1 oz	70	270
neufchatel	1 oz	74	113
neufchatel	1 pkg (3 oz)	221	339
REDUCED FAT			
Fleur De Lait Alouette C'est Light			
Herbs & Garlic	1 oz	70	120
Spinach	1 oz	65	90
Strawberry	1 oz	75	30
Vegetables Julienne	1 oz	60	110
Fleur De Lait Chavrie	1 oz	50	150
Fleur De Lait Ultra Light			
Chives & Onions	1 oz	60	130
Fresh Vegetables	1 oz	60	130
Garlic & Spices	1 oz	60	120
Mixed Berry	1 oz	80	65
Nacho	1 oz	70	175
Plain	1 oz	60	110
Strawberry	1 oz	70	70
Philadelphia Brand Light	1 oz	60	160
Weight Watchers	2 tbsp	35	40

FOOD	PORTION	CALORIES	SODIUM
REGULAR			
Fleur De Lait	1 oz	100	40
Philadelphia Brand	1 oz	100	90
With Chives	1 oz	90	125
With Pimentos	1 oz	90	150
cream cheese	1 oz	99	84
cream cheese	1 pkg (3 oz)	297	251
SOFT			
Philadelphia Brand	1 oz	100	100
With Chives & Onions	1 oz	100	100
With Herb And Garlic	1 oz	100	160
With Olives & Pimento	1 oz	90	160
With Pineapple	1 oz	90	90
With Smoked Salmon	1 oz	90	180
With Strawberries	1 oz	90	75
WHIPPED			
Philadelphia Brand	1 oz	100	85
With Chives	1 oz	90	150
With Onions	1 oz	90	170
With Smoked Salmon	1 oz	90	170

CRESS
(*see also* WATERCRESS)

FOOD	PORTION	CALORIES	SODIUM
garden, cooked	½ cup	16	5
garden, raw	½ cup	8	4

CROAKER

FOOD	PORTION	CALORIES	SODIUM
FRESH			
atlantic, breaded & fried	3 oz	188	296
atlantic, raw	3 oz	89	47

FOOD	PORTION	CALORIES	SODIUM
CROISSANT			
All Butter (Sara Lee)	1	170	240
Petite Size	1	120	160
Croissant Sandwich Quartet (Pepperidge Farm)	1	170	250
Petite, All Butter (Pepperidge Farm)	1	120	170
croissant	1 (2 oz)	235	452
TAKE-OUT			
w/ egg & cheese	1	369	551
w/ egg, cheese & bacon	1	413	889
w/ egg, cheese & ham	1	475	1080
w/ egg, cheese & sausage	1	524	1115
CROUTONS			
Cheddar & Romano Cheese (Pepperidge Farm)	½ oz	60	200
Cheese & Garlic (Pepperidge Farm)	½ oz	70	180
Croutettes (Kellogg's)	1 cup (1 oz)	100	370
Onion & Garlic (Pepperidge Farm)	½ oz	70	160
Seasoned (Pepperidge Farm)	½ oz	70	180
Sour Cream & Chive (Pepperidge Farm)	½ oz	70	170
CUCUMBER			
FRESH			
raw	1 (11 oz)	39	6
raw, sliced	½ cup	7	1
TAKE-OUT			
cucumber salad	3.5 oz	50	480

FOOD	PORTION	CALORIES	SODIUM
CUMIN			
seed	1 tsp	8	4
CURRANTS			
DRIED			
zante	½ cup	204	6
FRESH			
black	½ cup	36	1
JUICE			
black currant nectar	3½ oz	55	5
red currant nectar	3½ oz	54	tr
CUSK			
FRESH			
fillet, baked	3 oz	106	38
CUSTARD			
Custard (Royal)	mix for 1 serving	60	75
Flan Caramel Custard (Royal)	mix for 1 serving	60	55
baked	1 cup	305	209
CUTTLEFISH			
steamed	3 oz	134	632
DANDELION GREENS			
fresh, cooked	½ cup	17	23
raw, chopped	½ cup	13	21

FOOD	PORTION	CALORIES	SODIUM

DANISH PASTRY

FROZEN

Apple

(Pepperidge Farm)	1	220	130
(Sara Lee)	1	120	120
Danish Twist (Sara Lee)	1 slice (1.9 oz)	190	200
Free & Light (Sara Lee)	1 slice (2 oz)	130	120

Cheese

(Pepperidge Farm)	1	240	230
(Sara Lee)	1	130	130
Danish Twist (Sara Lee)	1 slice (1.9 oz)	200	270

Cinnamon Raisin

(Pepperidge Farm)	1	250	170
(Sara Lee)	1	150	140

Raspberry

(Pepperidge Farm)	1	220	140
Danish Twist (Sara Lee)	1 slice (1.9 oz)	200	220

READY-TO-EAT

cheese	1 (3 oz)	353	320
cinnamon	1 (3 oz)	349	326
fruit	1 (2.3 oz)	235	233
fruit	1 (3.3 oz)	335	333
plain	1 (2 oz)	220	218
plain ring	1 (12 oz)	1305	1302

REFRIGERATED

Caramel Danish w/ Nuts (Pillsbury)	1	160	240
Cinnamon Raisin Danish w/ Icing (Pillsbury)	1	150	230
Orange Danish w/ Icing (Pillsbury)	1	150	250

FOOD	PORTION	CALORIES	SODIUM

DATES

DRIED			
Dole Chopped	½ cup	280	3
Dole Pitted	½ cup	280	0
Dromedary Chopped	¼ cup	130	0
Dromedary Pitted	5	100	0
chopped	1 cup	489	5
whole	10	228	2

DEER
(*see* VENISON)

DIETING AIDS
(*see* NUTRITIONAL SUPPLEMENTS)

DILL

seed	1 tsp	6	tr
sprigs, fresh	1 cup	4	5
sprigs, fresh	5	0	1
weed, dry	1 tsp	3	2

DINNER
(*see also* MEXICAN FOOD, ORIENTAL FOOD, PASTA DINNERS, POT PIE)

FROZEN			
Armour Classics			
Chicken & Noodles	11 oz	230	660
Chicken Fettucini	11 oz	260	660
Chicken Mesquite	9.5 oz	370	660
Chicken Parmigiana	11.5 oz	370	1060
Chicken w/ Wine & Mushroom Sauce	10.75 oz	280	900
Glazed Chicken	10.75 oz	300	960

FOOD	PORTION	CALORIES	SODIUM
Armour Classics *(cont.)*			
Meat Loaf	11.25 oz	360	1170
Salisbury Parmigiana	11.5 oz	410	1120
Salisbury Steak	11.25 oz	350	1430
Swedish Meatballs	11.25 oz	330	1140
Turkey w/ Dressing & Gravy	11.5 oz	320	1280
Veal Parmigiana	11.25 oz	400	1320
Armour Lite			
Beef Pepper Steak	11.25 oz	220	970
Beef Stroganoff	11.25 oz	250	510
Chicken Ala King	11.25 oz	290	630
Chicken Burgundy	10 oz	210	780
Chicken Marsala	10.5 oz	250	930
Chicken Oriental	10 oz	180	660
Salisbury Steak	11.5 oz	300	980
Shrimp Creole	11.25 oz	260	900
Sweet & Sour Chicken	11 oz	240	820
Banquet			
Beans & Frankfurters Dinner	10 oz	350	1310
Beef Platter	9 oz	230	770
Boneless Chicken Drumsnacker Platter	7 oz	290	1580
Boneless Chicken Nugget Platter	6 oz	340	790
Boneless Chicken Pattie Platter	6.75 oz	310	820
Chicken & Dumplings	10 oz	270	1080
Cookin' Bag Turkey Chili	4 oz	80	15
Fish Platter	8 oz	270	650
Fried Chicken Dinner	9 oz	520	1130
Ham Platter	8.25 oz	200	1050
Italian Style Dinner	9 oz	180	790

FOOD	PORTION	CALORIES	SODIUM
Meat Loaf Dinner	9.5 oz	340	1220
Mexican Style Combination Dinner	11 oz	360	1290
Mexican Style Dinner	11 oz	410	1330
Noodles & Chicken	10 oz	170	740
Salisbury Steak Dinner	9 oz	280	1050
Southern Fried Chicken Platter	8.75 oz	400	3640
Veal Parmagian	9.25 oz	330	1140
Western Style Dinner	9 oz	300	1280
White Meat, Fried Chicken Platter	8.75 oz	390	1620
White Meat, Hot'n Spicy Fried Chicken Platter	9 oz	440	2280
Banquet Entree			
Chicken And Noodles	8.5 oz	240	1120
Gravy And Turkey w/ Dressing	7 oz	220	1410
Banquet Extra Helping			
Beef Dinner	15.5 oz	430	1220
Chicken Nuggets w/ Barbecue Sauce	10 oz	540	2330
Chicken Nuggets w/ Sweet & Sour Sauce	10 oz	540	2330
Fried Chicken, All White Meat	14.25 oz	760	1770
Fried Chicken Dinner	14.25 oz	790	1490
Meat Loaf	16.25 oz	640	3320
Mexican Style Dinner	19 oz	680	3930
Salisbury Steak Dinner	16.25 oz	590	2760
Southern Fried Chicken Dinner	13.25 oz	790	2390
Turkey Dinner	17 oz	460	2030
Budget Gourmet			
Beef Cantonese	1 pkg	260	750
Beef Stroganoff	1 pkg	290	570

FOOD	PORTION	CALORIES	SODIUM
Budget Gourmet *(cont.)*			
Breast of Chicken In Wine Sauce	1 pkg	250	830
Chicken And Egg Noodle w/ Broccoli	1 pkg	440	980
Chicken Au Gratin	1 pkg	250	870
Chicken Cacciatore	1 pkg	470	1210
Chicken Marsala	1 pkg	270	700
Chicken With Fettucini	1 pkg	400	700
French Recipe Chicken	1 pkg	240	1000
Glazed Turkey	1 pkg	270	760
Ham & Asparagus Au Gratin	1 pkg	290	1170
Mandarin Chicken	1 pkg	300	670
Orange Glazed Chicken	1 pkg	250	350
Oriental Beef	1 pkg	290	810
Pepper Steak w/ Rice	1 pkg	330	600
Roast Chicken w/ Herb Gravy	1 pkg	270	1010
Roast Sirloin Supreme	1 pkg	320	630
Scallops And Shrimp Marinara	1 pkg	330	730
Seafood Newburg	1 pkg	350	630
Sirloin Beef In Herb Sauce	1 pkg	270	720
Sirloin Cheddar Melt	1 pkg	390	860
Sirloin Salisbury Steak	1 pkg	260	700
Sirloin Salisbury Steak Dinner	1 pkg	450	1030
Sirloin Tips In Burgundy Sauce	1 pkg	340	750
Sirloin Tips With Country Vegetables	1 pkg	300	810
Sliced Turkey Breast With Herb Gravy	1 pkg	290	1050
Swedish Meatballs With Noodles	1 pkg	580	1040

FOOD	PORTION	CALORIES	SODIUM
Sweet & Sour Chicken	1 pkg	340	630
Swiss Steak With Zesty Tomato Sauce	1 pkg	410	1000
Turkey A La King With Rice	1 pkg	390	750
Veal Parmigiana	1 pkg	490	1450
Yankee Pot Roast	1 pkg	360	780
Budget Gourmet Light And Healthy			
Chicken Breast Parmigiana	1 pkg	260	420
Herbed Chicken Breast With Fettucini	1 pkg	240	430
Italian Style Meatloaf	1 pkg	270	480
Pot Roast	1 pkg	210	440
Sirloin Beef in Wine Sauce	1 pkg	230	570
Sirloin Salisbury Steak	1 pkg	260	510
Special Recipe, Sirloin of Beef	1 pkg	250	550
Stuffed Turkey Breast	1 pkg	230	520
Teriyaki Chicken Breast	1 pkg	310	440
Dining Light			
Chicken Ala King	9 oz	240	780
Chicken w/ Noodles	9 oz	240	570
Salisbury Steak	9 oz	200	1000
Sauce & Swedish Meatballs	9 oz	280	660
Healthy Choice			
Barbecue Beef Ribs	11 oz	330	530
Beef Pepper Steak	11 oz	290	530
Breast of Turkey	10.5 oz	290	420
Cacciatore Chicken	12.5 oz	310	430
Chicken a L' Orange	9 oz	240	220
Chicken & Pasta Divan	11.5 oz	310	510
Chicken And Vegetables	11.5 oz	210	490
Chicken Dijon	11 oz	260	420

FOOD	PORTION	CALORIES	SODIUM
Healthy Choice *(cont.)*			
Chicken Oriental	11.25 oz	230	460
Chicken Parmigiana	11.5 oz	270	240
Glazed Chicken	8.5 oz	220	390
Herb Roasted Chicken	12.3 oz	290	430
Lemon Pepper Fish	10.7 oz	300	370
Mandarin Chicken	11 oz	260	400
Mesquite Chicken	10.5 oz	340	290
Roasted Turkey & Mushroom Gravy	8.5 oz	200	380
Salisbury Steak	11.5 oz	300	480
Salisbury Steak w/ Mushroom Gravy	11 oz	280	500
Salsa Chicken	11.25 oz	240	450
Seafood Newburg	8 oz	200	440
Shrimp Creole	11.25 oz	230	430
Shrimp Marinara	10.25 oz	260	320
Sirloin Beef w/ Barbecue Sauce	11 oz	300	320
Sirloin Tips	11.75 oz	280	370
Sliced Turkey w/ Gravy And Dressing	10 oz	270	530
Sole Au Gratin	11 oz	270	470
Sole w/ Lemon Butter	8.25 oz	230	430
Sweet & Sour Chicken	11.5 oz	280	260
Turkey Tetrazzini	12.6 oz	340	490
Yankee Pot Roast	11 oz	250	360
Kid Cuisine			
Chicken Nuggets	6.8 oz	360	660
Chicken Sandwiches	8.2 oz	470	830
Fish Sticks	7 oz	360	1050
Fried Chicken	7.5 oz	430	890

FOOD	PORTION	CALORIES	SODIUM
Hot Dogs w/ Buns	6.7 oz	450	880
Mexican Style	5.7 oz	290	610
Mega Meal Chicken Nuggets	8.4 oz	470	1010
Mega Meal Fried Chicken	10.8 oz	720	1400
Mega Meal Hot Dog w/ Bun	8.25 oz	500	1260
Le Menu			
Beef Sirloin Tips	11½ oz	400	760
Beef Stroganoff	10 oz	430	980
Chicken A La King	10¼ oz	330	830
Chicken Cordon Bleu	11 oz	460	850
Chicken In Wine Sauce	10 oz	280	680
Chicken Parmigiana	11¾ oz	410	1030
Chopped Sirloin Beef	12¼ oz	430	1010
Ham Steak	10 oz	300	1500
Pepper Steak	11½ oz	370	1020
Salisbury Steak	10½ oz	370	880
Sliced Breast of Turkey w/ Mushroom Gravy	10½ oz	300	1020
Sweet & Sour Chicken	11¼ oz	400	1020
Veal Parmigiana	11½ oz	390	840
Yankee Pot Roast	10 oz	330	700
Le Menu Entree LightStyle			
Chicken A La King	8¼ oz	24	670
Chicken Dijon	8 oz	240	500
Empress Chicken	8¼ oz	210	690
Glazed Turkey	8¼ oz	260	720
Herb Roast Chicken	7¾ oz	260	500
Swedish Meatballs	8 oz	260	700
Traditional Turkey	8 oz	200	610
Le Menu LightStyle			
Glazed Chicken Breast	10 oz	230	480

FOOD	PORTION	CALORIES	SODIUM
Le Menu LightStyle *(cont.)*			
Herb Roasted Chicken	10 oz	240	400
Salisbury Steak	10 oz	280	400
Sliced Turkey	10 oz	210	540
Sweet And Sour Chicken	10 oz	250	530
Turkey Divan	10 oz	260	420
Veal Marsala	10 oz	230	700
Lean Cuisine			
Beefsteak Ranchero	9¼ oz	260	530
Breaded Breast Of Chicken Parmesan	10⅞	270	540
Breast of Chicken Marsala With Vegetables	8⅛ oz	190	450
Chicken A l'Orange With Almond Rice	8 oz	280	290
Chicken & Vegetables Vermicelli	11¾ oz	250	490
Chicken Cacciatore With Vermicelli	10⅞ oz	280	570
Chicken In Barbecue Sauce	8¾ oz	260	500
Chicken Italiano	9 oz	290	490
Chicken Oriental With Vegetables And Vermicelli	9 oz	280	480
Chicken Tenderloins In Herb Cream Sauce	9½ oz	240	490
Chicken Tenderloins In Peanut Sauce	9 oz	290	530
Fiesta Chicken	8½ oz	240	560
Filet of Fish Divan	10⅜ oz	210	490
Filet of Fish Florentine	9⅝ oz	220	590
Glazed Chicken With Vegetable Rice	8½ oz	260	570
Homestyle Turkey With Vegetables And Pasta	9⅜ oz	230	550

FOOD	PORTION	CALORIES	SODIUM
Oriental Beef With Vegetables And Rice	8⅝ oz	290	590
Salisbury Steak With Gravy And Scalloped Potatoes	9½ oz	240	580
Sliced Turkey Breast In Mushroom Sauce	8 oz	220	550
Sliced Turkey Breast With Dressing	7⅞ oz	200	590
Stuffed Cabbage With Meat In Tomato Sauce	10¾ oz	210	560
Swedish Meatballs In Gravy With Pasta	9⅛ oz	290	590
Turkey Dijon	9½ oz	230	590
Morton			
Beans & Franks w/ Sauce	8.5 oz	300	1270
Fish w/ Mashed Potatoes And Carrots	9.25 oz	350	860
Glazed Ham	8 oz	230	1120
Gravy & Charbroiled Beef Patty	9 oz	270	1310
Gravy & Salisbury Steak	9 oz	270	1270
Tomato Sauce & Meatloaf	9 oz	280	1360
Veal Parmagian	8.75 oz	230	1330
Swanson			
Beans & Franks	10½ oz	440	900
Beef	11¼ oz	310	770
Beef In Barbecue Sauce	11 oz	460	860
Chopped Sirloin Beef	10¾ oz	340	790
Fish 'n' Chips	10 oz	500	960
Fried Chicken, Dark Meat	9¾ oz	560	1130
Fried Chicken, White Meat	10¼ oz	550	1460
Loin Of Pork	10¾ oz	280	790
Macaroni & Beef	12 oz	370	930
Meatloaf	10¾ oz	360	960

FOOD	PORTION	CALORIES	SODIUM
Swanson *(cont.)*			
Noodles & Chicken	10½ oz	280	740
Salisbury Steak	10¾ oz	400	880
Swedish Meatballs	8½ oz	360	790
Swiss Steak	10 oz	350	700
Turkey	11½ oz	350	1090
Veal Parmigiana	12¼ oz	430	1010
Western Style	11½ oz	430	1060
Swanson Homestyle			
Chicken Cacciatore	10.95 oz	260	1030
Chicken Nibbles	4¼ oz	340	730
Fish & Fries	6½ oz	340	670
Fried Chicken	7 oz	390	1100
Salisbury Steak	10 oz	320	980
Scalloped Potatoes And Ham	9 oz	300	1080
Seafood Creole With Rice	9 oz	240	810
Sirloin Tips In Burgundy Sauce	7 oz	160	550
Turkey With Dressing & Potatoes	9 oz	290	1010
Veal Parmigiana	10 oz	330	960
Swanson Hungry-Man			
Boneless Chicken	17¾ oz	700	1530
Chopped Beef Steak	16¾ oz	640	1600
Fried Chicken, Dark Meat	14¼ oz	860	1660
Fried Chicken, White Meat	14¼ oz	870	2150
Salisbury Steak	16½ oz	680	1730
Sliced Beef	15¼ oz	450	1060
Turkey	17 oz	550	1810
Veal Parmigiana	18¼ oz	590	1840
Ultra Slim-Fast			
Beef Pepper Steak	12 oz	270	590

FOOD	PORTION	CALORIES	SODIUM
Chicken Fettucini	12 oz	380	980
Chicken & Vegetable	12 oz	290	850
Country Style Vegetable & Beef Tips	12 oz	230	960
Mesquite Chicken	12 oz	360	300
Roasted Chicken In Mushroom Sauce	12 oz	280	830
Shrimp Creole	12 oz	240	730
Shrimp Marinara	12 oz	290	880
Sweet & Sour Chicken	12 oz	330	340
Turkey Medallions In Herb Sauce	12 oz	280	950
Weight Watchers			
Barbecue Glazed Chicken	7 oz	200	450
Beef Sirloin Tips	7.5 oz	210	560
Beef Stroganoff	8.5 oz	280	590
Chicken Ala King	9 oz	230	460
Chicken Cordon Bleu	7.7 oz	170	560
Chicken Kiev	7 oz	190	470
Homestyle Chicken And Noodles	9 oz	240	450
Imperial Chicken	8.5 oz	210	420
London Broil	7.5 oz	110	320
Oven Baked Fish	7 oz	150	260
Southern Baked Chicken	6.3 oz	170	520
Stuffed Turkey Breast	8.5 oz	270	520
Veal Patty Parmigiana	8.2 oz	150	550

DIP

FOOD	PORTION	CALORIES	SODIUM
Avocado Guacamole (Kraft)	2 tbsp	50	210
Bacon And Horseradish (Breakstone's)	2 tbsp	70	270

FOOD	PORTION	CALORIES	SODIUM
Bacon And Horseradish *(cont.)*			
(Kraft)	2 tbsp	60	200
(Kraft Premium)	2 tbsp	50	270
(Sealtest)	2 tbsp	70	270
Bacon & Onion			
(Kraft Premium)	1 tbsp	60	170
Gourmet (Breakstone's)	2 tbsp	70	270
Blue Cheese (Kraft Premium)	2 tbsp	50	210
Chesapeake Clam Gourmet (Breakstone's)	2 tbsp	50	200
Clam			
(Breakstone's)	2 tbsp	50	220
(Kraft)	2 tbsp	60	240
(Kraft Premium)	2 tbsp	45	210
(Sealtest)	2 tbsp	50	220
Creamy Cucumber (Kraft Premium)	2 tbsp	50	130
Creamy Onion (Kraft Premium)	2 tbsp	45	160
Cucumber And Onion			
(Breakstone's)	2 tbsp	50	160
(Sealtest)	2 tbsp	50	160
Fiesta			
Bean (Chi Chi's)	1 oz	32	156
Cheese (Chi Chi's)	1 oz	37	258
French Onion			
(Breakstone's)	2 tbsp	50	140
(Kraft)	2 tbsp	60	240
(Kraft Premium)	2 tbsp	45	150
(Sealtest)	2 tbsp	50	140
Green Onion (Kraft)	2 tbsp	60	170
Jalapeno Cheddar Gourmet (Breakstone's)	2 tbsp	70	90
Jalapeno Cheese (Kraft Premium)	1 tbsp	50	160

FOOD	PORTION	CALORIES	SODIUM
Jalapeno Pepper (Kraft)	2 tbsp	50	160
Mushroom And Herb Gourmet (Breakstone's)	2 tbsp	50	150
Nacho Cheese (Kraft Premium)	2 tbsp	55	200
Toasted Onion Gourmet (Breakstone's)	2 tbsp	50	170

DOCK

fresh, cooked	3½ oz	20	3
raw, chopped	½ cup	15	3

DOGFISH

raw	3½ oz	193	14

DOLPHINFISH

FRESH			
baked	3 oz	93	96
fillet, baked	5.6 oz	174	179

DOUGHNUTS
   (*see also* DUNKIN' DONUTS)

Donut Sticks (Little Debbie)	1 pkg (1.67 oz)	200	220
Old Fashion Donuts (Drake's)	1 (1.7 oz)	182	238
Powdered Sugar Donut Delites (Drake's)	7 (2.5 oz)	300	316
cake-type	1 (1.8 oz)	210	192
glazed	1 (2 oz)	235	222

DRESSING
   (*see* STUFFING/DRESSING)

DRINK MIXER
   (*see also* SODA, MINERAL/BOTTLED WATER)

FOOD	PORTION	CALORIES	SODIUM
Bloody Mary Mix			
(Libby's)	6 oz	40	1120
(Tabasco)	6 oz	56	788
whiskey sour mix	2 oz	55	66

DRUM

FRESH			
freshwater, baked	3 oz	130	82
freshwater fillet, baked	5.4 oz	236	148

DUCK

w/ skin, roasted	½ duck (13.4 oz)	1287	227
w/ skin, roasted	6 oz	583	103
w/o skin, roasted	½ duck (7.8 oz)	445	143
w/o skin, roasted	3.5 oz	201	65
wild, breast w/o skin, raw	½ breast (2.9 oz)	102	47
wild w/ skin raw	½ duck 9.5 oz)	571	152

DUMPLING

FROZEN			
Apple Dumpling (Pepperidge Farm)	1 (3 oz)	260	230

DURIAN

fresh	3½ oz	141	1

EEL

FRESH			
cooked	1 fillet (5.6 oz)	375	104
cooked	3 oz	200	55
raw	3 oz	156	43

FOOD	PORTION	CALORIES	SODIUM

EGG
(*see also* EGG DISHES, EGG SUBSTITUTES)

CHICKEN

FOOD	PORTION	CALORIES	SODIUM
fried w/ margarine	1	91	162
frozen	1	75	63
frozen	1 cup	363	307
hard cooked	1	77	62
hard cooked, chopped	1 cup	210	169
poached	1	74	140
raw	1	75	63
scrambled, plain	2	200	211
scrambled w/ whole milk & margarine	1	101	171
scrambled w/ whole milk & margarine	1 cup	365	616
white only	1	17	55
white only	1 cup	121	399

OTHER POULTRY

FOOD	PORTION	CALORIES	SODIUM
duck, raw	1	130	102

EGG DISHES

FROZEN
Great Starts

FOOD	PORTION	CALORIES	SODIUM
Egg, Sausage & Cheese	5½ oz	460	1310
Omelets w/ Cheese & Ham	7 oz	390	1220
Reduced Cholesterol, Eggs With Mini Oatbran Muffins	4¾ oz	250	400
Scrambled Eggs & Bacon With Home Fries	5.6 oz	340	690
Scrambled Eggs & Home Fries	4.6 oz	260	380
Scrambled Eggs & Sausage With Hash Browns	6½ oz	430	760

FOOD	PORTION	CALORIES	SODIUM
Great Starts *(cont.)*			
Scrambled Eggs With Cheese & Cinnamon Pancakes	3.4 oz	290	380
Kid Cuisine			
Egg Patties w/ Cheese	4.8 oz	200	650
Scrambled Eggs	4.1 oz	270	520
Quaker Scrambled Eggs			
& Sausage With Hash Browns	1 pkg (5.7 oz)	290	810
& Sausage With Pancakes	1 pkg (5.2 oz)	270	880
Cheddar Cheese & Fried Potatoes	1 pkg (5.9 oz)	250	910
HOME RECIPE			
deviled	2 halves	145	180
TAKE-OUT			
salad	½ cup	307	565
sandwich w/ cheese	1	340	804
sandwich w/ cheese & ham	1	348	1005

EGG SUBSTITUTES

FOOD	PORTION	CALORIES	SODIUM
Egg Beaters	¼ cup	25	80
Cheese Omelette	½ cup	110	480
Vegetable Omelette	½ cup	50	170
Egg Watchers	2 oz	50	100
Healthy Choice Cholesterol Free	¼ cup	30	90
frozen	1 cup	384	479
frozen	¼ cup	96	120
liquid	1½ oz	40	83
liquid	1 cup	211	444
powder	0.35 oz	44	79
powder	0.7 oz	88	158

FOOD	PORTION	CALORIES	SODIUM

EGGNOG

FOOD	PORTION	CALORIES	SODIUM
Borden Light	½ cup	130	80
eggnog	1 cup	342	138
eggnog	1 qt	1368	553
eggnog flavor mix, as prep w/ milk	9 oz	260	163

EGGPLANT

FRESH			
cubed, cooked	½ cup	13	2
raw, cut up	½ cup	11	1
FROZEN			
Parmigiana (Mrs. Paul's)	5 oz	240	600
TAKE-OUT			
Baba Ghannouj	¼ cup	55	95

ELDERBERRIES

JUICE			
elderberry	3½ oz	38	1

ELK

roasted	3 oz	124	52

ENDIVE

fresh	3½ oz	9	53
raw, chopped	½ cup	4	6

ENGLISH MUFFIN

FROZEN			
Great Starts			
Egg, Beefsteak & Cheese	5.9 oz	360	730

FOOD	PORTION	CALORIES	SODIUM
Great Starts *(cont.)*			
Egg, Canadian Bacon & Cheese	4.1 oz	290	770
Healthy Choice			
English Muffin Sandwich	1 (4.5 oz)	200	510
Turkey Sausage Omelet On English Muffin	1 (4.75 oz)	210	470
Western Style Omelet On English Muffin	1 (4.75 oz)	200	480
Weight Watchers Sandwich With Egg, Ham And Cheese	1 (4 oz)	230	590
HOME RECIPE			
cinnamon raisin	1	186	123
english muffin	1	158	122
honey bran	1	153	154
whole wheat	1	167	135
READY-TO-EAT			
Matthew's			
9 Grain & Nut	1	140	220
Cinnamon Raisin	1	160	290
Golden White	1	140	340
Whole Wheat	1	150	340
Pepperidge Farm			
Cinnamon Apple	1	140	210
Cinnamon Chip	1	160	180
Cinnamon Raisin	1	150	200
Plain	1	140	220
Sourdough	1	135	260
plain, toasted	1	140	378
TAKE-OUT			
w/ butter	1	189	386
w/ cheese & sausage	1	394	1036
w/ egg, cheese & bacon	1	487	1135

FOOD	PORTION	CALORIES	SODIUM
w/ egg, cheese & canadian bacon	1	383	785

EPPAW
| raw | ½ cup | 75 | 6 |

FALAFEL
| falafel | 1 (1.2 oz) | 57 | 50 |
| falafel | 3 (1.8 oz) | 170 | 150 |

FAST FOODS
(*see* individual names)

FAT
(*see also* BUTTER, BUTTER BLENDS, BUTTER SUBSTITUTES, MARGARINE, OIL)

Wesson Shortening	1 tbsp	100	0
beef tallow	1 tbsp	115	0
beef, cooked	1 oz	193	12
lamb, new zealand raw	1 oz	182	6
lard	1 cup	1849	tr
lard	1 tbsp	115	0
pork, cooked	1 oz	200	9
salt pork	1 oz	212	404

FEIJOA
| fresh | 1 (1.75 oz) | 25 | 2 |
| puree | 1 cup | 119 | 7 |

FENNEL
fresh, bulb	1 (8.2 oz)	72	122
fresh, sliced	1 cup	27	45
seed	1 tsp	7	2

FOOD	PORTION	CALORIES	SODIUM
FENUGREEK			
seed	1 tsp	12	2
FIBER			
Natural Delta Fiber	½ cup (1 oz)	20	20
FIGS			
CANNED			
in heavy syrup	3	75	1
in light syrup	3	58	1
water pack	3	42	1
DRIED			
cooked	½ cup	140	6
whole	10	477	20
FRESH			
fig	1 med	50	1
FILBERTS			
dried, blanched	1 oz	191	1
dried, unblanched	1 oz	179	1
dry roasted, unblanched	1 oz	188	1
oil roasted, unblanched	1 oz	187	1
FISH			
(*see also* individual names)			
FROZEN			
Gorton's			
Crispy Batter Dipped Fillets	2	290	550
Cripsy Batter Sticks	4	260	480
Crunch Fillets	2	230	420
Crunchy Sticks	4	210	240

FOOD	PORTION	CALORIES	SODIUM
Light Recipe, Lightly Breaded Fish Fillets	1 fillet	180	380
Light Recipe, Tempura Fillets	1 fillet	200	400
Microwave Fillets	2	340	400
Microwave Crispy Batter, Large Cut Fillets	1	320	680
Microwave Entree Fillets in Herb Butter	1 pkg	190	450
Microwave Larger Cut Fillets	1	320	500
Microwave Larger Cut Ranch Fillets	1	330	520
Microwave Sticks	6	340	420
Potato Crisp Fillets	2	300	360
Potato Crisp Sticks	4	260	390
Value Pack Portions	1 portion	180	490
Value Pack Sticks	4	190	420
Mrs. Paul's			
40 Crunchy Fish Sticks	4 (2.75 oz)	200	340
Batter Dipped Fish Fillets	2 fillets	330	650
Battered Fish Portions	2 portions	300	540
Battered Fish Sticks	4 sticks	210	590
Combination Seafood Platter	9 oz	600	408
Crispy Crunchy Breaded Fish Portions	2 portions	230	300
Crispy Crunchy Breaded Fish Sticks	4 sticks	140	340
Crispy Crunchy Fish Fillets	2 fillets	220	380
Crispy Crunchy Fish Sticks	4 sticks	190	560
Crunchy Batter Fish Fillets	2 fillets	280	730
Fish Cakes	2	190	690
Light Fillets In Butter Sauce	1 fillet	140	520
Light Seafood Entrees, Fish Dijon	8¾ oz	200	650

FOOD	PORTION	CALORIES	SODIUM
Mrs. Paul's *(cont.)*			
Light Seafood Entrees, Fish Florentine	8 oz	220	820
Light Seafood Entrees, Fish Mornay	9 oz	230	670
Microwave Buttered Fillet	1 fillet	80	130
Microwave Fillet Sandwich	1	280	460
Microwave Fillets	1 fillet	280	390
Microwave Fish Sticks	5	290	330
breaded fillet	1 (2 oz)	155	332
sticks	1 stick (1 oz)	76	163
MIX			
Beer Batter Fry (Golden Dipt)	1 oz	100	650
Cajun Style Fish Fry (Golden Dipt)	⅔ oz	60	470
Fish & Chips Batter Mix (Golden Dipt)	1¼ oz	120	910
Fish Fry (Golden Dipt)	⅔ oz	60	430
Seafood Frying Mix (Golden Dipt)	⅔ oz	60	600
Tempura Batter Mix (Golden Dipt)	1 oz	100	130
TAKE-OUT			
sandwich w/ tartar sauce	1	431	615
sandwich w/ tartar sauce & cheese	1	524	939

FLATFISH

FRESH			
cooked	1 fillet (4.5 oz)	148	133
cooked	3 oz	99	89
TAKE-OUT			
battered & fried	3.2 oz	211	484
breaded & fried	3.2 oz	211	484

FOOD	PORTION	CALORIES	SODIUM

FLAX

Seeds (Arrowhead)	1 oz	140	tr

FLOUNDER

FROZEN			
Crunchy Batter Fillets (Mrs. Paul's)	2 fillets	220	560
Fishmarket Fresh (Gorton's)	5 oz	110	170
Light Fillets (Mrs. Paul's)	1 fillet	240	450
Microwave Entree, Stuffed (Gorton's)	1 pkg	350	850

FLOUR

All Purpose			
(Ballard)	1 cup	400	0
(Ceresota)	1 cup	390	0
(Gold Medal)	1 cup	400	0
(Heckers)	1 cup	390	0
(Pillsbury Best)	1 cup	400	0
(Robin Hood)	1 cup	400	0
Unbleached (Pillsbury Best)	1 cup	400	0
Amaranth (Arrowhead)	2 oz	200	tr
Barley (Arrowhead)	2 oz	200	1
Better For Bread (Gold Medal)	1 cup	400	0
Bohemian Style Rye and Wheat (Pillsbury Best)	1 cup	400	0
Bread (Pillsbury Best)	1 cup	400	0
Brown Rice (Arrowhead)	2 oz	200	3
Buckwheat (Arrowhead)	2 oz	190	0
Garbanzo (Arrowhead)	2 oz	200	10
Medium Rye (Pillsbury Best)	1 cup	400	0

FOOD	PORTION	CALORIES	SODIUM
Millet (Arrowhead)	2 oz	185	1
Oat (Arrowhead)	2 oz	200	tr
Oat Blend (Gold Medal)	1 cup	390	0
Pastry (Arrowhead)	2 oz	180	1
Rye (Arrowhead)	2 oz	190	tr
Rye, Stone Ground (Robin Hood)	1 cup	360	10
Self-Rising			
(Aunt Jemima)	¼ cup	109	794
(Ballard)	1 cup	380	1290
(Gold Medal)	1 cup	380	1520
(Pillsbury Best)	1 cup	380	1290
(Robin Hood)	1 cup	380	1520
Shake & Blend (Pillsbury Best)	2 tbsp	50	0
Soy (Arrowhead)	2 oz	250	tr
Teff (Arrowhead)	2 oz	200	7
Unbleached			
(Gold Medal)	1 cup	400	0
(Robin Hood)	1 cup	400	0
White (Arrowhead)	2 oz	200	tr
Whole Wheat			
(Ceresota)	1 cup	400	0
(Gold Medal)	1 cup	350	0
(Heckers)	1 cup	400	0
(Pillsbury Best)	1 cup	400	10
Blend (Gold Medal)	1 cup	380	0
Stone Ground (Arrowhead)	2 oz	200	1
corn masa	1 cup	416	6
corn, whole grain	1 cup	422	6
cottonseed, lowfat	1 oz	94	10
peanut, defatted	1 cup	196	108
peanut, defatted	1 oz	92	50

FOOD	PORTION	CALORIES	SODIUM
peanut, lowfat	1 cup	257	0
potato	1 cup	628	61
rice, brown	1 cup	574	12
rice, white	1 cup	578	1
rye			
dark	1 cup	415	2
light	1 cup	374	2
medium	1 cup	361	3
sesame, lowfat	1 oz	95	11
triticale, whole grain	1 cup	440	3
white			
all-purpose	1 cup	455	2
bread	1 cup	495	2
cake	1 cup	395	2
self-rising	1 cup	442	1587
whole wheat	1 cup	407	6

FRANKFURTER
(see HOT DOG)

FRENCH BEANS

DRIED
cooked	1 cup	228	11

FRENCH FRIES
(see POTATO)

FRENCH TOAST

FROZEN
Aunt Jemima	3 oz	166	554
Cinnamon Swirl	3 oz	171	516

FOOD	PORTION	CALORIES	SODIUM
Great Starts			
Cinnamon Swirl With Sausage	5½ oz	390	530
French Toast With Sausage	5½ oz	380	550
Mini French Toast With Sausage	2½ oz	190	320
Oatmeal French Toast With Lite Links	4.65 oz	310	500
Healthy Starts French Toast With LeanLinks	6.5 oz	400	595
Kid Cuisine	4.11 oz	260	320
Quaker			
French Toast Sticks & Syrup	1 pkg (5.2 oz)	400	640
French Toast Wedges & Sausage	1 pkg (5.3 oz)	360	780
Weight Watchers French Toast With Cinnamon	2 slices	160	280
HOME RECIPE			
french toast	1 slice	155	257
TAKE-OUT			
w/ butter	2 slices	356	513

FROSTING
(*see* CAKE)

FRUCTOSE

Fructose (Estee)	1 tsp	12	0

FRUIT DRINKS

FROZEN			
Tree Top Apple			
Citrus, as prep	6 oz	90	10
Cranberry, as prep	6 oz	100	10
Grape, as prep	6 oz	100	10

FOOD	PORTION	CALORIES	SODIUM
Pear, as prep	6 oz	90	10
Raspberry, as prep	6 oz	80	10
citrus juice drink	12 oz	684	12
citrus juice drink, as prep	1 cup	114	7
fruit punch	1 can (12 oz)	678	34
fruit punch, as prep w/ water	1 cup	113	11
lemonade	1 can (6 oz)	397	8
lemonade, as prep w/ water	1 cup	100	8
limeade, as prep w/ water	1 cup	102	6
MIX			
Wylers Drink Mix			
Unsweetened Bunch O' Berries	8 oz	2	28
Unsweetened Lemonade	8 oz	3	19
Unsweetened Lemonade, Pink	8 oz	3	19
Unsweetened Tropical Punch	8 oz	2	tr
fruit punch, as prep w/ water	9 oz	97	38
lemonade powder, as prep w/ water	9 oz	113	19
lemonade powder w/ nutrasweet	1 pitcher (67 oz)	40	58
READY-TO-USE			
Crystal Geyser Juice Squeeze			
Orange & Passion Fruit	6 oz	70	15
Passion Fruit & Mango	6 oz	70	15
Pink Lemonade	6 oz	70	15
Dole New Breakfast Juice			
Pineapple Orange	6 oz	90	20
Pineapple Orange Banana	6 oz	90	10
Pineapple Orange Guava	6 oz	100	10
Pineapple Passion Banana	6 oz	100	10
Dole			
Pineapple Grapefruit	6 oz	90	25

FOOD	PORTION	CALORIES	SODIUM
Dole *(cont.)*			
Pineapple Orange	6 oz	90	20
Pineapple Orange Banana	6 oz	90	10
Pineapple Pink Grapefruit	6 oz	100	5
Juice & More			
Apple Cherry	8 oz	120	20
Apple Grape	8 oz	120	20
Apple Raspberry	8 oz	120	10
Juicy Juice			
Apple Grape	6 oz	90	10
Berry	6 oz	90	10
Berry	8.45 oz	130	15
Cherry	6 oz	90	10
Punch	6 oz	100	10
Punch	8.45 oz	140	10
Tropical	6 oz	110	10
Tropical	8.45 oz	150	10
Kern's			
Apricot Orange Nectar	6 oz	112	<10
Apricot Pineapple Nectar	6 oz	110	10
Banana Pineapple Nectar	6 oz	120	10
Coconut Pineapple Nectar	6 oz	120	40
Passionfruit Orange Nectar	6 oz	110	10
Strawberry Banana Nectar	6 oz	100	10
Tropical Nectar	6 oz	112	10
Libby's			
Passion Fruit Orange Nectar	8 oz	150	10
Strawberry Banana Nectar	8 oz	150	5
Mauna La'i			
Hawaiian Guava Fruit Drink	6 oz	100	10
Hawaiian Guava Passion Fruit Drink	6 oz	100	5

FOOD	PORTION	CALORIES	SODIUM
Newman's Own Roadside Virginia Lemonade	8 oz	100	0
Ocean Spray			
Cranapple	6 oz	130	10
Cranapple Low Calorie	6 oz	40	5
Cran-Blueberry	6 oz	120	10
Cran-Grape	6 oz	130	5
Cranicot	6 oz	110	5
Cran-Raspberry	6 oz	110	5
Cran-Raspberry Low Calorie	6 oz	40	10
Cran-Strawberry	6 oz	110	10
Cran-Tastic	6 oz	110	15
Pineapple Grapefruit Juice Cocktail	6 oz	110	5
S&W Apricot Pineapple			
Nectar	6 oz	120	10
Nectar Diet	6 oz	80	10
Smucker's			
Apple Cranberry Juice	8 oz	120	10
Orange Banana Juice	8 oz	120	10
Tree Top Apple			
Citrus	6 oz	90	10
Cranberry	6 oz	100	10
Grape	6 oz	100	10
Pear	6 oz	90	10
Raspberry	6 oz	80	10
White House Apple Cherry	6 oz	90	10
Wylers			
Lemonade	6 oz can	64	33
Tropical Punch	6 oz	82	9
cranberry apple drink	6 oz	123	4
cranberry apricot drink	6 oz	118	4

FOOD	PORTION	CALORIES	SODIUM
fruit punch	6 oz	87	41
orange grapefruit juice	1 cup	107	8
pineapple & grapefruit juice	1 cup	117	14
pineapple & orange drink	1 cup	125	9

FRUIT MIXED
(*see also* individual names)

CANNED			
Chunky Mixed			
Diet (S&W)	½ cup	40	5
Natural Style (S&W)	½ cup	90	5
Unsweetened (S&W)	½ cup	40	5
Fruit Cocktail			
(Hunt's)	4 oz	90	7
Diet (S&W)	½ cup	40	5
Heavy Syrup (S&W)	½ cup	90	15
Natural Lite (S&W)	½ cup	60	5
Natural Style (S&W)	½ cup	90	5
Unsweetened (S&W)	½ cup	40	5
Tropical Fruit Salad (Dole)	½ cup	70	10
fruit cocktail			
in heavy syrup	½ cup	93	7
juice pack	½ cup	56	4
water pack	½ cup	40	5
fruit salad			
in heavy syrup	½ cup	94	7
in light syrup	½ cup	73	7
juice pack	½ cup	62	7
water pack	½ cup	37	4
mixed fruit in heavy syrup	½ cup	92	5
tropical fruit salad in heavy syrup	½ cup	110	3

FOOD	PORTION	CALORIES	SODIUM
DRIED			
Fruit'n Nut Mix (Planters)	1 oz	150	90
mixed	11 oz pkg	712	52
FROZEN			
mixed fruit, sweetened	1 cup	245	8

FRUIT SNACKS

FOOD	PORTION	CALORIES	SODIUM
Fruit By The Foot			
Cherry	1	80	45
Grape	1	80	45
Strawberry	1	80	45
Fruit Roll-Ups			
Cherry	1 (½ oz)	50	40
Crazy Colors	1 (½ oz)	50	40
Fruit Punch	1 (½ oz)	50	40
Grape	1 (½ oz)	50	40
Raspberry	1 (½ oz)	50	40
Strawberry	1 (½ oz)	50	40
Garfield And Friends			
1-2 Punch	1 pkg	100	60
Cat Cooler	1 pkg	100	60
Fat Cat Funnies	1 (½ oz)	50	20
Fruit Party	1 (½ oz)	50	40
Very Strawberry	1 pkg	100	60
Hanna Barbera			
Flintstones	1 pkg (1 oz)	100	15
Jetsons	1 pkg (1 oz)	100	15
Yo Yogi!	1 pkg (1 oz)	100	15
Health Valley			
Bakes Apple	1 bar	100	25
Bakes Date	1 bar	100	25
Bakes Raisin	1 bar	100	20

FOOD	PORTION	CALORIES	SODIUM
Health Valley Fruit & Fitness Bars	2 bars	200	75
Almond & Date	1 bar	160	5
Health Valley Fat Free Fruit Bars 100% Organic			
Apple	1 bar	140	10
Apricot	1 bar	140	10
Date	1 bar	140	10
Raisin	1 bar	140	10
Health Valley Oat Bran Bakes			
Apricot	1 bar	100	15
Fig & Nut	1 bar	110	10
Health Valley Oat Bran Jumbo Fruit Bars			
Almond & Date	1 bar	170	10
Raisin & Cinnamon	1 bar	160	10
Shark Bites & Berry Bears			
Assorted Fruit	1 pkg	100	20
Fruit Punch	1 pkg	100	20
Squeezit			
Berry B. Wild	1 (6.75 oz)	90	0
Chucklin' Cherry	1 (6.75 oz)	90	5
Grumpy Grape	1 (6.75 oz)	90	0
Mean Green Puncher	1 (6.75 oz)	90	0
Silly Billy Strawberry	1 (6.75 oz)	90	0
Smarty Arty Orange	1 (6.75 oz)	90	50
Sunkist Fruit Flippits			
Cherry	0.8 oz	107	18
Strawberry	0.8 oz	107	18
Sunkist Fruit Roll			
Apricot	1	76	17
Cherry	1	75	18
Grape	1	76	13
Raspberry	1	75	20
Strawberry	1	74	11

FOOD	PORTION	CALORIES	SODIUM
Sunkist Fun Fruit			
Animals	.9 oz	100	10
Dinosaurs, Strawberry	.9 oz	100	10
Galactic Gems	0.9 oz	100	10
Mario Nintendo	0.9 oz	100	10
Meteorites	0.9 oz	100	10
Spooky Fruit	1 pkg	100	10
Strawberry	.9 oz	100	10
Wacky Players	0.9 oz	100	10
Surf's Up!			
Sun Splash	1 pkg	100	30
Tutti Frutti	1 pkg	100	20
Thunder Jets			
Assorted Fruit Squadron	1 pkg	100	30
Mach 1 Fruit Mix	1 pkg	100	30
Tiny Toons			
Bunch Of Berries	1 pkg (.9 oz)	100	10
Fruit Assortment	1 pkg (.9 oz)	100	10
Paaaarrrty Punch	1 pkg (.9 oz)	100	10
Weight Watchers			
Apple	½ oz	50	140
Cinnamon	½ oz	50	140
Peach	½ oz	50	140
Strawberry	½ oz	50	140

GARBANZOS
(see CHICKPEAS)

GARLIC

clove	1	4	1
powder	1 tsp	9	1

FOOD	PORTION	CALORIES	SODIUM

GEFILTE FISH

READY-TO-USE
sweet	1 piece (1.5 oz)	35	220

GELATIN

DRINKS
Orange Flavored Drinking Gelatin w/ Nutrasweet (Knox)	1 pkg	39	17

MIX
Apple (Royal)	½ cup	80	95
Blackberry (Royal)	½ cup	80	95
Cherry (Royal)	½ cup	80	95
Cherry Sugar Free (Royal)	½ cup	8	90
Concord Grape (Royal)	½ cup	80	130
Fruit Punch (Royal)	½ cup	80	90
Gelatin Desserts (Estee)	½ cup	8	0
Lemon (Royal)	½ cup	80	250
Lemon-Lime (Royal)	½ cup	80	95
Lime (Royal)	½ cup	80	125
Lime Sugar Free (Royal)	½ cup	8	100
Mixed Berry (Royal)	½ cup	80	90
Orange (Royal)	½ cup	80	95
Orange Sugar Free (Royal)	½ cup	10	90
Peach (Royal)	½ cup	80	95
Pineapple (Royal)	½ cup	80	95
Raspberry (Royal)	½ cup	80	125
Raspberry Sugar Free (Royal)	½ cup	8	90
Strawberry (Royal)	½ cup	80	105
Strawberry Banana, Sugar Free (Royal)	½ cup	8	85

FOOD	PORTION	CALORIES	SODIUM
Strawberry Orange (Royal)	½ cup	80	110
Strawberry Sugar Free (Royal)	½ cup	8	90
Tropical Fruit (Royal)	½ cup	80	110
fruit flavored	½ cup	70	55
low calorie	½ cup	8	9

GIBLETS

capon, simmered	1 cup (5 oz)	238	80
chicken, floured & fried	1 cup (5 oz)	402	164
chicken, simmered	1 cup (5 oz)	228	85
turkey, simmered	1 cup (5 oz)	243	85

GINGER

ground	1 tsp	6	1
root fresh	¼ cup	17	3
root fresh	5 slices	8	1
root fresh, sliced	¼ cup	17	3
root fresh, sliced	5 slices	8	1

GINKGO NUTS

canned	1 oz	32	87
dried	1 oz	99	4
raw	1 oz	52	1

GIZZARDS

chicken, simmered	1 cup (5 oz)	222	97
turkey, simmered	1 cup (5 oz)	236	79

GOAT

roasted	3 oz	122	73

FOOD	PORTION	CALORIES	SODIUM

GOOSE

FRESH

FOOD	PORTION	CALORIES	SODIUM
w/ skin, roasted	½ goose (1.7 lbs)	2362	543
w/ skin, roasted	6.6 oz	574	132
w/o skin, roasted	½ goose (1.3 lbs)	1406	447
w/o skin, roasted	5 oz	340	108

GOOSEBERRIES

FOOD	PORTION	CALORIES	SODIUM
fresh	1 cup	67	1
CANNED in light syrup	½ cup	93	3

GRANOLA

BARS
Fi-Bar

FOOD	PORTION	CALORIES	SODIUM
Coconut	1	120	30
Peanut Butter	1	130	30
Hershey Chocolate Covered			
Chocolate Chip	1 (1.2 oz)	170	50
Cocoa Creme	1 (1.2 oz)	180	50
Cookies & Creme	1 (1.2 oz)	170	50
Peanut Butter	1 (1.2 oz)	180	65
Nature Valley			
Cinnamon	1	120	70
Oat Bran Honey Graham	1	110	90
Oats n'Honey	1	120	65
Peanut Butter	1	120	70
Rice Bran Cinnamon Graham	1	90	75
New Trail Chocolate Covered Cookies and Creme	1	200	85

FOOD	PORTION	CALORIES	SODIUM
Quaker Chewy			
Chocolate Chip	1	128	90
Chunky Nut & Raisin	1	131	86
Cinnamon Raisin	1	128	92
Honey & Oats	1	125	95
Peanut Butter	1	128	116
Peanut Butter Chocolate Chip	1	131	112
Quaker Dipps			
Caramel Nut	1	148	81
Chocolate Chip	1	139	78
Chocolate Fudge	1	160	74
Peanut Butter	1	170	74
Peanut Butter Chocolate Chip	1	174	102
Sunbelt Chewy			
Chocolate Chip	1 bar (1.25 oz)	150	75
Oats & Honey	1 bar (1 oz)	130	35
With Almonds	1 bar (1 oz)	120	65
With Raisins	1 bar (1.25 oz)	150	65
Sunbelt Fudge Dipped Chewy			
Chocolate Chip	1 bar (1.5 oz)	210	55
Macaroon	1 bar (1.4 oz)	200	50
With Peanuts	1 bar (1.5 oz)	200	60
CEREAL			
Arrowhead Maple-Nut	2 oz	250	10
Erewhon			
Date Nut	1 oz	130	45
Honey Almond	1 oz	130	65
Maple	1 oz	130	55
Spiced Apple	1 oz	130	55
Sunflower Crunch	1 oz	130	60

FOOD	PORTION	CALORIES	SODIUM
Erewhon *(cont.)*			
With Bran	1 oz	130	10
Kellogg's Low Fat	⅓ cup (1 oz)	120	60
Nature Valley			
Cinnamon & Raisin	⅓ cup (1 oz)	120	90
Fruit & Nut	⅓ cup (1 oz)	130	75
Toasted Oat	⅓ cup (1 oz)	130	90
Quaker Sun Country			
100% Natural w/ Almonds	¼ cup	130	11
100% Natural With Raisins & Dates	¼ cup	123	9
With Raisins	¼ cup	125	10
Sunbelt			
Banana Almond	1 oz	130	25
Fruit & Nut	1 oz	120	20

GRAPEFRUIT

FOOD	PORTION	CALORIES	SODIUM
CANNED			
Sections			
In Light Syrup (S&W)	½ cup	80	0
Unsweetened (S&W)	½ cup	40	0
juice pack	½ cup	46	9
unsweetened	1 cup	93	3
water pack	½ cup	44	1
FRESH			
Dole	½	50	0
Ocean Spray			
Pink	½ med	50	0
White	½ med	45	0
pink	½	37	0
pink sections	1 cup	69	1

FOOD	PORTION	CALORIES	SODIUM
red	½	37	0
red sections	1 cup	69	1
white	½	39	0
white sections	1 cup	76	0
JUICE			
Crystal Geyser Juice Squeeze	6 oz	70	15
Libby's	6 oz	70	0
Ocean Spray	6 oz	60	10
Pink Grapefruit Juice Cocktail	6 oz	80	15
Pink Premium Grapefruit Juice	6 oz	60	10
Tree Top	6 oz	80	0
fresh	1 cup	96	2
frzn, as prep	1 cup	102	2
frzn, not prep	6 oz	302	6
sweetened	1 cup	116	4

GRAPES

CANNED			
Thompson Seedless Premium (S&W)	½ cup	100	5
thompson, seedless, in heavy syrup	½ cup	94	7
thompson, seedless, water pack	½ cup	48	7
FRESH			
Dole	1½ cup	85	3
grapes	10	36	1
JUICE			
Juicy Juice	6 oz	90	5
Juicy Juice	8.45 oz	130	10
Ocean Spray Concord Grape Concentrated, as prep	6 oz	100	10

FOOD	PORTION	CALORIES	SODIUM
S&W Concord Unsweetened	6 oz	100	9
Tree Top	6 oz	120	10
Wylers Drink Mix Unsweetened	8 oz	2	12
bottled	1 cup	155	7
frzn sweetened, as prep	1 cup	128	5
frzn sweetened, not prep	6 oz	386	15
grape drink	6 oz	84	12

GRAVY
(see also SAUCE)

FOOD	PORTION	CALORIES	SODIUM
CANNED			
Au Jus (Franco-American)	2 oz	10	330
Beef (Franco-American)	2 oz	25	340
Chicken (Franco-American)	2 oz	45	240
Chicken Giblet (Franco-American)	2 oz	30	310
Cream (Franco-American)	2 oz	35	220
Mushroom (Franco-American)	2 oz	25	290
Pork (Franco-American)	2 oz	40	330
Turkey (Franco-American)	2 oz	30	290
beef	1 can (10 oz)	155	1630
beef	1 cup	124	1305
chicken	1 cup	189	1375
mushroom	1 cup	120	1259
DRY			
Brown (Pillsbury)	¼ cup	15	300
Chicken (Pillsbury)	¼ cup	25	230
Home Style (Pillsbury)	¼ cup	15	300
au jus, as prep w/ water	1 cup	32	964
brown, as prep w/ water	1 cup	75	1076
chicken, as prep	1 cup	83	1133

FOOD	PORTION	CALORIES	SODIUM
mushroom, as prep	1 cup	70	1402
onion, as prep w/ water	1 cup	77	1013
pork, as prep	1 cup	76	1235
turkey, as prep	1 cup	87	1498

GREAT NORTHERN BEANS

CANNED			
Green Giant	½ cup	80	290
Trappey's	½ cup	80	410
great northern	1 cup	300	11
DRIED			
cooked	1 cup	210	4

GREEN BEANS

CANNED			
Almondine (Green Giant)	½ cup	45	300
Cut			
(Green Giant)	½ cup	16	300
Premium Blue Lake (S&W)	½ cup	20	385
Water Pack (S&W)	½ cup	20	5
Dilled (S&W)	½ cup	60	385
French (Green Giant)	½ cup	16	330
French Style Premium Blue Lake (S&W)	½ cup	20	385
Green Beans & Wax Beans (S&W)	½ cup	20	385
Kitchen Sliced (Green Giant)	½ cup	16	280
Whole			
Fancy Stringless (S&W)	½ cup	20	385
Vertical Pack (S&W)	½ cup	20	385

FOOD	PORTION	CALORIES	SODIUM
FROZEN			
Cut, In Butter Sauce (Green Giant)	½ cup	30	230
Green Giant	½ cup	14	10
Harvest Fresh, Cut (Green Giant)	½ cup	16	95
One Serve, In Butter Sauce (Green Giant)	1 pkg	60	370
SHELF STABLE			
Cut (Pantry Express)	½ cup	12	20

GROUPER

FRESH			
cooked	1 fillet (7.1 oz)	238	107
cooked	3 oz	100	45
raw	3 oz	78	45

GUAVA

Kern's Nectar	6 oz	110	10
Libby's			
Nectar	6 oz	110	15
Ripe Nectar	8 oz	140	20
fresh	1	45	2
guava sauce	½ cup	43	4

HADDOCK

FRESH			
cooked	1 fillet (5.3 oz)	168	131
cooked	3 oz	95	74
raw	3 oz	74	58
FROZEN			
Crunchy Batter Fillets (Mrs. Paul's)	2 fillets	190	580

FOOD	PORTION	CALORIES	SODIUM
Fishmarket Fresh (Gorton's)	5 oz	110	120
Light Fillets (Mrs. Paul's)	1 fillet	220	350
Microwave Entree, Haddock In Lemon Butter (Gorton's)	1 pkg	360	730
SMOKED			
smoked	1 oz	33	214
smoked	3 oz	99	649

HAKE

FOOD	PORTION	CALORIES	SODIUM
raw	3½ oz	84	101

HALIBUT

FOOD	PORTION	CALORIES	SODIUM
FRESH			
atlantic & pacific			
cooked	½ fillet (5.6 oz)	223	110
cooked	3 oz	119	59
raw	3 oz	93	46
greenland, baked	3 oz	203	87
greenland, baked	5.6 oz	380	163

HAM

(see also HAM DISHES, LUNCHEON MEATS/COLD CUTS, PORK, TURKEY)

FOOD	PORTION	CALORIES	SODIUM
Carl Buddig	1 oz	50	400
Hansel 'n Gretel			
Baked Virginia	1 oz	34	245
Cooked Fresh	1 oz	33	120
Deluxe	1 oz	31	245
Honey Valley	1 oz	31	260
Jalapeno	1 oz	25	260
Lessalt	1 oz	30	200
Lessalt Virginia	1 oz	32	190

FOOD	PORTION	CALORIES	SODIUM
Hansel 'n Gretel *(cont.)*			
Light AM	1 oz	27	200
Travane	1 oz	31	210
Russer Lil' Salt			
Cooked	1 oz	30	220
Smoked	1 oz	30	220
Weight Watchers			
Deli Thin Oven Roasted	5 slices (⅓ oz)	12	95
Deli Thin Oven Roasted Honey Ham	5 slices (⅓ oz)	12	95
Deli Thin Premium Smoked	5 slices (⅓ oz)	12	85
Oven Roasted Honey Ham	2 slices (¾ oz)	25	220
Oven Roasted Smoked	2 slices (¾ oz)	25	220
Premium Cooked	2 slices (¾ oz)	25	220
canned (13% fat), roasted	3 oz	192	800
canned, extra lean (4% fat)	3 oz	116	965
center slice, lean & fat	4 oz	229	1566
chopped	1 oz	65	389
chopped, canned	1 oz	68	387
ham & cheese loaf	1 oz	73	762
ham & cheese spread	1 oz	69	339
ham & cheese spread	1 tbsp	37	179
ham salad spread	1 oz	61	259
ham salad spread	1 tbsp	32	137
minced	1 oz	75	353
sliced, extra lean (5% fat)	1 oz	37	405
sliced, regular (11% fat)	1 oz	52	373
steak, boneless, extra lean	1 oz	35	360

FOOD	PORTION	CALORIES	SODIUM

HAM DISHES

FROZEN

Handy Pocket Cheese Sauce & Ham (Weight Watchers)	1 (4 oz)	200	490
Ovenstuffs Ham/Turkey Deli Melt	1 (4.75 oz)	360	1050

HOME RECIPE

croquettes	1 (3.1)	217	475
salad	½ cup	287	671

TAKE-OUT

sandwich w/ cheese	1	353	772

HAMBURGER
(see also BEEF)

FROZEN
Kid Cuisine

Beef Patty Sandwich/Cheese	6.25 oz	430	550
Mega Meal Double Beef Patty Sandwich w/ Cheese	9.1 oz	480	1040

MicroMagic

Cheeseburger	1 pkg (4.75 oz)	450	790
Hamburger	1 pkg (4 oz)	350	500

TAKE-OUT
double patty

w/ bun	1 reg	544	554
w/ catsup, cheese, mayonnaise, mustard, pickle, tomato & bun	1 lg	706	1149
w/ catsup, mayonnaise, onion, pickle, tomato & bun	1 reg	649	920
w/ catsup, mustard, mayonnaise, onion, pickle, tomato & bun	1 lg	540	791
w/ catsup, mustard, onion, pickle & bun	1 reg	576	742

FOOD	PORTION	CALORIES	SODIUM
double patty *(cont.)*			
w/ cheese & bun	1 reg	457	635
w/ cheese & double bun	1 reg	461	892
w/ cheese, catsup, mayonnaise, onion, pickle, tomato & bun	1 reg	416	1051
single patty			
w/ bacon, catsup, cheese, mustard, onion, pickle & bun	1 lg	609	1044
w/ bun	1 lg	400	474
w/ bun	1 reg	275	387
w/ catsup, cheese, ham, mayonnaise, pickle, tomato & bun	1 lg	745	1713
w/ catsup, mustard, mayonnaise, onion, pickle, tomato & bun	1 reg	279	504
w/ cheese & bun	1 lg	608	1589
w/ cheese & bun	1 reg	320	500
triple patty			
w/ catsup, mustard, pickle & bun	1 lg	693	713
w/ cheese & bun	1 lg	769	1211

HEART

beef, simmered	3 oz	148	54
chicken, simmered	1 cup (5 oz)	268	69
lamb, braised	3 oz	158	54
turkey, simmered	1 cup (5 oz)	257	79
veal, braised	3 oz	158	50

FOOD	PORTION	CALORIES	SODIUM

HERBAL TEA
(*see* TEA/HERBAL TEA)

HERBS/SPICES
(*see also* INDIVIDUAL NAMES)

FOOD	PORTION	CALORIES	SODIUM
All Purpose Seafood (Golden Dipt)	¼ tsp	2	85
Blackened Redfish (Golden Dipt)	¼ tsp	2	140
Broiled Fish (Golden Dipt)	¼ tsp	2	125
Cajun Style Shrimp & Crab (Golden Dipt)	¼ tsp	2	200
Cleopatra's Secret (Nile Spice)	⅛ tsp	0	20
Desert Spice (Nile Spice)	⅛ tsp	0	5
Ginger Curry (Nile Spice)	⅛ tsp	0	5
Lemon Pepper Seafood (Golden Dipt)	¼ tsp	8	115
Maya Maize Popcorn Seasoning (Nile Spice)	½ tsp	0	25
Mrs. Dash			
Extra Spicy	1 tsp	12	4
Garlic & Herb	1 tsp	12	2
Lemon & Herb	1 tsp	12	4
Low Pepper Blend	1 tsp	12	4
Original	1 tsp	12	4
Table Blend	1 tsp	12	4
Nile Spice	⅛ tsp	0	20
curry powder	1 tsp	6	1
poultry seasoning	1 tsp	5	tr
pumpkin pie spice	1 tsp	6	1

FOOD	PORTION	CALORIES	SODIUM
HERRING			
FRESH			
atlantic, cooked	1 fillet (5 oz)	290	165
atlantic, cooked	3 oz	172	98
atlantic, raw	3 oz	134	76
pacific, baked	3 oz	213	81
pacific fillet, baked	5.1 oz	360	137
READY-TO-USE			
atlantic, kippered	1 fillet (1.4 oz)	87	367
atlantic, pickled	½ oz	39	131
HICKORY NUTS			
dried	1 oz	187	0
HOMINY			
canned	½ cup	57	168
HONEY			
Burleson's			
Clover	1 tbsp	60	1
Creamed	1 tbsp	60	1
Natural	1 tbsp	60	1
Pure	1 tbsp	60	1
Raw	1 tbsp	60	1
Rocky Mountain Clover	1 tbsp	60	1
Golden Blossom	1 tsp	20	tr
honey	1 cup	1030	17
honey	1 tbsp	65	1

FOOD	PORTION	CALORIES	SODIUM
HONEYDEW			
Dole	1/10	50	50
cubed	1 cup	60	17
fresh	1/10	46	13
HORSE			
roasted	3 oz	149	47
HORSERADISH			
Gold's			
Hot	1 tsp	4	60
Red	1 tsp	4	75
White	1 tsp	4	55
Kraft			
Cream Style	1 tbsp	12	85
Horseradish, Mustard	1 tbsp	14	135
Prepared	1 tbsp	10	140
Sauceworks Horseradish	1 tbsp	50	105

HOT CAKES
(*see* PANCAKES)

HOT DOG
(*see also* MEAT SUBSTITUTES, SAUSAGE)

FOOD	PORTION	CALORIES	SODIUM
CHICKEN			
Health Valley Weiners	1	96	90
chicken	1 (1.5 oz)	116	617
MEAT			
Nathan's Famous			
Natural Casing Franks	1	158	422
Skinless Franks	1	176	463

FOOD	PORTION	CALORIES	SODIUM
beef	1 (1.5)	142	462
beef	1 (2 oz)	180	585
beef & pork	1 (1.5 oz)	144	504
beef & pork	1 (2 oz)	183	639
pork, cheesefurter smokie	1 (1.5 oz)	141	465
TAKE-OUT			
corndog	1	460	972
w/ bun, chili	1	297	480
w/ bun, plain	1	242	671
TURKEY			
Health Valley Weiners	1	96	112
turkey	1 (1.5 oz)	102	642

HUMMUS

hummus	1 cup	420	599
hummus	⅓ cup	140	200

HYACINTH BEANS

DRIED			
cooked	1 cup	228	13

ICE CREAM AND FROZEN DESSERT

All Flavors, Avari Creme Glace	1 oz	10	35
Almond Praline Light (Edy's)	4 oz	140	50
Banana-Politan Light (Edy's)	4 oz	110	50
Berry Berry Berry (Mocha Mix)	3.5 oz	209	99
Black Cherry (Sealtest Free)	½ cup	100	45
Fat Free (Borden)	½ cup	90	40
Blueberry Sorbet & Cream (Haagen-Dazs)	4 oz	190	35

FOOD	PORTION	CALORIES	SODIUM
Bordeaux Cherry (Healthy Choice)	4 oz	120	50
Butter Almond (Breyers)	½ cup	170	125
Butter Crunch (Sealtest)	½ cup	150	90
Butter Pecan			
(Breyers)	½ cup	180	125
(Frusen Gladje)	½ cup	280	160
(Haagen-Dazs)	4 oz	390	100
(Sealtest)	½ cup	160	125
Light (Edy's)	4 oz	140	50
Cafe Au Lait Light (Edy's)	4 oz	110	50
Candy Bar Light (Edy's)	4 oz	140	50
Caramel Almond Crunch Bar (Haagen-Dazs)	1	240	65
Caramel Nut Ice Milk (Light N'Lively)	½ cup	120	85
Caramel Nut Sundae (Haagen-Dazs)	4 oz	310	100
Cherry Vanilla (Breyers)	½ cup	150	45
Chocolate			
(Breyers)	½ cup	160	30
(Frusen Gladje)	½ cup	240	65
(Haagen-Dazs)	4 oz	270	50
(Healthy Choice)	4 oz	130	70
(Sealtest)	½ cup	140	50
(Sealtest Free)	½ cup	100	50
(Ultra Slim-Fast)	4 oz	100	45
Chocolate American Dream (Edy's)	3 oz	90	45
Chocolate Brownie Light (Ben & Jerry's)	4 oz	230	121
Chocolate Chip (Sealtest)	½ cup	150	50

FOOD	PORTION	CALORIES	SODIUM
Chocolate Chip American Dream (Edy's)	3 oz	100	45
Chocolate Chip Ice Milk (Light N'Lively)	½ cup	120	35
Chocolate Chip Ice Milk (Weight Watchers)	½ cup	120	80
Chocolate Chip Light (Edy's)	4 oz	120	50
Chocolate Chocolate Chip (Frusen Gladje)	½ cup	270	60
Chocolate Chocolate Chip (Haagen-Dazs)	4 oz	290	40
Chocolate Chocolate Mint (Haagen-Dazs)	4 oz	300	50
Chocolate Dark Chocolate Bar (Haagen-Dazs)	1	390	60
Chocolate Dip Bar (Weight Watchers)	1 (2 oz)	110	45
Chocolate Fat Free (Borden)	½ cup	100	50
Chocolate Fat Free Frozen Dessert (Weight Watchers)	½ cup	80	75
Chocolate Fudge (Ultra Slim-Fast)	4 oz	120	65
Chocolate Fudge Mousse Light (Edy's)	4 oz	130	50
Chocolate Fudge Swirl Dessert Bar (Sealtest Free)	1	90	30
Chocolate Fudge Twirl Ice Milk (Breyers Light)	½ cup	130	60
Chocolate Ice Milk (Breyers Light)	½ cup	120	55
Chocolate Marshmallow Sundae (Sealtest)	½ cup	150	40
Chocolate Mousse Bar Sugar Free (Weight Watchers)	1 (1.75 oz)	35	30
Chocolate Swirl Fat Free Frozen Dessert (Weight Watchers)	½ cup	90	75
Chocolate Treat Bar Sugar Free (Weight Watchers)	1 (2.75 oz)	90	75

FOOD	PORTION	CALORIES	SODIUM
Coffee			
(Breyers)	½ cup	150	50
(Haagen-Dazs)	4 oz	270	55
(Sealtest)	½ cup	140	50
Ice Milk (Light n'Lively)	½ cup	100	40
Cookies n' Cream			
(Breyers)	½ cup	170	60
(Healthy Choice)	4 oz	130	80
American Dream (Edy's)	3 oz	100	45
Ice Milk (Light n'Lively)	½ cup	110	65
Light (Edy's)	4 oz	120	50
Deep Chocolate (Haagen-Dazs)	4 oz	290	70
Deep Chocolate Fudge (Haagen-Dazs)	4 oz	290	90
Double Fudge Bar (Weight Watchers)	1 (1.75 oz)	60	50
Dreamy Caramel Cream Light (Edy's)	4 oz	140	50
Dutch Chocolate (Mocha Mix)	3.5 oz	210	135
English Toffee Crunch Bar (Weight Watchers)	1 (2 oz)	120	60
French Vanilla (Sealtest)	½ cup	140	50
Fresh Lites (Dole)			
Cherry	1 bar	25	10
Chocolate Chip	1 bar	60	30
Lemon	1 bar	25	20
Pineapple Orange	1 bar	25	33
Raspberry	1 bar	25	5
Fruit N' Cream Bar (Dole)			
Peach	1 bar	90	15
Raspberry	1 bar	90	20
Strawberry	1 bar	90	20

FOOD	PORTION	CALORIES	SODIUM
Fruit N' Juice Bar (Dole)			
Peach, Passion Fruit	1 bar	70	10
Pineapple	1 bar	70	5
Pineapple, Orange, Banana	1 bar	70	10
Raspberry	1 bar	70	15
Strawberry	1 bar	70	10
Fudge Bar (Ultra Slim-Fast)	1	90	50
Fudge Pop Bar (Haagen-Dazs)	1	210	50
Fudge Royale (Sealtest)	½ cup	140	55
Heavenly Hash			
(Mocha Mix)	3.5 oz	244	116
(Sealtest)	½ cup	150	50
Ice Milk (Breyers Light)	½ cup	150	55
Ice Milk (Light N'Lively)	½ cup	120	35
Honey Vanilla (Haagen-Dazs)	4 oz	250	55
Keylime Sorbet & Cream (Haagen-Dazs)	4 oz	190	30
Lifesavers Ice Pops	1	35	0
Sugar Free	1	12	5
Lime Sherbet (Sealtest)	½ cup	130	30
Macadamia Brittle (Haagen-Dazs)	4 oz	280	60
Malt Ball 'N' Fudge Light (Edy's)	4 oz	140	50
Maple Walnut (Sealtest)	½ cup	160	40
Marble Fudge Light (Edy's)	4 oz	120	50
Mint Chocolate (Breyers)	½ cup	170	45
Mocha Almond Fudge			
(Mocha Mix)	3.5 oz	229	113
American Dream (Edy's)	3 oz	110	45
Light (Edy's)	4 oz	140	50
Neapolitan			
(Healthy Choice)	4 oz	120	60

FOOD	PORTION	CALORIES	SODIUM
(Mocha Mix)	3.5 oz	208	120
Fat Free Frozen Dessert (Weight Watchers)	½ cup	80	75
ONE-ders (Weight Watchers)			
Brownies 'n Creme	4 oz	130	115
Chocolate Chip	4 oz	120	80
Heavenly Hash	4 oz	130	90
Pralines 'n Creme	4 oz	130	90
Strawberry	4 oz	110	75
Orange & Cream Pop (Haagen-Dazs)	1	130	25
Orange Sherbet (Sealtest)	½ cup	130	30
Orange Sorbet & Cream (Haagen-Dazs)	4 oz	190	35
Orange Vanilla Treat Bar, Sugar Free, Fat Free (Weight Watchers)	1 (1.75 oz)	30	40
Peach			
(Breyers)	½ cup	130	35
(Mocha Mix)	3.5 oz	198	96
(Sealtest Free)	½ cup	100	45
(Ultra Slim-Fast)	4 oz	100	55
Fat Free (Borden)	½ cup	90	40
Peanut Butter & Chocolate Light (Edy's)	4 oz	130	50
Peanut Butter Crunch Bar (Haagen-Dazs)	1	270	55
Peanut Fudge Sundae (Sealtest)	½ cup	140	50
Pecan Pralines 'n Creme Ice Milk (Weight Watchers)	½ cup	130	90
Praline Almond Ice Milk (Breyers Light)	½ cup	130	70
Praline & Caramel (Healthy Choice)	4 oz	130	70

FOOD	PORTION	CALORIES	SODIUM
Pralines And Caramel (Ultra Slim-Fast)	4 oz	120	95
Rainbow Sherbet (Sealtest)	½ cup	130	30
Raspberry			
Sorbet (Frusen Gladje)	½ cup	140	10
Sorbet & Cream (Haagen-Dazs)	4 oz	180	35
Truffle Light (Edy's)	4 oz	110	50
Red Raspberry Sherbet (Sealtest)	½ cup	130	30
Rocky Road			
(Healthy Choice)	4 oz	140	70
American Dream (Edy's)	3 oz	110	45
Light (Edy's)	4 oz	130	50
Rum Raisin (Haagen-Dazs)	4 oz	250	45
Sorbet (Dole)			
Mandarin Orange	4 oz	110	10
Peach	4 oz	110	10
Pineapple	4 oz	110	10
Raspberry	4 oz	110	10
Strawberry	4 oz	100	10
Strawberry			
(Breyers)	½ cup	130	40
(Frusen Gladje)	½ cup	230	60
(Haagen-Dazs)	4 oz	250	40
(Healthy Choice)	4 oz	110	50
(Sealtest)	½ cup	130	40
(Sealtest Free)	½ cup	100	40
American Dream (Edy's)	3 oz	70	40
Fat Free (Borden)	½ cup	90	40
Ice Milk (Breyers Light)	½ cup	110	50
Light (Edy's)	4 oz	110	50

FOOD	PORTION	CALORIES	SODIUM
Swirl (Mocha Mix)	3.5 oz	209	98
SunTops (Dole)			
Grape	1 bar	40	5
Lemonade	1 bar	40	5
Orange	1 bar	40	5
Sundae Cone			
(Borden)	1	210	110
(Meadow Gold)	1	210	110
Swiss Chocolate Candy Almond (Frusen Gladje)	½ cup	270	60
Toasted Almond (Mocha Mix)	3.5 oz	229	117
Toasted Almond American Dream (Edy's)	3 oz	110	45
Toffee Fudge Parfait Ice Milk (Breyers Light)	½ cup	140	90
Triple Chocolate Stripes (Sealtest)	½ cup	140	50
Vanilla			
(Breyers)	½ cup	150	50
(Frusen Gladje)	½ cup	230	70
(Haagen-Dazs)	4 oz	260	55
(Healthy Choice)	4 oz	120	60
(Mocha Mix)	3.5 oz	209	117
(Sealtest)	½ cup	140	50
(Sealtest Free)	½ cup	100	45
(Ultra Slim-Fast)	4 oz	90	55
Vanilla American Dream (Edy's)	3 oz	80	45
Vanilla Chocolate Sandwich (Ultra Slim-Fast)	1	140	220
Vanilla Chocolate Strawberry (Edy's)	4 oz	110	50
Vanilla Chocolate Strawberry American Dream (Edy's)	3 oz	80	45

FOOD	PORTION	CALORIES	SODIUM
Vanilla Cookie Crunch Bar (Ultra Slim-Fast)	1	90	70
Vanilla Crunch Bar (Haagen-Dazs)	1	220	55
Vanilla Fat Free (Borden)	½ cup	90	50
Vanilla Fat Free Frozen Dessert (Weight Watchers)	½ cup	80	75
Vanilla Fudge (Haagen-Dazs)	4 oz	270	100
Vanilla Fudge Cookie (Ultra Slim-Fast)	4 oz	110	90
Vanilla Fudge Royale (Sealtest Free)	½ cup	100	50
Vanilla Fudge Swirl Dessert Bar (Sealtest Free)	1	80	30
Vanilla Fudge Twirl (Breyers)	½ cup	160	55
Vanilla Fudge Twirl Ice Milk (Light N'Lively)	½ cup	110	45
Vanilla Ice Milk (Light N'Lively)	½ cup	100	40
Vanilla Light (Edy's)	4 oz	100	50
Vanilla Milk Chocolate Almond Bar (Haagen-Dazs)	1	370	55
Vanilla Milk Chocolate Bar (Haagen-Dazs)	1	360	55
Vanilla Milk Chocolate Brittle Bar (Haagen-Dazs)	1	370	160
Vanilla Oatmeal Sandwich (Ultra Slim-Fast)	1	150	160
Vanilla Old Fashioned (Healthy Choice)	4 oz	120	60
Vanilla Peanut Butter Swirl (Haagen-Dazs)	4 oz	280	120
Vanilla Red Raspberry Parfait Ice Milk (Breyers Light)	½ cup	130	50
Vanilla Sandwich (Ultra Slim-Fast)	1	140	220

FOOD	PORTION	CALORIES	SODIUM
Vanilla Sandwich Bar Fat Free (Weight Watchers)	1 (2.5 oz)	130	170
Vanilla Strawberry Royale (Sealtest Free)	½ cup	100	35
Vanilla Strawberry Swirl Dessert Bar (Sealtest Free)	1	80	40
Vanilla Swiss Almond (Frusen Gladje)	½ cup	270	65
Vanilla Swiss Almond (Haagen-Dazs)	4 oz	290	55
Vanilla With Chocolate Covered Almonds Ice Milk (Light N'Lively)	½ cup	120	45
Vanilla With Orange Sherbet (Sealtest)	½ cup	130	40
Vanilla With Raspberry Twirl Ice Milk (Light N'Lively)	½ cup	110	35
Vanilla With Red Raspberry Sherbet (Sealtest)	½ cup	130	40
Wild Berry Swirl (Healthy Choice)	4 oz	120	60
french vanilla, soft serve	1 cup	377	153
french vanilla, soft serve	½ gal	3014	1228
orange sherbet	1 cup	270	88
orange sherbet	½ gal	2158	706
orange sherbet (home recipe)	½ cup	120	30
vanilla 10% fat	1 cup	269	116
vanilla 10% fat	½ gal	2153	929
vanilla 16% fat	1 cup	349	108
vanilla 16% fat	½ gal	2805	868
vanilla ice milk	1 cup	184	105
vanilla ice milk	½ gal	1469	836
vanilla ice milk, soft serve	1 cup	223	163
vanilla ice milk, soft serve	½ gal	1787	1303

FOOD	PORTION	CALORIES	SODIUM
TAKE-OUT			
cone, vanilla ice milk, soft serve	1 (4.6 oz)	164	92
sundae, caramel	1 (5.4 oz)	303	195
sundae, hot fudge	1 (5.4 oz)	284	182
sundae, strawberry	1 (5.4 oz)	269	92

ICE CREAM CONES AND CUPS

Comet Cups	1	18	5
Comet Sugar Cone	1	50	40
Comet Waffle Cone	1	70	30
Keebler Sugar Cones	1	45	35
Keebler Vanilla Cups	1	15	20

ICE CREAM TOPPINGS
(*see also* SYRUP)

Butterscotch			
(Kraft)	1 tbsp	60	70
(Smucker's)	2 tbsp	140	75
Special Recipe (Smucker's)	2 tbsp	160	40
Caramel			
(Kraft)	1 tbsp	60	45
(Smucker's)	2 tbsp	140	110
Chocolate			
(Kraft)	1 tbsp	50	15
(Smucker's)	2 tbsp	130	35
Magic Shell (Smucker's)	2 tbsp	190	25
Chocolate Fudge			
(Hershey)	2 tbsp	100	30
(Smucker's)	2 tbsp	130	50
Magic Shell (Smucker's)	2 tbsp	190	50

FOOD	PORTION	CALORIES	SODIUM
Chocolate Nut Magic Shell (Smucker's)	2 tbsp	200	40
Dark Chocolate Special Recipe (Smucker's)	2 tbsp	130	45
Hot Caramel (Smucker's)	2 tbsp	150	75
Hot Fudge			
(Kraft)	1 tbsp	70	50
(Smucker's)	2 tbsp	110	55
Light (Smucker's)	2 tbsp	70	35
Special Recipe (Smucker's)	2 tbsp	150	60
Hot Toffee Fudge (Smucker's)	2 tbsp	110	55
Marshmallow			
(Smucker's)	2 tbsp	120	0
Creme (Kraft)	1 oz	90	20
Peanut Butter Caramel (Smucker's)	2 tbsp	150	120
Pecans in Syrup (Smucker's)	2 tbsp	130	0
Pineapple			
(Kraft)	1 tbsp	50	0
(Smucker's)	2 tbsp	130	0
Strawberry			
(Kraft)	1 tbsp	50	5
(Smucker's)	2 tbsp	120	0
Swiss Milk Chocolate Fudge (Smucker's)	2 tbsp	140	70
Walnuts in Syrup (Smucker's)	2 tbsp	130	0

ICED TEA
(*see* TEA/HERBAL TEA)

ICING
(*see* CAKE)

FOOD	PORTION	CALORIES	SODIUM

INSTANT BREAKFAST
(*see* BREAKFAST DRINKS)

JACKFRUIT
fresh	3½ oz	70	2

JAM/JELLY/PRESERVES

ALL FRUIT			
Apple Butter, Simply Fruit (Smucker's)	1 tsp	12	0
Simply Fruit Spread, All Flavors (Smucker's)	1 tsp	16	0
REDUCED CALORIE			
All Flavors			
Jelly (Estee)	1 tsp	2	10
Preserves (Louis Sherry)	1 tsp	2	10
Apricot Pineapple Preserves (S&W)	1 tsp	4	0
Blueberry Jam (S&W)	1 tsp	4	0
Concord Grape Jelly (S&W)	1 tsp	4	0
Grape Jelly (Kraft)	1 tsp	6	5
Grape Spread (Weight Watchers)	1 tsp	8	0
Imitation, Single Serving			
Blackberry Jelly (Smucker's)	⅜ oz pkg	4	<10
Cherry Jelly (Smucker's)	⅜ oz pkg	4	<10
Grape Jelly (Smucker's)	⅜ oz pkg	4	<10
Low Sugar Spread, All Flavors (Smucker's)	1 tsp	8	<10
Orange Marmalade (S&W)	1 tsp	4	0
Raspberry Spread (Weight Watchers)	1 tsp	8	0
Red Raspberry Jam (S&W)	1 tsp	4	0

FOOD	PORTION	CALORIES	SODIUM
Red Tart Cherry Preserves (S&W)	1 tsp	4	0
Slenderella Fruit Spread, All Flavors	1 tsp	7	0
Strawberry			
Jam (S&W)	1 tsp	4	0
Preserves (Kraft)	1 tsp	6	5
Spread (Weight Watchers)	1 tsp	8	0
REGULAR			
All Flavors			
Jam (Kraft)	1 tsp	17	0
Jelly (Kraft)	1 tsp	17	0
Preserves (Kraft)	1 tsp	17	0
Apple Butter			
(White House)	1 oz	50	5
Autumn Harvest (Smucker's)	1 tsp	12	0
Natural (Smucker's)	1 tsp	12	0
Apple Cider Butter (Smucker's)	1 tsp	12	0
Blueberry Jam (Whistling Wings)	1 oz	50	2
Jam, All Flavors (Smucker's)	1 tsp	18	0
Jelly			
All Flavors (Smucker's)	1 tsp	18	tr
Single Serving, All Flavors (Smucker's)	½ oz	38	<10
Orange Marmalade (Smucker's)	1 tsp	18	0
Peach Butter (Smucker's)	1 tsp	15	0
Preserves			
All Flavors (Smucker's)	1 tsp	18	0
Single Serving, All Flavors (Smucker's)	½ oz	38	<10
Pumpkin Butter, Autumn Harvest (Smucker's)	1 tsp	12	14

FOOD	PORTION	CALORIES	SODIUM
Raspberry Jam (Whistling Wings)	1 oz	60	1
apple jelly	3½ oz	259	15
orange jam	3½ oz	243	11
red currant jelly	3½ oz	265	4
rose hip jam	3½ oz	250	5

JAPANESE FOOD
(see ORIENTAL FOOD)

JAVA PLUM

fresh	1	5	1
fresh	1 cup	82	18

JELLY
(see JAM/JELLY/PRESERVES)

JEW'S EAR

pepeao, dried	½ cup	36	8
pepeao, raw, sliced	1 cup	25	9

JUJUBE

fresh	3½ oz	105	3

KALE

FRESH

Dole, chopped	½ cup	17	15
chopped, cooked	½ cup	21	15
raw, chopped	½ cup	21	15
scotch, chopped, cooked	½ cup	18	29

FROZEN

chopped, cooked	½ cup	20	10

FOOD	PORTION	CALORIES	SODIUM

KEFIR

kefir	3½ oz	66	46

KIDNEY

beef, simmered	3 oz	122	114
lamb, braised	3 oz	117	128
veal, braised	3 oz	139	93

KIDNEY BEANS

CANNED Goya, Spanish Style	7.5 oz	140	760
Green Giant Dark Red	½ cup	90	250
Light Red	½ cup	90	250
Hunt's Red	4 oz	100	400
S&W Dark Red Lite, 50% Less Salt	½ cup	120	355
S&W Water Pack	½ cup	90	0
Trappey's, New Orleans Style	½ cup	100	410
Van Camp's Dark Red	1 cup	182	830
Light Red	1 cup	184	650
New Orleans Style Red	1 cup	178	940
kidney beans	1 cup	208	889
red	1 cup	216	873
DRIED Arrowhead Red	2 oz	190	3
california red, cooked	1 cup	219	7
cooked	1 cup	225	4
red, cooked	1 cup	225	4
royal red, cooked	1 cup	218	8

FOOD	PORTION	CALORIES	SODIUM

KIWIS

FOOD	PORTION	CALORIES	SODIUM
Dole	2	90	0
fresh	1 med	46	4

KOHLRABI

FRESH

FOOD	PORTION	CALORIES	SODIUM
raw, sliced	½ cup	19	14
sliced, cooked	½ cup	24	17

KUMQUATS

FOOD	PORTION	CALORIES	SODIUM
fresh	1	12	1

LAMB
(see also LAMB DISHES)

FRESH

FOOD	PORTION	CALORIES	SODIUM
cubed, lean only			
braised	3 oz	190	60
broiled	3 oz	158	65
ground, broiled	3 oz	240	69
leg lean & fat, Choice, roasted	3 oz	219	56
loin chop w/ bone			
lean & fat, Choice, broiled	1 chop (2.3 oz)	201	49
lean only, Choice, broiled	1 chop (1.6 oz)	100	39
rib chop			
lean & fat, Choice, broiled	3 oz	307	64
lean only, Choice, broiled	3 oz	200	73
shank			
lean & fat, Choice, braised	3 oz	206	61
lean & fat, Choice, roasted	3 oz	191	55
shoulder chop w/ bone			
lean & fat, Choice, braised	1 chop (2.5 oz)	244	51

FOOD	PORTION	CALORIES	SODIUM
lean only, Choice, braised	1 chop (1.9 oz)	152	41
sirloin, lean & fat, Choice, roasted	3 oz	248	58
FROZEN			
new zealand			
lean & fat, cooked	3 oz	259	39
lean only, cooked	3 oz	175	43

LAMB DISHES

TAKE-OUT			
curry	¾ cup	345	258
stew	¾ cup	124	140

LECITHIN
(*see* SOY)

LEEKS

DRIED			
freeze-dried	1 tbsp	1	0
FRESH			
chopped, cooked	¼ cup	8	3
cooked	1 (4.4 oz)	38	13
raw	1 (4.4 oz)	76	25
raw, chopped	¼ cup	16	5

LEMON

Dole	1	18	10
lemon	1 med	22	3
peel	1 tbsp	0	0
wedge	1	5	1
JUICE			
bottled	1 tbsp	3	3

FOOD	PORTION	CALORIES	SODIUM
fresh	1 tbsp	4	0
frzn	1 tbsp	3	0

LEMONADE
(*see* FRUIT DRINKS)

LENTILS

CANNED

Health Valley Fast Menu Hearty Lentils Garden Vegetables	7½ oz	150	200
Organic Lentils With Tofu Weiners	7½ oz	170	260

DRIED
Arrowhead

Green	2 oz	190	10
Red	2 oz	195	12
cooked	1 cup	231	4

SPROUTS

raw	½ cup	40	4

LETTUCE

Dole Butter Lettuce	1 head	21	8
Dole Iceberg	⅙ med head	20	10
Dole Leaf, shredded	1½ cup	12	40
Dole Romaine, shredded	1½ cup	18	40
bibb	1 head (6 oz)	21	8
boston	1 head (6 oz)	21	8
boston	2 leaves	2	1
iceberg	1 head (19 oz)	70	48
iceberg	1 leaf	3	2

FOOD	PORTION	CALORIES	SODIUM
looseleaf, shredded	½ cup	5	3
romaine, shredded	½ cup	4	2

LIMA BEANS

CANNED
S&W Small Fancy	½ cup	80	390
Trappey's			
Baby Green	½ cup	90	410
Baby White	½ cup	90	410
large	1 cup	191	809
lima beans	½ cup	93	309

DRIED
baby, cooked	1 cup	229	5
cooked	½ cup	104	14
large, cooked	1 cup	217	4

FROZEN
Green Giant			
Harvest Fresh	½ cup	80	170
In Butter Sauce	½ cup	100	390
cooked	½ cup	94	26
fordhook, cooked	½ cup	85	45

LIME

FRESH
| lime | 1 | 20 | 1 |

JUICE
| bottled | 1 tbsp | 3 | 2 |
| fresh | 1 tbsp | 4 | 0 |

FOOD	PORTION	CALORIES	SODIUM

LING

FRESH

baked	3 oz	95	147
fillet, baked	5.3 oz	168	261

LINGCOD

baked	3 oz	93	64
fillet, baked	5.3 oz	164	114

LIQUOR/LIQUEUR

(see also BEER AND ALE, DRINK MIXER, MALT, WINE)

bloody mary	5 oz	116	332
bourbon & soda	4 oz	105	16
coffee liquer	1½ oz	174	4
coffee w/ cream liqueur	1½ oz	154	43
creme de menthe	1½ oz	186	3
daiquiri	2 oz	111	1
gin	1½ oz	110	1
gin & tonic	7.5 oz	171	10
manhattan	2 oz	128	2
martini	2½ oz	156	2
piña colada	4½ oz	262	9
rum	1½ oz	97	0
screwdriver	7 oz	174	2
sloe gin fizz	2½ oz	132	1
tequila sunrise	5½ oz	189	7
tom collins	7½ oz	121	39
vodka	1½ oz	97	0
whiskey	1½ oz	105	0
whiskey sour	3 oz	123	10

FOOD	PORTION	CALORIES	SODIUM
whiskey sour mix, as prep	3.6 oz	169	48
whiskey sour mix, not prep	1 pkg (.6 oz)	64	46

LIVER
(see also PATÉ)

beef, braised	3 oz	137	59
beef, pan-fried	3 oz	184	90
chicken, stewed	1 cup (5 oz)	219	71
goose, raw	1 (3.3 oz)	125	132
lamb, braised	3 oz	187	48
lamb, fried	3 oz	202	105
pork, braised	3 oz	141	42
sheep, raw	3½ oz	131	95
turkey, simmered	1 cup (5 oz)	237	89
veal, braised	3 oz	140	45
veal, fried	3 oz	208	112

LOBSTER

FRESH
northern, cooked	1 cup	142	551
northern, cooked	3 oz	83	323
spiny, steamed	1 (5.7 oz)	233	370
spiny, steamed	3 oz	122	193

TAKE-OUT
newburg	1 cup	485	127

LOGANBERRIES
frzn	1 cup	80	1

LONGANS
fresh	1	2	0

FOOD	PORTION	CALORIES	SODIUM

LOQUATS

fresh	1	5	0

LOTUS

root, raw, sliced	10 slices	45	33
root, sliced, cooked	10 slices	59	40
seeds, dried	1 oz	94	1

LOX
(*see* SALMON)

LUNCHEON MEATS/COLD CUTS
(*see also* CHICKEN, HAM, MEAT SUBSTITUTES, TURKEY)

Carl Buddig			
Beef	1 oz	40	430
Corned Beef	1 oz	40	380
Pastrami	1 oz	40	320
Hansel 'n Gretel Healthy Deli			
Bologna Beef & Pork	1 oz	41	200
Cooked Corn Beef	1 oz	35	210
Italian Roast Beef	1 oz	31	140
Pastrami Round	1 oz	34	195
Regular Roast Beef	1 oz	30	130
St. Paddy's Corned Beef	1 oz	24	290
Russer Lil' Salt			
Bologna	1 oz	70	200
Bologna Beef	1 oz	80	200
Braunschweiger	1 oz	70	200
Cooked Salami	1 oz	60	200
Old Fashioned Loaf	1 oz	60	200
P&P Loaf	1 oz	60	200

FOOD	PORTION	CALORIES	SODIUM
Weight Watchers Bologna	2 slices (¾ oz)	35	220
barbecue loaf, pork & beef	1 oz	49	378
beerwurst beef	1 slice (1/16″ × 2¾″)	20	62
beerwurst beef	1 slice (4″ × 1/8″)	75	214
beerwurst pork	1 slice (2¾″ × 1/16″)	14	74
beerwurst pork	1 slice (4″ × 1/8″)	55	285
berliner pork & beef	1 oz	65	368
bologna			
beef	1 oz	88	278
beef & pork	1 oz	89	289
pork	1 oz	70	336
braunschweiger pork	1 oz	102	324
braunschweiger pork	1 slice (2½″ × ¼″)	65	206
corned beef loaf	1 oz	43	270
dutch brand loaf, pork & beef	1 oz	68 ·	354
headcheese pork	1 oz	60	356
honey loaf, pork & beef	1 oz	36	374
honey roll, sausage beef	1 oz	42	304
lebanon bologna, beef	1 oz	60	379
liver cheese, pork	1 oz	86	347
luncheon meat			
beef	1 oz	87	377
pork & beef	1 oz	100	367
pork canned	1 oz	95	365
luncheon sausage, pork & beef	1 oz	74	335
luxury loaf, pork	1 oz	40	347

FOOD	PORTION	CALORIES	SODIUM
mortadella, beef & pork	1 oz	88	353
mother's loaf, pork	1 oz	80	320
new england sausage, pork & beef	1 oz	46	346
olive loaf, pork	1 oz	67	421
peppered loaf, pork & beef	1 oz	42	432
pepperoni, pork & beef	1 slice (.2 oz)	27	112
pepperoni, pork & beef	1 (9 oz)	1248	5120
pickle & pimiento loaf, pork	1 oz	74	394
picnic loaf, pork & beef	1 oz	66	330
salami			
cooked, beef & pork	1 oz	71	302
hard, pork	1 pkg (4 oz)	460	2554
hard, pork	1 slice (⅓ oz)	41	226
hard, pork & beef	1 pkg (4 oz)	472	2101
hard, pork & beef	1 slice (⅓ oz)	42	186
sandwich spread, pork & beef	1 oz	67	287
sandwich spread, pork & beef	1 tbsp	35	152
summer sausage, thuringer cervelat	1 oz	98	412
TAKE-OUT			
submarine w/ salami, ham, cheese, lettuce, tomato, onion & oil	1	456	1650

LUPINES

DRIED			
cooked	1 cup	197	7

LYCHEES

fresh	1	6	0

FOOD	PORTION	CALORIES	SODIUM
MACADAMIA NUTS			
Candy, Glazed (Mauna Loa)	1 oz	170	80
Chocolate Covered (Mauna Loa)	1 oz	170	21
Honey Roasted (Mauna Loa)	1 oz	200	80
Macadamia Nut Brittle (Mauna Loa)	1 oz	150	140
Roasted & Salted (Mauna Loa)	1 oz	210	75
dried	1 oz	199	1
oil roasted	1 oz	204	3
MACARONI (see PASTA)			
MACE			
ground	1 tsp	8	1
MACKEREL			
CANNED			
Jack (Empress)	4 oz	140	480
jack	1 can (12.7 oz)	563	1368
jack	1 cup	296	720
FRESH			
atlantic, cooked	3 oz	223	71
atlantic, raw	3 oz	174	76
jack, baked	3 oz	171	94
jack fillet, baked	6.2 oz	354	194
king, baked	3 oz	114	172
king fillet, baked	5.4 oz	207	312
pacific, baked	3 oz	171	94
pacific fillet, baked	6.2 oz	354	194
spanish, cooked	3 oz	134	56

FOOD	PORTION	CALORIES	SODIUM
spanish, cooked	1 fillet (5.1 oz)	230	96
spanish, raw	3 oz	118	50

MALT

Schaefer	12 oz	165	20
Schlitz	12 oz	177	21

MALTED MILK

Kraft			
Instant Chocolate	3 tsp	90	45
Instant Natural	3 tsp	90	100
chocolate, as prep w/ milk	1 cup	229	172
chocolate flavor powder	3 heaping tsp (¾ oz)	79	53
natural flavor, as prep w/ milk	1 cup	237	223
natural flavor powder	3 heaping tsp (¾ oz)	87	103

MAMMY-APPLE

fresh	1	431	127

MANGO

fresh	1	135	4
JUICE			
Kern's Nectar	6 oz	110	10
Libby's Nectar	6 oz	110	0

MARGARINE
  (*see also* BUTTER BLENDS, BUTTER SUBSTITUTES)

REDUCED CALORIE			
Fleischmann's			
Diet	1 tbsp	50	50

FOOD	PORTION	CALORIES	SODIUM
Extra Light Corn Oil Spread	1 tbsp	50	55
Mazola			
Diet	1 cup	815	2160
Diet	1 tbsp	50	130
Light Corn Oil Spread	1 cup	835	1690
Light Corn Oil Spread	1 tbsp	50	100
Parkay Diet Soft	1 tbsp	50	110
Smart Beat	1 tbsp	25	110
Unsalted	1 tbsp	25	0
Weight Watchers			
Extra Light Sweet Unsalted Tub	1 tbsp	50	0
Extra Light Tub	1 tbsp	50	130
Light Stick	1 tbsp	60	130
diet	1 cup	800	2226
diet	1 tsp	17	46
REGULAR			
Blue Bonnet	1 tbsp	100	95
Fleischmann's	1 tbsp	100	95
Light Corn Oil Stick	1 tbsp	80	70
Sweet, Unsalted	1 tbsp	100	0
Land O'Lakes	1 tsp	35	35
Premium Corn Oil	1 tsp	35	35
Spread With Sweet Cream	1 tsp	30	35
Spread With Sweet Cream, Unsalted	1 tsp	30	0
Mazola	1 cup	1650	1650
Mazola	1 tbsp	100	100
Mazola Unsalted	1 cup	1635	8
Mazola Unsalted	1 tbsp	100	1
Nucanola	1 tbsp	90	90

FOOD	PORTION	CALORIES	SODIUM
Parkay	1 tbsp	100	105
corn	1 stick (4 oz)	815	1070
corn	1 tsp	34	44
salted	1 stick (4 oz)	815	1069
salted	1 tsp	39	44
unsalted	1 stick (4 oz)	809	2
unsalted	1 tsp	34	tr
SOFT			
Blue Bonnet	1 tbsp	100	95
Chiffon	1 tbsp	90	95
Stick	1 tbsp	100	105
Unsalted	1 tbsp	90	0
Fleischmann's	1 tbsp	100	95
Light Corn Oil Spread	1 tbsp	80	70
Sweet, Unsalted	1 tbsp	100	0
Land O'Lakes			
Spread With Sweet Cream	1 tsp	25	25
Tub	1 tsp	35	35
Parkay			
Soft	1 tbsp	100	105
Spread	1 tbsp	60	110
corn	1 cup	1626	2449
corn	1 tsp	34	51
safflower	1 cup	1626	2449
safflower	1 tsp	34	51
soybean, salted	1 cup	1626	2449
soybean, salted	1 tsp	34	51
soybean, unsalted	1 cup	1626	63
soybean, unsalted	1 tsp	34	1
tub, salted	1 cup	1626	2449

FOOD	PORTION	CALORIES	SODIUM
tub, salted	1 tsp	34	51
tub, unsalted	1 cup	1626	63
tub, unsalted	1 tsp	34	1
SQUEEZE			
Parkay Squeeze	1 tbsp	90	110
soybean & cottonseed	1 tsp	34	37
WHIPPED			
Blue Bonnet Whipped Spread	1 tbsp	80	100
Chiffon	1 tbsp	70	80
Fleischmann's			
Lightly Salted	1 tbsp	70	60
Unsalted	1 tbsp	70	0
Miracle Brand	1 tbsp	60	70
Stick	1 tbsp	70	65
Parkay	1 tbsp	70	70
Stick	1 tbsp	70	65

MARJORAM

dried	1 tsp	2	tr

MARSHMALLOW

Funmallows			
(Kraft)	1	30	15
Miniature (Kraft)	10	18	5
Jet-Puffed (Kraft)	1	25	5
Marshmallow Fluff	1 heaping tsp	59	12
Miniature (Kraft)	10	18	5
marshmallow	1 oz	90	25

MATZO

Daily Thin Tea (Manischewitz)	1	103	1

FOOD	PORTION	CALORIES	SODIUM
Dietetic Thins (Manischewitz)	1	91	tr
Egg n' Onion (Manischewitz)	1	112	180
Matzo Farfel (Manischewitz)	1 cup	180	2
Matzo Meal (Manischewitz)	1 cup	514	3
Unsalted (Manischewitz)	1	110	1
Whole Wheat w/ Bran (Manischewitz)	1	110	1

MAYONNAISE
(*see also* MAYONNAISE-TYPE SALAD DRESSING, RELISH)

FOOD	PORTION	CALORIES	SODIUM
REDUCED CALORIE			
Best Foods			
Cholesterol Free	1 cup	760	1210
Cholesterol Free	1 tbsp	50	80
Light	1 cup	760	1815
Light	1 tbsp	50	115
Estee	1 tbsp	50	80
Hellmann's			
Cholesterol Free	1 cup	760	1210
Cholesterol Free	1 tbsp	50	80
Light	1 cup	760	1815
Light	1 tbsp	50	115
Kraft			
Free	1 tbsp	12	190
Light	1 tbsp	50	110
Smart Beat			
Canola Oil	1 tbsp	40	110
Corn Oil	1 tbsp	40	110
Weight Watchers			
Fat Free	1 tbsp	12	125
Light	1 tbsp	50	100
Low Sodium	1 tbsp	50	45

FOOD	PORTION	CALORIES	SODIUM
reduced calorie	1 cup	556	1193
reduced calorie	1 tbsp	34	75
REGULAR			
Best Foods Real	1 cup	1570	1255
Best Foods Real	1 tbsp	100	80
Hellman's	1 cup	1570	1255
Hellman's	1 tbsp	100	80
Kraft			
Real	1 tbsp	100	70
Sandwich Spread	1 tbsp	50	95
mayonnaise	1 cup	1577	1250
mayonnaise	1 tbsp	99	78

MAYONNAISE-TYPE SALAD DRESSING
(*see also* MAYONNAISE, RELISH)

FOOD	PORTION	CALORIES	SODIUM
REDUCED CALORIE			
Miracle Whip			
Free	1 tbsp	20	210
Light	1 tbsp	45	125
Smart Beat	1 tbsp	12	130
Weight Watchers Fat Free Whipped Dressing	1 tbsp	16	115
reduced calorie w/o cholesterol	1 cup	1084	794
reduced calorie w/o cholesterol	1 tbsp	68	49
REGULAR			
Miracle Whip	1 tbsp	70	85
Coleslaw Dressing	1 tbsp	70	105
Spin Blend	1 tbsp	60	110
Cholesterol-Free	1 tbsp	40	110
home recipe	1 cup	400	1872
home recipe	1 tbsp	25	117
mayonnaise-type salad dressing	1 cup	916	1670

FOOD	PORTION	CALORIES	SODIUM

MEAT SUBSTITUTES
(see also CHICKEN SUBSTITUTES)

FOOD	PORTION	CALORIES	SODIUM
Jaclyn's			
Salisbury Steak Style Dinner	11 oz	260	320
Sirloin Strips Style Dinner	12 oz	290	320
Spring Creek Soysage	1 patty (1.6 oz)	63	237
simulated meat product	1 oz	88	3
simulated sausage	1 link (25 g)	64	222
simulated sausage	1 patty (38 g)	97	137

MELON
(see also individual names)

FROZEN

FOOD	PORTION	CALORIES	SODIUM
melon balls	1 cup	55	53

MEXICAN FOOD
(see also BEANS, CHIPS, DINNER, PEPPERS, SALSA, SNACKS)

FOOD	PORTION	CALORIES	SODIUM
CANNED			
Enchilada Sauce Mild (Rosarita)	2.5 oz	25	230
Enchiladas (Gebhardt)	2	310	460
Picante			
Chunky Hot (Rosarita)	3 tbsp	18	515
Chunky Medium (Rosarita)	3 tbsp	16	650
Chunky Mild (Rosarita)	3 tbsp	25	630
Hot (Chi Chi's)	1 oz	11	263
Mild (Chi Chi's)	1 oz	11	191
Taco Sauce			
Hot (Chi Chi's)	1 oz	17	247
Mild (Chi Chi's)	1 oz	18	165
Thick And Smooth, Hot (Ortega)	1 tbsp	8	105
Thick And Smooth, Mild (Ortega)	1 tbsp	8	115

FOOD	PORTION	CALORIES	SODIUM
Tamales			
(Derby)	2	160	570
(Gebhardt)	2	290	730
(Wolf Brand)	7.5 oz	328	1181
Jumbo (Gebhardt)	2	400	1025
With Sauce (Van Camp's)	1 cup	293	1132
FROZEN			
Banquet			
Beef & Bean Burrito	9.5 oz	390	1460
Beef Enchilada & Tamale w/ Chili Gravy	10 oz	300	1390
Chimichanga	9.5 oz	480	1480
Enchilada Beef	11 oz	370	1200
Enchilada Cheese	11 oz	340	1310
Enchilada Chicken	11 oz	340	1370
Tamale Beef	11 oz	420	1420
Budget Gourmet			
Beef Mexicana	1 pkg	520	1280
Chicken Enchilada Suiza	1 pkg	290	810
Chicken Mexicana	1 pkg	560	1170
Sirloin Enchilada Ranchero	1 pkg	280	750
Healthy Choice			
Enchilada Beef	12.75 oz	350	430
Enchilada Chicken	12.75 oz	330	440
Enchiladas Chicken	9.5 oz	280	510
Fajitas Beef	7 oz	210	250
Fajitas Chicken	7 oz	200	310
Le Menu Entree LightStyle Enchilada Chicken	8 oz	280	530
Lean Cuisine			
Enchanadas Beef And Bean	9¼ oz	240	480
Enchanadas Chicken	9⅞ oz	290	500

FOOD	PORTION	CALORIES	SODIUM
Patio			
Fiesta Dinner	12 oz	460	1990
Mexican Dinner	13.25	540	1940
Tamale Dinner	13 oz	470	1850
Patio Britos			
Beef & Bean	1 (3 oz)	210	290
Nacho Beef	1 (3 oz)	220	350
Nacho Cheese	1 (3.63 oz)	250	330
Spicy Chicken & Cheese	1 (3 oz)	210	280
Patio Burritos			
Hot Beef & Bean Red Chili	1 (5 oz)	340	810
Medium Beef & Bean	1 (5 oz)	370	830
Mild Beef & Bean Green Chili	1 (5 oz)	330	770
Patio Enchilada			
Beef Dinner	13.25 oz	520	1810
Cheese Dinner	12 oz	370	1970
Swanson			
Enchiladas Beef	13¾ oz	480	1350
Mexican Style Combination	14¼ oz	490	1760
Mexican Style Hungry-Man	20¼ oz	820	2080
Weight Watchers			
Enchiladas Ranchero Beef	9.12 oz	190	500
Enchiladas Ranchero Cheese	8.87 oz	260	550
Enchiladas Suiza Chicken	9 oz	230	530
Fajitas Chicken	6.75 oz	210	490
MIX			
Masa Harina De Maiz (Quaker)	2 tortillas	137	5
Masa Trigo (Quaker)	2 tortillas	149	794
Menudo Mix (Gebhardt)	1 tsp	5	310
Taco Meat Seasoning Mix, Mild (Ortega)	1 filled taco	90	999

FOOD	PORTION	CALORIES	SODIUM
READY-TO-USE			
Taco Shells			
(Gebhardt)	1	50	tr
(Rosarita)	1 shell	50	tr
Tortilla, Wheat Flour (Mariachi)	1	112	174
Tostada Shells (Rosarita)	1 shell	60	tr
tortilla corn	1 (1 oz)	65	1
TAKE-OUT			
burrito			
w/ apple	1 lg (5.4 oz)	484	443
w/ apple	1 sm (2.6 oz)	231	211
w/ beans	2 (7.6 oz)	448	986
w/ beans & cheese	2 (6.5 oz)	377	1166
w/ beans & chili peppers	2 (7.2 oz)	413	1043
w/ beans & meat	2 (8.1 oz)	508	1335
w/ beans, cheese & beef	2 (7.1 oz)	331	990
w/ beans, cheese & chili peppers	2 (11.8 oz)	663	2060
w/ beef	2 (7.7 oz)	523	1492
w/ beef & chili peppers	2 (7.1 oz)	426	1116
w/ beef, cheese & chili peppers	2 (10.7 oz)	634	2091
w/ cherry	1 lg (5.4 oz)	484	443
w/ cherry	1 sm (2.6 oz)	231	211
chimichanga			
w/ beef	1 (6.1 oz)	425	910
w/ beef & cheese	1 (6.4 oz)	443	956
w/ beef & red chili peppers	1 (6.7 oz)	424	1169
w/ beef, cheese & red chili peppers	1 (6.3 oz)	364	895
enchilada			
w/ cheese	1 (5.7 oz)	320	784
w/ cheese & beef	1 (6.7 oz)	324	1320

FOOD	PORTION	CALORIES	SODIUM
enchirito w/ cheese, beef & beans	1 (6.8 oz)	344	1251
frijoles w/ cheese	1 cup (5.9 oz)	226	882
nachos			
w/ cheese	6 to 8 (4 oz)	345	816
w/ cheese & jalapeno peppers	6 to 8 (7.2 oz)	607	1736
w/ cheese, beans, ground beef & peppers	6 to 8 (8.9 oz)	568	1800
w/ cinnamon & sugar	6 to 8 (3.8 oz)	592	439
taco	1 sm (6 oz)	370	802
taco salad	1½ cup	279	763
w/ chili con carne	1½ cup	288	886
tostada			
w/ beans & cheese	1 (5.1 oz)	223	543
w/ beans, beef & cheese	1 (7.9 oz)	334	870
w/ beef & cheese	1 (5.7 oz)	315	896
w/ guacamole	2 (9.2 oz)	360	789

MILK
(*see also* CHOCOLATE, COCOA, MILK DRINKS)

FOOD	PORTION	CALORIES	SODIUM
CANNED			
condensed, sweetened	1 cup	982	389
condensed, sweetened	1 oz	123	49
evaporated	½ cup	169	122
evaporated, skim	½ cup	99	147
DRIED			
Lactose Reduced, as prep (Nutra/Balance)	8 oz	80	125
Sanalac, as prep	8 oz	80	125
buttermilk	1 tbsp	25	34
nonfat, instantized	1 pkg (3.2 oz)	244	499

FOOD	PORTION	CALORIES	SODIUM
LIQUID, LOWFAT			
CalciMilk	1 cup	102	123
Lactaid 1%	1 cup	102	123
1%	1 cup	102	123
1%	1 qt	409	493
1%, protein fortified	1 cup	119	143
1%, protein fortified	1 qt	477	574
2%	1 cup	121	122
2%	1 qt	485	487
buttermilk	1 cup	99	257
buttermilk	1 qt	396	1028
LIQUID, REGULAR			
Farmland, 75% Cholesterol Reduced	8 oz	150	125
buffalo	3½ oz	112	40
camel	3½ oz	80	30
goat	1 cup	168	122
goat	1 qt	672	486
human	1 cup	171	42
indian buffalo	1 cup	236	127
low sodium	1 cup	149	6
sheep	1 cup	264	108
whole	1 cup	150	120
LIQUID, SKIM			
Farmland, Skim Plus	8 oz	100	150
Lactaid Nonfat	1 cup	86	126
Lite-Line	1 cup	100	150
Viva	1 cup	100	150
Weight Watchers	1 cup	90	140
skim	1 cup	86	125

FOOD	PORTION	CALORIES	SODIUM
skim	1 qt	342	505
skim, protein fortified	1 cup	100	144
skim, protein fortified	1 qt	400	578

MILK DRINKS
(*see also* BREAKFAST DRINKS, CHOCOLATE, COCOA)

FOOD	PORTION	CALORIES	SODIUM
Chocolate Milk			
1% (Lactaid)	1 cup	158	152
2% (Hershey)	1 cup	190	130
Quik (Nestle)			
Banana Lowfat Milk	8 oz	190	115
Chocolate	¾ oz	90	25
Chocolate, as prep w/ 2% milk	8 oz	210	150
Chocolate, as prep w/ skim milk	8 oz	170	150
Chocolate, as prep w/ whole milk	8 oz	230	140
Chocolate Lowfat Milk	8 oz	200	150
Strawberry	¾ oz	80	0
Strawberry, as prep w/ 2% milk	8 oz	200	120
Strawberry, as prep w/ skim milk	8 oz	160	125
Strawberry, as prep w/ whole milk	8 oz	220	120
Strawberry Lowfat Milk	8 oz	200	120
Vanilla Lowfat Milk	8 oz	200	115
Quik Ready to Drink (Nestle)			
Chocolate	8 oz	230	120
Lite Chocolate Lowfat	8 oz	130	150
Strawberry	8 oz	230	140
Quik Sugar Free (Nestle)			
Chocolate	1 heaping tsp	18	35

FOOD	PORTION	CALORIES	SODIUM
Chocolate, as prep w/ 2% milk	8 oz	140	150
Quik Syrup (Nestle)			
Chocolate	1⅔ tbsp	100	45
Chocolate, as prep w/ 2% milk	8 oz	220	160
Chocolate, as prep w/ skim milk	8 oz	220	160
Chocolate, as prep w/ whole milk	8 oz	240	160
Strawberry	1⅔ tbsp	100	0
Strawberry, as prep w/ 2% milk	8 oz	220	120
Strawberry, as prep w/ skim milk	8 oz	180	130
Strawberry, as prep w/ whole milk	8 oz	240	120
Whole Chocolate Milk (Hershey)	8 oz	210	120
chocolate milk	1 cup	208	149
chocolate milk	1 qt	833	596
chocolate milk 1%	1 cup	158	152
chocolate milk 1%	1 qt	630	607
chocolate milk 2%	1 cup	179	150
strawberry flavor mix, as prep w/ whole milk	9 oz	234	128

MILK SUBSTITUTES
   (*see also* COFFEE WHITENERS)

FOOD	PORTION	CALORIES	SODIUM
Spring Creek			
!Honey Vanilla	1 oz	23	7
Original	1 oz	21	6
Plain	1 oz	15	4
imitation milk	1 cup	150	191
imitation milk	1 qt	600	764

FOOD	PORTION	CALORIES	SODIUM
MILKSHAKE			
Chocolate (MicroMagic)	1 (10.5 oz)	290	90
Chocolate Fudge (Weight Watchers)	1 pkg	70	150
Orange Sherbet (Weight Watchers)	1 pkg	70	210
chocolate	10 oz	360	273
strawberry	10 oz	319	234
thick shake			
chocolate	10.6 oz	356	333
vanilla	11 oz	350	299
vanilla	10 oz	314	232
MILLET			
Millet Hulled (Arrowhead)	1 oz	90	tr
cooked	½ cup	143	2
MINERAL/BOTTLED WATER			
Crystal Geyser Sparkling			
Cola Berry	6 oz	0	30
Lemon	6 oz	0	30
Lime	6 oz	0	30
Mineral	6 oz	0	30
Natural Wild Cherry	6 oz	0	30
Orange	6 oz	0	30
Evian	1 liter	0	5
San Pellegrino	1 liter (33.8 oz)	0	41
Saratoga Sparkling	8 oz	0	tr
MISO			
miso	½ cup	284	5036

FOOD	PORTION	CALORIES	SODIUM
MOLASSES			
Brer Rabbit			
Dark	2 tbsp	110	20
Light	2 tbsp	110	15
blackstrap	2 tbsp	85	38
molasses	2 tbsp	85	38
MONKFISH			
baked	3 oz	82	20
MOOSE			
roasted	3 oz	114	58
MOTH BEANS			
DRIED			
cooked	1 cup	207	17
MOUSSE			
FROZEN			
Chocolate			
(Sara Lee)	1 slice (2.7 oz)	260	100
(Weight Watchers)	1 (2.5 oz)	160	160
Light (Sara Lee)	1 (3 oz)	170	60
Praline Pecan (Weight Watchers)	1 (2.71 oz)	180	180
San Francisco Chocolate Mousse (Pepperidge Farm)	1	490	75
HOME RECIPE			
orange	½ cup	87	24
MIX			
Amaretto (Estee)	½ cup	70	50

FOOD	PORTION	CALORIES	SODIUM
Chocolate Mousse No-Bake (Royal)	⅛ pie	130	190
Dark Chocolate, as prep (Knorr)	½ cup	90	50
Milk Chocolate, as prep (Knorr)	½ cup	90	50
Orange Chocolate (Estee)	½ cup	70	50
Unflavored, as prep (Knorr)	½ cup	80	45
White Chocolate Almond Mousse (Weight Watchers)	½ cup	70	105
White Chocolate, as prep (Knorr)	½ cup	80	50

MUFFIN

FROZEN

FOOD	PORTION	CALORIES	SODIUM
Almond & Date Oat Bran Fancy Fruit (Health Valley)	1	180	80
Apple Oat Bran (Sara Lee)	1	190	300
Apple Spice			
(Healthy Choice)	1 (2.5 oz)	190	90
(Sara Lee)	1	220	280
Fat Free (Health Valley)	1	140	110
Banana Fat Free (Health Valley)	1	130	110
Banana Nut			
(Healthy Choice)	1 (2.5 oz)	180	80
(Pepperidge Farm)	1	170	220
Blueberry			
(Healthy Choice)	1 (2.5 oz)	190	110
(Pepperidge Farm)	1	170	250
(Sara Lee)	1	200	290
Free & Light (Sara Lee)	1	120	140
Cheese Streusel (Sara Lee)	1	220	170
Chocolate Chunk (Sara Lee)	1	220	210
Cholesterol Free Multi Grain Muesli (Pepperidge Farm)	1	200	230

FOOD	PORTION	CALORIES	SODIUM
Oatbran With Apple (Pepperidge Farm)	1	190	200
Raisin Bran (Pepperidge Farm)	1	170	280
Cinnamon Swirl (Pepperidge Farm)	1	190	170
Corn (Pepperidge Farm)	1	180	260
Golden Corn (Sara Lee)	1	240	310
Oat Bran (Sara Lee)	1	210	320
Oat Bran Fancy Fruit Blueberry (Health Valley)	1	140	100
Raisin (Health Valley)	1	180	90
Raisin Bran (Sara Lee)	1	220	400
Raisin Spice Fat Free (Health Valley)	1	140	100
Rice Bran, Fancy Fruit, Raisin (Health Valley)	1	210	125
HOME RECIPE			
blueberry	1 (1.5 oz)	135	198
bran	1 (1.5 oz)	125	189
MIX			
Apple Cinnamon (Betty Crocker)	1	120	140
No Cholesterol Recipe (Betty Crocker)	1	110	140
Banana Nut (Betty Crocker)	1	120	140
No Cholesterol Recipe (Betty Crocker)	1	110	140
Blueberry Streusel Bake Shop (Betty Crocker)	1	210	230
Cinnamon Streusel (Betty Crocker)	1	200	240
Corn Muffin (Dromedary)	1	120	270

FOOD	PORTION	CALORIES	SODIUM
Corn Muffin *(cont.)*			
(Flako)	1	120	360
Oat Bran			
(Betty Crocker)	1	190	240
(Estee)	1	100	65
No Cholesterol Recipe (Betty Crocker)	1	180	240
Twice The Blueberries (Betty Crocker)	1	120	140
No Cholesterol Recipe (Betty Crocker)	1	110	140
Wild Blueberry (Betty Crocker)	1	120	150
No Cholesterol Recipe (Betty Crocker)	1	110	150
Light (Betty Crocker)	1	70	140
Light, No Cholesterol Recipe (Betty Crocker)	1	70	140
blueberry	1 (1.5 oz)	140	225
bran	1 (1.5 oz)	140	385
corn	1 (1.5 oz)	145	291

MULBERRIES

fresh	1 cup	61	14

MULLET

striped, cooked	3 oz	127	61
striped, raw	3 oz	99	55

MUNG BEANS

DRIED			
Arrowhead Red	2 oz	50	2
cooked	1 cup	213	4

FOOD	PORTION	CALORIES	SODIUM
SPROUTS			
cooked	½ cup	13	6
raw	½ cup	16	3
MUNGO BEANS			
DRIED			
cooked	1 cup	190	13
MUSHROOMS			
CANNED			
Button			
(Empress)	2 oz	14	260
Sliced (Empress)	2 oz	14	260
Mushrooms			
(B In B)	¼ cup	12	240
w/ Garlic (B In B)	¼ cup	12	200
Oriental Straw Mushrooms (Green Giant)	¼ cup	12	290
Pieces & Stems (Empress)	2 oz	14	260
Pieces And Stems (Green Giant)	¼ cup	12	220
Sliced (Green Giant)	¼ cup	12	220
Straw Mushrooms, Broken (Empress)	2 oz	10	180
Whole (Green Giant)	¼ cup	12	220
chanterelle	3½ oz	12	165
DRIED			
chanterelle	3½ oz	89	32
shitake	4 (½ oz)	44	2
FRESH			
chanterelle	3½ oz	11	3
enoki, raw	1 (4")	2	0
morel	3½ oz	9	2

FOOD	PORTION	CALORIES	SODIUM
raw	1 (½ oz)	5	1
raw, sliced	½ cup	9	1
shitake, cooked	4 (2.5 oz)	40	3
sliced, cooked	½ cup	21	2
whole, cooked	1 (.4 oz)	3	0
FROZEN			
Breaded Mushrooms (Ore Ida)	2.67 oz	120	440

MUSKRAT

roasted	3 oz	199	81

MUSSELS

FRESH			
blue, cooked	3 oz	147	313
blue, raw	1 cup	129	429
blue, raw	3 oz	73	243

MUSTARD

Grey Poupon			
Country Dijon	1 tsp	6	120
Dijon	1 tsp	6	120
Parisian	1 tsp	6	55
Heinz			
Mild Yellow	1 tbsp	8	175
Spicy Brown	1 tbsp	14	115
Kraft			
Horseradish Mustard	1 tbsp	14	135
Pure Prepared	1 tbsp	4	160
dry mustard seed, yellow	1 tsp	15	tr
yellow, ready-to-use	1 tsp	5	63

FOOD	PORTION	CALORIES	SODIUM

MUSTARD GREENS

FRESH

chopped, cooked	½ cup	11	11
raw, chopped	½ cup	7	7

FROZEN

chopped, cooked	½ cup	14	19

NATTO

natto	½ cup	187	6

NAVY BEANS

CANNED

Trappey's	½ cup	90	410
Jalapeno	½ cup	90	480
navy	1 cup	296	1173

DRIED

cooked	1 cup	259	2

NECTARINE

Dole	1	70	0
fresh	1	67	0

NEUFCHATEL CHEESE
(*see* CREAM CHEESE)

NONDAIRY CREAMERS
(*see* COFFEE WHITENERS)

NONDAIRY WHIPPED TOPPINGS
(*see* WHIPPED TOPPINGS)

NOODLES
(*see also* PASTA DINNERS)

FOOD	PORTION	CALORIES	SODIUM
CANNED			
Van Camp's Noodle Weenee	1 cup	245	1245
DRY			
Chinese (Azumaya)	4 oz	293	530
Chow Mein			
Narrow (La Choy)	½ cup	150	320
Wide (La Choy)	½ cup	150	300
Egg			
(Golden Grain)	2 oz	210	10
(Mueller's)	2 oz	220	8
Japanese (Azumaya)	4 oz	289	542
Noodle Trio (Mueller's)	2 oz	220	18
Rice (La Choy)	½ cup	130	420
cellophane	1 cup	492	14
chow mein	1 cup	237	197
egg	½ cup	145	8
egg, cooked	1 cup	212	11
japanese			
soba	2 oz	192	451
soba, cooked	½ cup	56	34
somen	2 oz	203	1049
somen, cooked	½ cup	115	142
spinach/egg	1 cup	145	27
spinach/egg, cooked	1 cup	211	20
DRY MIX			
Kraft Egg Noodle With Chicken Dinner	¾ cup	240	1050
La Choy Ramen Noodles			
Beef, as prep	1 cup	200	865
Chicken, as prep	1 cup	200	740
Lipton Noodles And Sauce			
Alfredo	½ cup	131	530

FOOD	PORTION	CALORIES	SODIUM
Beef	½ cup	120	513
Butter	½ cup	142	461
Butter And Herb	½ cup	136	458
Carbonara Alfredo	½ cup	126	465
Cheese	½ cup	136	470
Chicken	½ cup	125	391
Chicken Broccoli	½ cup	124	425
Creamy Chicken	½ cup	125	390
Parmesan	½ cup	138	409
Romanoff	½ cup	136	504
Sour Cream And Chive	½ cup	142	442
Stroganoff	½ cup	110	406
Tomato Alfredo	½ cup	126	562
Noodle Roni			
Parmesano	½ cup	240	140
Romanoff	½ cup	240	730
Ultra Slim-Fast Noodles			
& Beef	2.3 oz	230	1070
& Cheese	2.3 oz	230	770
& Chicken Sauce	2.3 oz	220	980
& Tomato Herb Sauce	2.3 oz	220	1090
TAKE-OUT			
noodle pudding	½ cup	132	222

NUTMEG

ground	1 tsp	12	tr

NUTRITIONAL SUPPLEMENTS
(*see also* BREAKFAST BAR, BREAKFAST DRINKS)

FOOD	PORTION	CALORIES	SODIUM
DIET			
Dynatrim			
Dutch Chocolate, as prep w/ 1% milk	8 oz	220	300
Strawberry Royale, as prep w/ 1% milk	8 oz	220	300
Figurines			
Chocolate	1 bar	100	45
Chocolate Caramel	1 bar	100	55
Chocolate Peanut Butter	1 bar	100	45
S'Mores	1 bar	100	54
Vanilla	1 bar	100	45
Slim-Fast Nutrition Bar			
Dutch Chocolate	1	130	90
Peanut Butter	1	140	100
Slim-Fast Powder			
Chocolate, as prep w/ skim milk	8 oz	190	210
Strawberry, as prep w/ skim milk	8 oz	190	220
Vanilla, as prep w/ skim milk	8 oz	190	220
Ultra Slim-Fast			
Cafe Mocha, as prep w/ skim milk	8 oz	200	280
Chocolate Royale, as prep w/ skim milk	8 oz	200	230
Dutch Chocolate, as prep w/ water	8 oz	220	260
French Vanilla, as prep w/ skim milk	8 oz	190	250
French Vanilla, as prep w/ water	8 oz	220	260
Fruit Juice Mix, as prep w/ fruit juice	8 oz	200	80
Hot Cocoa, as prep w/ water	8 oz	190	140

FOOD	PORTION	CALORIES	SODIUM
Piña Colada, as prep w/ skim milk	8 oz	180	250
Strawberry, as prep w/ skim milk	8 oz	190	250
Strawberry Supreme, as prep w/ water	8 oz	220	260
Ultra Slim-Fast Crunch Bar			
Cocoa Almond	1	110	30
Cocoa Raspberry	1	100	30
Vanilla Almond	1	110	30
Ultra Slim-Fast Ready-to-Drink			
Chocolate Royale	11 oz	230	220
Chocolate Royale	12 oz	250	240
French Vanilla	11 oz	230	190
French Vanilla	12 oz	220	240
Strawberry Supreme	12 oz	220	240
REGULAR			
EggPro	4 oz	200	105
Fi-Bar			
Apple	1 (1 oz)	90	12
Cocoa Almond	1	130	20
Cocoa Peanut	1	130	20
Cranberry & Wild Berries	1 (1 oz)	100	20
Lemon	1 (1 oz)	90	12
Mandarin Orange	1 (1 oz)	99	12
Raspberry	1 (1 oz)	100	20
Strawberry	1 (1 oz)	100	20
Vanilla Almond	1	130	20
Vanilla Peanut	1	130	20
Fi-Bar Treat Yourself Right			
Almond	1	152	38
Peanutty Butter	1	152	56

FOOD	PORTION	CALORIES	SODIUM
Gookinaid Lemonade	1 cup	45	70
Meal On The Go			
Apple	1 bar (3 oz)	294	114
Banana w/ Pecans	1 bar (3 oz)	289	109
Original	1 bar (3 oz)	286	119
Nutra/Balance Frozen Pudding			
Butterscotch	4 oz	225	220
Chocolate	4 oz	225	220
Tapioca	4 oz	225	220
Vanilla	4 oz	225	220
NutraShake			
Chocolate	4 oz	200	55
Strawberry	4 oz	200	55
Vanilla	4 oz	200	55
NutraShake With Fibre			
Strawberry	6 oz	300	110
Vanilla	6 oz	300	110

NUTS MIXED
(*see also* individual names)

FOOD	PORTION	CALORIES	SODIUM
Cashews & Peanuts Honey Roasted (Planters)	1 oz	170	170
Mixed Nuts, Lightly Salted (Planters)	1 oz	170	80
Peanuts & Cashews Honey Roasted (Planters)	1 oz	170	140
dry roasted			
w/ peanuts	1 oz	169	3
w/ peanuts, salted	1 oz	169	223
oil roasted			
w/ peanuts	1 oz	175	3
w/ peanuts, salted	1 oz	175	217
w/o peanuts	1 oz	175	3

FOOD	PORTION	CALORIES	SODIUM
w/o peanuts, salted	1 oz	175	233

OHELOBERRIES

fresh	1 cup	39	2

OIL
(see also FAT)

FOOD	PORTION	CALORIES	SODIUM
Mazola	1 cup	1955	0
Mazola	1 tbsp	120	0
Mazola No Stick	2.5 sec spray	2	0
Orville Redenbacher's	1 tbsp	120	0
Planters			
Peanut	1 tbsp	120	0
Popcorn	1 tbsp	120	0
Smart Beat	1 tbsp	120	0
Canola	1 tbsp	120	0
Weight Watchers			
Butter Spray	1 sec spray	2	0
Cooking Spray	1 sec spray	2	0
Wesson			
Canola	1 tbsp	120	0
Corn	1 tbsp	120	0
Lite Cooking Spray	.5 sec spray	0	0
Olive	1 tbsp	120	0
Sunflower	1 tbsp	120	0
Vegetable	1 tbsp	120	0
olive	1 cup	1909	tr
olive	1 tbsp	119	0
peanut	1 cup	1909	tr
peanut	1 tbsp	119	tr
soybean	1 cup	1927	tr
soybean	1 tbsp	120	0

FOOD	PORTION	CALORIES	SODIUM

OKRA

FRESH

raw	8 pods	36	8
raw, sliced	½ cup	19	4
sliced, cooked	8 pods	27	5
sliced, cooked	½ cup	25	4

FROZEN

Breaded Okra (Ore Ida)	3 oz	170	600
sliced, cooked	1 pkg (10 oz)	94	8
sliced, cooked	½ cup	34	3

OLIVES

California Ripe	3 sm	4	29
Ripe, Extra Large, (S&W)	3.5 oz	163	760
Ripe, Pitted, Large (S&W)	3.5 oz	163	760
green	3 extra lg	15	312
green	4 med	15	312
ripe	1 colossal	12	136
ripe	1 jumbo	7	75
ripe	1 lg	5	38
ripe	1 sm	4	28

ONION

CANNED

Lightly Spiced Cocktail Onions (Vlasic)	1 oz	4	365
Whole Small (S&W)	½ cup	35	345
chopped	½ cup	21	416
whole	1 (2.2 oz)	12	234

FOOD	PORTION	CALORIES	SODIUM
DRIED			
flakes	1 tbsp	16	1
powder	1 tsp	7	1
FRESH			
Antioch Farms Vidalia	1 med	60	10
Dole	1 med	60	10
Dole Green Onions, chopped	1 tbsp	2	0
chopped, cooked	½ cup	47	3
raw, chopped	1 tbsp	4	0
raw, chopped	½ cup	30	2
scallions, raw, chopped	1 tbsp	2	1
scallions, raw, sliced	½ cup	16	8
FROZEN			
Chopped (Ore Ida)	2 oz	20	5
Crispy Onion Rings (Mrs. Paul's)	2½ oz	190	230
Onion Ringers (Ore Ida)	2 oz	150	90
chopped, cooked	1 tbsp	4	2
chopped, cooked	½ cup	30	12
rings	7 (2.5 oz)	285	263
rings, cooked	2 (.7 oz)	81	75
whole, cooked	3½ oz	28	8
TAKE-OUT			
rings, breaded & fried	8 to 9	275	430

ORANGE

CANNED			
Mandarin			
(Empress)	5.5 oz	100	10
Natural Style (S&W)	½ cup	60	10
Segments (Dole)	½ cup	70	10

FOOD	PORTION	CALORIES	SODIUM
Mandarin *(cont.)*			
Selected Sections in Heavy Syrup (S&W)	½ cup	76	10
Unsweetened (S&W)	½ cup	28	10
Pineapple Mandarin Segments (Dole)	½ cup	60	5
FRESH			
Dole	1	50	0
california, navel	1	65	1
california, valencia	1	59	0
florida	1	69	1
peel	1 tbsp	6	0
sections	1 cup	85	0
JUICE			
Libby's	6 oz	80	0
Ocean Spray	6 oz	80	15
S&W 100% Unsweetened	6 oz	83	2
Tree Top	6 oz	90	5
canned	1 cup	104	6
chilled	1 cup	110	2
fresh	1 cup	111	2
frzn, as prep	1 cup	112	2
frzn, not prep	6 oz	339	7
orange drink	6 oz	94	31

OREGANO

| ground | 1 tsp | 5 | tr |

ORGAN MEATS

(see BRAINS, GIBLETS, GIZZARDS, HEART, KIDNEY, LIVER, SWEETBREADS)

FOOD	PORTION	CALORIES	SODIUM

ORIENTAL FOOD
(*see also* DINNER, NOODLES, RICE)

CANNED
La Choy Bi-Pack

FOOD	PORTION	CALORIES	SODIUM
Beef Pepper	¾ cup	80	950
Chow Mein Chicken	¾ cup	80	970
Chow Mein Pork	¾ cup	80	950
Chow Mein Shrimp	¾ cup	70	860
Sweet & Sour Chicken	¾ cup	120	440
Teriyaki Chicken	¾ cup	85	850
La Choy Dinner Chow Mein Chicken	½ pkg	300	1800

La Choy Entree

FOOD	PORTION	CALORIES	SODIUM
Beef Pepper Oriental	¾ cup	100	1340
Chow Mein Beef	¾ cup	40	960
Chow Mein Chicken	¾ cup	70	850
Chow Mein Meatless	¾ cup	25	860
Chow Mein Shrimp	¾ cup	35	940
Sweet And Sour Chicken	¾ cup	240	1420
Sweet And Sour Pork	¾ cup	250	1540
chow mein chicken	1 cup	95	725

FRESH

FOOD	PORTION	CALORIES	SODIUM
Won Ton Wraps (Azumaya)	1	23	50

FROZEN
Chun King

FOOD	PORTION	CALORIES	SODIUM
Beef Pepper Oriental	13 oz	319	1300
Chicken Chow Mein	13 oz	370	1560
Crunchy Walnut Chicken	13 oz	310	1700
Egg Rolls, Chicken	1 (3.6 oz)	220	600
Egg Rolls, Meat & Shrimp	1 (3.6 oz)	220	680
Egg Rolls, Shrimp	1 (3.6 oz)	200	480

FOOD	PORTION	CALORIES	SODIUM
Chun King *(cont.)*			
Fried Rice w/ Chicken	8 oz	260	1460
Fried Rice w/ Pork	8 oz	270	1210
Imperial Chicken	13 oz	300	1540
Restaurant Style Egg Rolls, Pork	1 (3 oz)	180	450
Sweet & Sour Pork	13 oz	400	1460
Dining Light Chicken Chow Mein	9 oz	180	650
Healthy Choice Chicken Chow Mein	8.5 oz	220	440
La Choy Restaurant Style Egg Roll			
Pork	1 (3 oz)	150	480
Shrimp	1 (3 oz)	130	260
Almond Chicken	1 (3 oz)	120	290
Sweet & Sour Chicken	1 (3 oz)	150	280
La Choy Snack Egg Roll			
Chicken	2	90	140
Lobster	1 (1.45 oz)	75	150
Meat & Shrimp	1 (1.45 oz)	80	115
Shrimp	1 (1.45 oz)	75	120
Lean Cuisine Chicken Chow Mein With Rice	9 oz	240	530
HOME RECIPE			
chop suey w/ beef & pork	1 cup	300	1053
chow mein chicken	1 cup	255	718
MIX			
Kikkoman Teriyaki, Baste & Glaze	1 tbsp	24	310
La Choy Dinner Classics			
Egg Foo Young	2 patties + 3 oz sauce	170	1390
Pepper Steak	¾ cup	180	760
Sweet & Sour	¾ cup	310	860

FOOD	PORTION	CALORIES	SODIUM
TAKE-OUT			
chicken teriyaki	¾ cup	399	2190
chop suey w/ pork	1 cup	375	1378
chow mein, pork	1 cup	425	1673
chow mein, shrimp	1 cup	221	1658
wonton	1 cup	205	322
wonton, fried	½ cup (1 oz)	111	147

OYSTERS

FOOD	PORTION	CALORIES	SODIUM
CANNED			
Bumble Bee, Whole	½ cup (3.5 oz)	100	390
Empress, Whole	4 oz	100	390
eastern	1 cup	170	277
eastern	3 oz	58	95
FRESH			
eastern, cooked	3 oz	117	190
eastern, cooked	6 med	58	94
eastern, raw	1 cup	170	277
eastern, raw	6 med	58	94
pacific, raw	1 med	41	53
pacific, raw	3 oz	69	90
steamed	1 med	41	53
steamed	3 oz	138	180
TAKE-OUT			
battered & fried	6 (4.9 oz)	368	677
breaded & fried	6 (4.9 oz)	368	677
eastern, breaded & fried	3 oz	167	355
eastern, breaded & fried	6 medium	173	367
oysters rockefeller	3 oysters	66	80
stew	1 cup	278	928

FOOD	PORTION	CALORIES	SODIUM

PANCAKE/WAFFLE SYRUP
(see also SYRUP*)*

FOOD	PORTION	CALORIES	SODIUM
Aunt Jemima	2 tbsp	110	30
Butter Lite	2 tbsp	50	90
Lite	2 tbsp	50	90
Brer Rabbit			
Dark	2 tbsp	120	0
Light	2 tbsp	120	0
Estee	1 tbsp	8	35
Golden Griddle	1 cup	885	225
Golden Griddle	1 tbsp	50	55
Karo	1 tbsp	60	35
Weight Watchers	1 tbsp	25	40
maple	2 tbsp	122	19

PANCAKES

FOOD	PORTION	CALORIES	SODIUM
FROZEN			
Blueberry			
(Aunt Jemima)	3.48 oz	220	826
(Kid Cuisine)	3.47 oz	210	410
Microwave (Pillsbury)	3	250	540
Buttermilk			
(Aunt Jemima)	3.48 oz	210	860
(Kid Cuisine)	4.17 oz	180	410
(Weight Watchers)	2 (2.5 oz)	140	270
Batter, as prep (Aunt Jemima)	3.6 oz	180	778
Microwave (Pillsbury)	3	260	590
Harvest Wheat Microwave (Pillsbury)	3	240	420
Lite Buttermilk (Aunt Jemima)	3.48 oz	140	660
Lite Pancakes & Lite Links (Quaker)	1 pkg (6 oz)	310	970

FOOD	PORTION	CALORIES	SODIUM
& Lite Syrup (Quaker)	1 pkg (6 oz)	260	860
Original (Aunt Jemima)	3.48 oz	211	801
Batter, as prep (Aunt Jemima)	3.6 oz	183	763
Microwave (Pillsbury)	3	240	550
Pancakes And Sausages (Great Starts)	6 oz	460	920
& Sausages (Quaker)	1 pkg (6 oz)	420	1140
With Bacon (Great Starts)	4½ oz	400	1000
w/ LeanLinks (Healthy Starts)	6 oz	360	490
Rolled Pancakes w/ Apples (Kid Cuisine)	3.85 oz	210	310
Silver Dollar Pancakes And Sausage (Great Starts)	3¾ oz	310	680
Whole Wheat Pancakes With Lite Links (Great Starts)	5½ oz	350	600
HOME RECIPE plain	1 (4" diam)	60	115
MIX Apple Cinnamon Shake 'N Pour (Bisquick)	3 (4" diam)	240	880
Blueberry (Hungry Jack)	3 (4" diam)	320	820
Shake 'N Pour (Bisquick)	3 (4" diam)	270	840
Buckwheat Pancake & Waffle Mix (Aunt Jemima)	3 (4" diam)	230	820
Buttermilk (Betty Crocker)	3 (4" diam)	280	810
(Hungry Jack)	3 (4" diam)	240	820
Complete (Hungry Jack)	3 (4" diam)	180	710
Complete Packets (Hungry Jack)	3 (4" diam)	180	680

FOOD	PORTION	CALORIES	SODIUM
Buttermilk *(cont.)*			
Complete Pancake & Waffle Mix (Aunt Jemima)	3 (4" diam)	230	950
Pancake & Waffle Mix (Aunt Jemima)	3 (4" diam)	220	760
Shake 'N Pour (Bisquick)	3 (4" diam)	250	880
Complete Pancake & Waffle Mix (Aunt Jemima)	3 (4" diam)	250	1020
Extra Lights (Hungry Jack)	3 (4" diam)	210	490
Complete (Hungry Jack)	3 (4" diam)	190	700
Original Pancake & Waffle Mix (Aunt Jemima)	3 (4" diam)	200	660
Shake 'N Pour (Bisquick)	3 (4" diam)	250	880
(Estee)	3, 3" pancakes	100	135
not prep (Health Valley)	1 oz	100	170
Panshakes (Hungry Jack)	3 (4" diam)	250	880
Whole Wheat Pancake & Waffle Mix (Aunt Jemima)	3 (4" diam)	270	950
TAKE-OUT			
buckwheat	1 (4" diam)	55	125
potato	1 (4" diam)	78	238
w/ butter & syrup	3	519	1103

PANCREAS
(*see* SWEETBREADS)

PAPAYA

FRESH			
cubed	1 cup	54	4
papaya	1	117	8

FOOD	PORTION	CALORIES	SODIUM
JUICE			
Goya Nectar	6 oz	110	10
Kern's Nectar	6 oz	110	10
Libby's Nectar	6 oz	110	10
nectar	1 cup	142	14

PAPRIKA

paprika	1 tsp	6	1

PARSLEY

Dole, chopped	1 tbsp	10	4
dry	1 tbsp	1	2
dry	1 tsp	1	1
fresh, chopped	½ cup	11	17

PARSNIPS

FRESH			
cooked	1 (5.6 oz)	130	17
cooked, sliced	½ cup	63	8
raw, sliced	½ cup	50	7

PASSION FRUIT

purple	1	18	5
juice, yellow	1 cup	149	15

PASTA
(*see also* NOODLES, PASTA DINNERS, PASTA SALAD)

DRY			
Dinosaurs (Mueller's)	2 oz	210	3
Egg (Prince)	2 oz	221	3
Elbow Style (Weight Watchers)	2 oz	160	35

FOOD	PORTION	CALORIES	SODIUM
Jungle Animals (Mueller's)	2 oz	210	3
Lasagna			
No Boil (DeFino)	1 oz	102	2
Spinach Whole Wheat (Health Valley)	2 oz	170	15
Whole Wheat (Health Valley)	2 oz	170	10
Whole Wheat (Health Valley)	2oz	170	10
Lasagne (Mueller's)	2 oz	210	4
Monsters (Mueller's)	2 oz	210	3
Outer Space (Mueller's)	2 oz	210	3
Pasta			
(Anthony)	2 oz	210	0
(Gioia)	2 oz	210	0
(Golden Grain)	2 oz	203	26
(Luxury)	2 oz	210	0
(Merlino's)	2 oz	210	0
(Penn Dutch)	2 oz	210	0
(Prince)	2 oz	210	0
(Red Cross)	2 oz	210	0
(Ronco)	2 oz	210	0
(Vimco)	2 oz	210	0
Rainbow (Prince)	2 oz	210	5
Ribbons, No Boil (DeFino)	2 oz	204	3
Spaghetti			
(Mueller's)	2 oz	210	3
Amaranth (Health Valley)	2 oz	170	10
Oat Bran (Health Valley)	2 oz	120	2
Spinach, Whole Wheat (Health Valley)	2 oz	170	15
Whole Wheat (Health Valley)	2 oz	170	10
Spaghettini (Weight Watchers)	2 oz	160	35

FOOD	PORTION	CALORIES	SODIUM
Spinach Egg (Prince)	2 oz	220	65
Teddy Bears (Mueller's)	2 oz	210	3
Twists Tri Color (Mueller's)	2 oz	210	10
corn, cooked	1 cup	176	1
elbows	1 cup	389	8
elbows, cooked	1 cup	197	1
protein-fortified, cooked	1 cup	188	6
shells	1 cup	389	4
shells, cooked	1 cup	197	1
spaghetti	2 oz	211	4
spaghetti, cooked	1 cup	197	1
spaghetti, protein-fortified, cooked	1 cup	229	7
spinach spaghetti	2 oz	212	20
spinach spaghetti, cooked	1 cup	183	20
spirals	1 cup	389	8
spirals, cooked	1 cup	197	1
vegetable	1 cup	308	36
vegetable, cooked	1 cup	171	9
whole wheat	1 cup	365	8
whole wheat, cooked	1 cup	174	4
whole wheat spaghetti	2 oz	198	5
whole wheat spaghetti, cooked	1 cup	174	4
FRESH			
plain, made w/ egg, cooked	2 oz	75	3
spinach, made w/ egg, cooked	2 oz	74	3
HOME RECIPE			
made w/ egg, cooked	2 oz	74	47
made w/o egg, cooked	2 oz	71	42

FOOD	PORTION	CALORIES	SODIUM

PASTA DINNERS
(*see also* DINNER, PASTA SALAD)

CANNED
Franco-American

FOOD	PORTION	CALORIES	SODIUM
Beef RavioliO's In Meat Sauce	½ can (7½ oz)	250	920
CircusO's Pasta In Tomato & Cheese Sauce	½ can (7⅜ oz)	170	860
CircusO's Pasta With Meatballs in Tomato Sauce	½ can (7⅜ oz)	210	950
Macaroni & Cheese	½ can (7⅜ oz)	170	870
Spaghetti In Tomato Sauce w/ Cheese	½ can (7⅜ oz)	180	840
Spaghetti w/ Meatballs In Tomato Sauce	½ can (7⅜ oz)	220	870
SpaghettiO's In Tomato & Cheese Sauce	½ can (7⅜ oz)	170	860
SpaghettiO's With Meatballs	½ can (7⅜ oz)	220	950
SpaghettiO's w/ Sliced Franks	½ can (7⅜ oz)	220	1000
SportyO's In Tomato & Cheese Sauce	½ can (7½ oz)	170	860
SportyO's Pasta With Meatballs In Tomato Sauce	½ can (7⅜ oz)	210	950
TeddyO's In Tomato & Cheese Sauce	½ can (7½ oz)	170	900
TeddyO's Pasta With Meatballs	½ can (7⅜ oz)	210	950
Healthy Choice			
Lasagne w/ Meat Sauce	½ can (7.5 oz)	220	530
Spaghetti Rings	½ can (7.5 oz)	140	460
Spaghetti w/ Meat Sauce	½ can (7.5 oz)	150	390
Van Camp's Spaghetti Weenee	1 cup	243	1128
DRY MIX			
Golden Grain Macaroni & Cheese	½ cup	310	620

FOOD	PORTION	CALORIES	SODIUM
Kraft			
Dinomac Macaroni And Cheese Dinner	¾ cup	310	560
Egg Noodle & Cheese Dinner	¾ cup	340	670
Mild American Style Spaghetti Dinner	1 cup	300	630
Spaghetti With Meat Sauce Dinner	1 cup	360	880
Spirals Macaroni & Cheese Dinner	¾ cup	340	600
Tangy Italian Style Spaghetti Dinner	1 cup	310	670
Teddy Bears Macaroni And Cheese Dinner	¾ cup	310	560
Wild Wheels Macaroni & Cheese Dinner	¾ cup	310	560
Kraft Macaroni & Cheese			
Deluxe Dinner	¾ cup	260	590
Dinner	¾ cup	290	530
Dinner Family Size	¾ cup	290	490
Kraft Pasta & Cheese			
3-Cheese With Vegetables	½ cup	180	630
Cheddar Broccoli	½ cup	180	620
Chicken With Herbs	½ cup	170	550
Fettuccini Alfredo	½ cup	180	590
Parmesan	½ cup	180	630
Sour Cream With Chives	½ cup	180	360
Lipton Pasta & Sauce			
Cheddar Broccoli	½ cup	132	458
Creamy Garlic	½ cup	146	447
Creamy Mushroom	½ cup	143	424
Herb Tomato	½ cup	130	356
Ultra Slim-Fast Macaroni & Cheese	2.3 oz	230	770

FOOD	PORTION	CALORIES	SODIUM
Velveeta			
Bits Of Bacon Shells And Cheese Dinner	½ cup	240	690
Shells and Cheese Dinner	¾ cup	210	170
Touch of Mexico Shells And Cheese Dinner	½ cup	210	630
FROZEN			
Banquet			
Entree, Spaghetti w/ Meat Sauce	8.5 oz	220	1180
Macaroni & Cheese	6.5 oz	290	760
Macaroni & Cheese	9 oz	240	1270
Spaghetti & Meat Sauce	8.75 oz	160	650
Budget Gourmet			
Cheese Lasagna With Vegetables	1 pkg	290	780
Cheese Manicotti	1 pkg	430	700
Cheese Raviolo	1 pkg	290	930
Cheese Tortellini	1 pkg	210	560
Italian Sausage Lasagna	1 pkg	430	850
Lasagne With Meat Sauce	1 pkg	300	760
Linguini With Scallops And Clams	1 pkg	290	710
Linguini With Shrimp And Clams	1 pkg	270	1170
Macaroni & Cheese	1 pkg	240	570
Pasta Alfredo With Broccoli	1 pkg	230	700
Shrimp With Fettucini	1 pkg	370	750
Three Cheese Lasagne	1 pkg	390	350
Ziti In Marinara Sauce	1 pkg	200	600
Dining Light			
Cheese Cannelloni	9 oz	310	650
Cheese Lasagna	9 oz	260	800

FOOD	PORTION	CALORIES	SODIUM
Fettucini	9 oz	290	1020
Lasagne	9 oz	240	800
Spaghetti	9 oz	220	440
Green Giant Garden Gourmet			
Creamy Mushroom	1 pkg	220	860
Pasta Dijon	1 pkg	260	630
Pasta Florentine	1 pkg	230	840
Rotini Cheddar	1 pkg	230	570
Green Giant One Serve			
Cheese Tortellini	1 pkg	260	660
Macaroni And Cheese	1 pkg	230	590
Pasta Marinara	1 pkg	180	440
Pasta Parmesan With Green Peas	1 pkg	170	510
Green Giant Pasta Accents			
Creamy Cheddar	½ cup	100	310
Garden Herb	½ cup	80	220
Garlic Seasoning	½ cup	110	280
Pasta Primavera	½ cup	110	180
Healthy Choice			
Baked Cheese Ravioli	9 oz	240	460
Cheese Manicotti	9.25 oz	230	450
Chicken Fettucini	8.5 oz	240	370
Fettucini Alfredo	8 oz	240	370
Fettucini w/ Turkey and Vegetables	12.5 oz	350	480
Lasagna w/ Meat Sauce	10 oz	260	420
Linguini w/ Shrimp	9.5 oz	230	420
Macaroni & Cheese	9 oz	280	520
Pasta Primavera	11 oz	280	360
Pasta w/ Shrimp	12.5 oz	270	490

FOOD	PORTION	CALORIES	SODIUM
Healthy Choice (cont.)			
Rigatoni In Meat Sauce	9.5 oz	240	470
Rigatoni w/ Chicken	12.5 oz	360	430
Spaghetti w/ Meat Sauce	10 oz	280	480
Stuffed Pasta Shells in Tomato Sauce	12 oz	330	470
Teriyaki Pasta w/ Chicken	12.6 oz	350	370
Zesty Tomato Sauce over Ziti Pasta	12 oz	350	530
Zucchini Lasagna	11.5 oz	240	390
Kid Cuisine			
Macaroni & Cheese w/ Mini Franks	9 oz	360	920
Mega Meal Macaroni & Cheese	12.45 oz	470	1270
Mini-Cheese Ravioli	8.75 oz	290	780
Spaghetti w/ Meat Sauce	9.25 oz	310	760
Le Menu Entree LightStyle			
Garden Vegetables Lasagna	10½ oz	260	500
Lasagna With Meat Sauce	10 oz	290	510
Meat Sauce & Cheese Tortellini	8 oz	250	480
Spaghetti With Beef Sauce And Mushrooms	9 oz	280	450
Le Menu LightStyle			
3-Cheese Stuffed Shells	10 oz	280	690
Cheese Tortellini	10 oz	230	460
Le Menu Manicotti With Three Cheeses	11¾ oz	390	870
Lean Cuisine			
Beef Cannelloni With Mornay Sauce	9⅝ oz	210	590
Cheese Cannelloni With Tomato Sauce	9⅛ oz	270	590
Cheese Ravioli	8½ oz	240	590

FOOD	PORTION	CALORIES	SODIUM
Chicken Fettucini	9 oz	280	530
Lasagne With Meat Sauce	10¼ oz	260	590
Linguini With Clam Sauce	9⅝ oz	280	560
Macaroni And Beef In Tomato Sauce	10 oz	240	590
Macaroni And Cheese	9 oz	290	550
Rigatoni Bake With Meat Sauce And Cheese	9¾ oz	250	430
Spaghetti And Meatballs	9½ oz	280	490
Spaghetti With Meat Sauce	11½ oz	290	500
Tuna Lasagna With Spinach Noodles And Vegetables	9¾ oz	240	520
Zucchini Lasagna	11 oz	260	550
Morton			
Macaroni & Cheese	6.5 oz	290	760
Spaghetti & Meat Sauce	8.5 oz	170	930
Mrs. Paul's Light Seafood Entree			
Seafood Lasagne	9½ oz	290	750
Seafood Rotini	9 oz	240	570
Mrs. Paul's Seafood Rotini	9 oz	240	570
Swanson			
Macaroni & Cheese	12¼ oz	370	1070
Macaroni & Cheese	7 oz	200	740
Spaghetti & Meatballs	12½ oz	390	1100
Swanson Homestyle			
Lasagne With Meat Sauce	10½ oz	400	1070
Macaroni & Cheese	10 oz	390	1150
Spaghetti With Italian Style Meatballs	13 oz	490	940
Ultra Slim-Fast			
Pasta Primavera	12 oz	340	730
Spaghetti With Beef & Mushroom Sauce	12 oz	370	990

FOOD	PORTION	CALORIES	SODIUM
Weight Watchers			
Angel Hair Pasta	10 oz	200	330
Baked Cheese Ravioli	9 oz	240	370
Cheese Manicotti	9.25 oz	260	510
Cheese Tortellini	9 oz	310	570
Chicken Fettucini	8.25 oz	280	590
Fettucini Alfredo	8 oz	230	550
Garden Lasagne	11 oz	260	430
Italian Cheese Lasagna	11 oz	290	510
Lasagne	10.25 oz	240	510
Spaghetti With Meat Sauce	10 oz	240	490
HOME RECIPE			
macroni & cheese	1 cup	430	1086
spaghetti w/ meatballs & tomato sauce	1 cup	330	1009
SHELF STABLE			
Healthy Choice			
Lasagne w/ Meat Sauce	7.5 oz cup	220	530
Spaghetti Rings	7.5 oz cup	140	460
Spaghetti w/ Meat Sauce	7.5 oz cup	150	390
TAKE-OUT			
lasagna	1 piece (2.5" x 2.5")	374	668
macaroni & cheese	1 cup	230	730
manicotti	¾ cup (6.4 oz)	273	414
rigatoni w/ sausage sauce	¾ cup	260	106
spaghetti w/ meatballs & cheese	1 cup	407	696

FOOD	PORTION	CALORIES	SODIUM

PASTA SALAD

MIX
Kraft

Garden Primavera Pasta Salad And Dressing	½ cup	170	450
Homestyle Pasta Salad And Dressing	½ cup	240	300
Light Italian Pasta Salad And Dressing	½ cup	130	420
Light Rancher's Choice Pasta Salad And Dressing	½ cup	170	350
Pasta Salad And Dressing, Broccoli And Vegetables	½ cup	210	290
Lipton Robust Italian	½ cup	126	118

Suddenly Salad

Classic Pasta, as prep	½ cup	160	530
Creamy Macaroni, as prep	½ cup	200	280
Creamy Macaroni, as prep, lowfat recipe	½ cup	140	310
Italian Pasta, as prep	½ cup	60	480
Pasta Primavera, as prep	½ cup	190	340
Pasta Primavera, as prep, lowfat recipe	½ cup	150	370
Tortellini Italiano, as prep	½ cup	160	450

TAKE-OUT

elbow macaroni salad	3.5 oz	160	590
italian style pasta salad	3.5 oz	140	480
mustard macaroni salad	3.5 oz	190	560
pasta salad w/ vegetables	3.5 oz	140	210

PATÉ

CANNED

liver	1 oz	90	198

FOOD	PORTION	CALORIES	SODIUM
liver	1 tbsp	41	91

PEACH

FOOD	PORTION	CALORIES	SODIUM
Clingstone			
Halves (S&W)	½ cup	100	10
Halves, Diet (S&W)	½ cup	30	5
Halves, Unsweetened (S&W)	½ cup	30	5
Sliced, Diet (S&W)	½ cup	30	5
Sliced, Unsweetened (S&W)	½ cup	30	5
Freestone			
Halves, Diet (S&W)	½ cup	30	10
Halves in Heavy Syrup (S&W)	½ cup	100	10
Slices, Diet (S&W)	½ cup	30	10
Sliced in Heavy Syrup (S&W)	½ cup	100	10
Halves (Hunt's)	4 oz	90	7
Sliced Yellow Cling, Natural Style (S&W)	½ cup	90	10
Slices (Hunt's)	4 oz	90	7
Yellow Cling			
Natural Lite (S&W)	½ cup	50	10
Sliced, Premium in Heavy Syrup (S&W)	½ cup	100	10
Whole, Spiced, in Heavy Syrup (S&W)	½ cup	90	10
halves in heavy syrup	1 half	60	5
halves in light syrup	1 half	44	4
halves, juice pack	1 half	34	3
halves, water pack	1 half	18	3
spiced, in heavy syrup	1 cup	180	9
spiced, in heavy syrup	1 fruit	66	3
DRIED			
halves	1 cup	383	12

FOOD	PORTION	CALORIES	SODIUM
halves	10	311	9
halves, cooked w/ sugar	½ cup	139	3
halves, cooked w/o sugar	½ cup	99	3
FRESH			
Dole	2	70	0
peach	1	37	0
sliced	1 cup	73	1
FROZEN			
slices, sweetened	1 cup	235	16
JUICE			
Dole Pure & Light	6 oz	100	20
Goya Nectar	6 oz	110	30
Kern's Nectar	6 oz	110	5
Libby's			
Nectar	6 oz	100	5
Ripe Nectar	8 oz	130	5
Smucker's	8 oz	120	10
nectar	1 cup	134	17

PEANUT BUTTER

FOOD	PORTION	CALORIES	SODIUM
Arrowhead			
Creamy	2 tbsp	190	tr
Crunchy	2 tbsp	190	tr
Erewhon			
Chunky	2 tbsp	190	75
Chunky Unsalted	2 tbsp	190	10
Creamy	2 tbsp	190	75
Creamy Unsalted	2 tbsp	190	10
Estee			
Chunky	1 tbsp	100	3
Creamy	1 tbsp	100	3

FOOD	PORTION	CALORIES	SODIUM
Health Valley			
Chunky, No Salt	2 tbsp	170	2
Creamy, No Salt	2 tbsp	170	2
Jif			
Creamy	2 tbsp	180	155
Extra Crunchy	2 tbsp	180	130
Jif Simply			
Creamy	2 tbsp	180	65
Extra Crunchy	2 tbsp	180	50
Peter Pan			
Creamy	2 tbsp	190	150
Creamy, Salt Free	2 tbsp	190	0
Crunchy	2 tbsp	190	150
Crunchy, Salt Free	2 tbsp	190	0
Reese's Peanut Butter Flavored Chips	¼ cup	230	90
Skippy			
Creamy	1 cup	1540	1240
Creamy, w/ 2 slices white bread	1 sandwich	340	430
Super Chunk	1 cup	1540	1120
Super Chunk	2 tbsp	190	130
Super Chunk, w/ 2 slices white bread	1 sandwich	340	410
Smucker's			
Goober Grape	2 tbsp	180	120
Honey Sweetened	2 tbsp	200	155
Natural	2 tbsp	200	125
Natural No-Salt Added	2 tbsp	200	<10
chunky	1 cup	1520	1255
chunky	2 tbsp	188	156
chunky w/o salt	1 cup	1520	44
chunky w/o salt	2 tbsp	188	5

FOOD	PORTION	CALORIES	SODIUM
smooth	1 cup	1517	1234
smooth	2 tbsp	188	153
smooth w/o salt	1 cup	1517	44
smooth w/o salt	2 tbsp	188	5

PEANUTS

FOOD	PORTION	CALORIES	SODIUM
Cocktail			
Lightly Salted (Planters)	1 oz	170	80
Unsalted (Planters)	1 oz	170	0
Dry Roasted			
Lightly Salted (Planters)	1 oz	160	110
Unsalted (Planters)	1 oz	170	250
Fresh Roast			
Lightly Salted (Planters)	1 oz	160	120
Salted (Planters)	1 oz	170	110
Honey Roasted			
(Little Debbie)	1 pkg (1.13 oz)	190	15
(Weight Watchers)	.7 oz	100	100
Dry Roasted (Planters)	1 oz	160	90
Peanuts (Planters)	½ oz bag	80	55
Salted (Little Debbie)	1 pkg (1.25 oz)	220	115
Spanish			
(Planters)	1 oz	170	100
Raw (Planters)	1 oz	160	5
cooked	½ cup	102	240
dry roasted	1 cup	855	1187
dry roasted	1 oz	164	228
oil roasted	1 cup	837	624
oil roasted	1 oz	163	121
oil roasted w/o salt	1 cup	837	9
oil roasted w/o salt	1 oz	163	2
spanish, oil roasted	1 oz	162	121

FOOD	PORTION	CALORIES	SODIUM
spanish, oil roasted w/o salt	1 oz	162	2
unroasted	1 oz	159	5
valencia oil, roasted	1 cup	848	1111
valencia oil, roasted	1 oz	165	216
valencia oil, roasted w/o salt	1 cup	848	9
valencia oil, roasted w/o salt	1 oz	165	2
virginia oil, roasted	1 cup	826	619
virginia oil, roasted	1 oz	161	121

PEAR

FOOD	PORTION	CALORIES	SODIUM
CANNED			
Bartlett Halves, Peeled, Unsweetened (S&W)	½ cup	35	10
Halves (Hunt's)	4 oz	90	6
Peeled, Diet (S&W)	½ cup	35	10
Quartered, Peeled, Diet (S&W)	½ cup	35	10
Sliced, Natural Light, Bartlett (S&W)	½ cup	60	10
Sliced, Natural Style (S&W)	½ cup	80	10
halves in heavy syrup	1 cup	188	13
halves in heavy syrup	1 half	68	4
halves in light syrup	1 half	45	4
halves, juice pack	1 cup	123	10
halves, water pack	1 half	22	41
DRIED			
halves	1 cup	472	10
halves	10	459	10
halves, cooked w/ sugar	½ cup	196	4
halves, cooked w/o sugar	½ cup	163	4

FOOD	PORTION	CALORIES	SODIUM
FRESH			
Dole	1	100	1
asian	1 (4.3 oz)	51	0
pear	1	98	1
sliced w/ skin	1 cup	97	1
JUICE			
Goya Nectar	6 oz	120	15
Kern's Nectar	6 oz	110	5
Libby's Nectar	6 oz	110	0
nectar	1 cup	149	9

PEAS

FOOD	PORTION	CALORIES	SODIUM
CANNED			
Field Peas			
(Trappey's)	½ cup	90	410
With Snaps (Trappey's)	½ cup	90	410
Petit Pois (S&W)	½ cup	70	330
Sweet			
(Green Giant)	½ cup	50	320
(S&W)	½ cup	70	330
Water Pack (S&W)	½ cup	40	5
Veri-Green Sweet (S&W)	½ cup	70	320
green	½ cup	59	186
green, low sodium	½ cup	59	2
DRIED			
Arrowhead Split Peas, Green	2 oz	200	17
split, cooked	1 cup	231	4
FRESH			
Dole Sugar Peas	½ cup	30	3
edible-pod, cooked	½ cup	34	3

FOOD	PORTION	CALORIES	SODIUM
edible-pod, raw	½ cup	30	3
green, cooked	½ cup	67	2
green, raw	½ cup	58	3
FROZEN			
Chinese Pea Pods (Chun King)	1.5 oz	20	<10
Harvest Fresh			
Early June (Green Giant)	½ cup	60	140
Sugar Snap (Green Giant)	½ cup	30	100
Sweet (Green Giant)	½ cup	50	95
In Butter Sauce (Green Giant)	½ cup	80	410
Le Suer Early (Green Giant Select)	½ cup	60	115
In Butter Sauce (Green Giant)	½ cup	80	440
One Serve, In Butter Sauce (Green Giant)	1 pkg	90	500
Snow Pea Pods (La Choy)	½ pkg (3 oz)	35	10
Sugar Snap Sweet Peas (Green Giant Select)	½ cup	30	0
Sweet Peas (Green Giant)	½ cup	50	95
edibile-pod, cooked	1 pkg (10 oz)	132	12
edible-pod, cooked	½ cup	42	4
green, cooked	½ cup	63	70
SHELF STABLE			
Mini Sweet (Green Giant)	½ cup	60	240
SPROUTS			
raw	½ cup	77	12

PECANS

FOOD	PORTION	CALORIES	SODIUM
Halves (Planters)	1 oz	190	0
Pieces (Planters)	1 oz	190	0
dried	1 oz	190	0

FOOD	PORTION	CALORIES	SODIUM
dry roasted	1 oz	187	0
dry roasted, salted	1 oz	187	260
halves, dried	1 cup	721	1
oil roasted	1 oz	195	0
oil roasted, salted	1 oz	195	252

PECTIN

FOOD	PORTION	CALORIES	SODIUM
Slim Set	1 pkg	208	42
Slim Set	1 tbsp	3	1

PEPPER

FOOD	PORTION	CALORIES	SODIUM
Spice Lemon Pepper (Nile Spice)	⅛ tsp	0	5
black	1 tsp	5	1
cayenne	1 tsp	6	1
red	1 tsp	6	1
white	1 tsp	7	tr

PEPPERS

FOOD	PORTION	CALORIES	SODIUM
CANNED			
Hot Banana Pepper Rings (Vlasic)	1 oz	4	465
Hot Cherry (Vlasic)	1 oz	10	425
Jalapeno, Mexican Hot (Vlasic)	1 oz	8	380
Mexican, Tiny Hot (Vlasic)	1 oz	6	430
Mild Cherry (Vlasic)	1 oz	8	410
Mild Greek Pepperoncini Salad Peppers (Vlasic)	1 oz	4	450
green halves	½ cup	13	958
jalapeno, chopped	½ cup	17	995
red halves	½ cup	13	958
DRIED			
green	1 tbsp	1	1

FOOD	PORTION	CALORIES	SODIUM
red	1 tbsp	1	1
FRESH			
Dole Bell	1 med	25	0
chili, green hot, raw	1	18	3
chili, green hot, raw, chopped	½ cup	30	5
chili, red hot, raw	1 (1.6 oz)	18	3
chili, red, raw, chopped	½ cup	30	5
green, chopped, cooked	½ cup	19	1
green, cooked	1 (2.6 oz)	20	1
green, raw	1 (2.6 oz)	20	1
green, raw, chopped	½ cup	13	1
red, chopped, cooked	½ cup	19	1
red, cooked	1 (2.6 oz)	20	1
red, raw	1 (2.6 oz)	20	1
red, raw, chopped	½ cup	13	1
yellow, raw	1 (6.5 oz)	50	3
yellow, raw	10 strips	14	1
FROZEN			
green, chopped, not prep	1 oz	6	1
red, chopped	1 oz	6	1

PERCH

FOOD	PORTION	CALORIES	SODIUM
FRESH			
cooked	1 fillet (1.6 oz)	54	36
cooked	3 oz	99	67
ocean perch, atlantic, cooked	1 fillet (1.8 oz)	60	48
ocean perch, atlantic, cooked	3 oz	103	82
ocean perch, atlantic, raw	3 oz	80	64
raw	3 oz	77	52
red, raw	3½ oz	114	80

FOOD	PORTION	CALORIES	SODIUM
FROZEN			
Fishmarket Fresh Ocean Perch (Gorton's)	5 oz	140	100

PERSIMMONS

dried japanese	1	93	1
fresh	1	32	0
fresh japanese	1	118	3

PHEASANT

FRESH			
breast w/o skin, raw	½ breast (6.4 oz)	243	60
leg w/o skin, raw	1 (3.6 oz)	143	48
w/ skin, raw	½ pheasant (14 oz)	723	161
w/o skin, raw	½ pheasant (12.4 oz)	470	131

PHYLLO DOUGH

Ekizian	½ lb	865	573

PICKLES

Bread & Butter			
Chips (Vlasic)	1 oz	30	160
Chunks (Vlasic)	1 oz	25	120
Stixs (Vlasic)	1 oz	18	110
Deli			
Bread & Butter (Vlasic)	1 oz	25	120
Dill Halves (Vlasic)	1 oz	4	290
Half-The-Salt			
Hamburger Dill Chips (Vlasic)	1 oz	2	175
Kosher Crunchy Dills (Vlasic)	1 oz	4	125

FOOD	PORTION	CALORIES	SODIUM
Half-The-Salt *(cont.)*			
Kosher Dill Spears (Vlasic)	1 oz	4	120
Sweet Butter Chips (Vlasic)	1 oz	30	80
Hot & Spicy Garden Mix (Vlasic)	1 oz	4	380
Kosher			
Baby Dills (Vlasic)	1 oz	4	210
Crunchy Dills (Vlasic)	1 oz	4	210
Dill Gherkins (Vlasic)	1 oz	4	210
Dill Spears (Vlasic)	1 oz	4	175
Snack Chunks (Vlasic)	1 oz	4	220
No Garlic Dill Spears (Vlasic)	1 oz	4	210
Original Dills (Vlasic)	1 oz	2	375
Polish Snack, Chunk Dills (Vlasic)	1 oz	4	300
Zesty			
Crunchy Dills (Vlasic)	1 oz	4	250
Dill Snack Chunks (Vlasic)	1 oz	4	290
Dill Spears (Vlasic)	1 oz	4	230
dill	1 (2.3 oz)	12	833
dill, low sodium	1 (2.3 oz)	12	12
dill, low sodium, sliced	1 slice	1	1
dill, sliced	1 slice	1	77
gherkins	3½ oz	21	960
kosher dill	1 (2.3 oz)	12	833
polish dill	1 (2.3 oz)	12	833
quick sour	1 (1.2 oz)	4	423
quick sour, low sodium	1 (1.2 oz)	4	6
quick sour, sliced	1 slice	1	85
sweet	1 (1.2 oz)	41	328
sweet gherkin	1 sm (½ oz)	20	107
sweet, low sodium	1 (1.2 oz)	41	6
sweet, sliced	1 slice	7	56

FOOD	PORTION	CALORIES	SODIUM

PIE
(*see also* PIECRUST)

CANNED FILLING

FOOD	PORTION	CALORIES	SODIUM
Mincemeat, Old Fashioned (S&W)	½ cup	206	206
pumpkin pie mix	1 cup	282	280

FROZEN
Apple

FOOD	PORTION	CALORIES	SODIUM
(Banquet)	1 slice (3.3 oz)	250	290
(Weight Watchers)	1 slice (3.5 oz)	165	90
Homestyle (Sara Lee)	1 slice (4 oz)	280	220
Homestyle High (Sara Lee)	1 slice (4.9 oz)	400	450
Streusel, Free & Light (Sara Lee)	1 slice (2.9 oz)	170	140
Banana (Banquet)	1 slice (2.3 oz)	180	150
Blackberry (Banquet)	1 slice (3.3 oz)	270	350
Blueberry (Banquet)	1 slice (3.3 oz)	270	350
Homestyle (Sara Lee)	1 slice (4 oz)	300	210
Cherry (Banquet)	1 slice (3.3 oz)	250	260
Homestyle (Sara Lee)	1 slice (4 oz)	270	270
Streusel, Free & Light (Sara Lee)	1 slice (3.6 oz)	160	140
Chocolate (Banquet)	1 slice (2.3 oz)	190	110
Mocha (Weight Watchers)	1 slice (2.75 oz)	180	150
Coconut (Banquet)	1 slice (2.3 oz)	190	120
Dutch Apple Homestyle (Sara Lee)	1 slice (4 oz)	300	310
Hyannis Boston Cream (Pepperidge Farm)	1	230	125
Lemon (Banquet)	1 slice (2.3 oz)	170	120

FOOD	PORTION	CALORIES	SODIUM
Mince Homestyle (Sara Lee)	1 slice (4 oz)	300	340
Mincemeat (Banquet)	1 slice (3.3 oz)	260	370
Mississippi Mud (Pepperidge Farm)	1	310	45
Peach			
(Banquet)	1 slice (3.3 oz)	245	280
Homestyle (Sara Lee)	1 slice (3.4 oz)	280	170
Pecan Homestyle (Sara Lee)	1 slice (3.4 oz)	400	290
Pumpkin			
(Banquet)	1 slice (3.3 oz)	200	350
Homestyle (Sara Lee)	1 slice (4 oz)	240	250
Raspberry Homestyle (Sara Lee)	1 slice (4 oz)	280	150
Strawberry (Banquet)	1 slice (2.3 oz)	170	120
HOME RECIPE			
pecan	⅙ of 9" pie	575	305
MIX			
Boston Cream Classic Dessert (Betty Crocker)	⅛ pie	270	390
Key Lime Pie Filling (Royal)	mix for 1 serving	50	120
Lemon Meringue No-Bake (Royal)	⅛ pie	210	170
Lemon Pie Filling (Royal)	mix for 1 serving	50	120
READY-TO-USE			
apple	⅙ of 9" pie	405	476
blueberry	⅙ of 9" pie	380	423
cherry	⅙ of 9" pie	410	480
creme	⅙ of 9" pie	455	369
custard	⅙ of 9" pie	330	436
lemon meringue	⅙ of 9" pie	355	395
peach	⅙ of 9" pie	405	423
pumpkin	⅙ of 9" pie	320	325

FOOD	PORTION	CALORIES	SODIUM
SNACK			
Apple			
(Drake's)	1 (2 oz)	210	135
(Little Debbie)	1 pkg (3 oz)	310	200
Blueberry (Drake's)	1 (2 oz)	210	135
Cherry (Drake's)	1 (2 oz)	220	135
Dutch Apple (Little Debbie)	1 pkg (2.17 oz)	270	160
Lemon (Drake's)	1 (2 oz)	210	115
Marshmallow			
Banana (Little Debbie)	1 pkg (1.38 oz)	170	85
Chocolate (Little Debbie)	1 pkg (1.38 oz)	170	75
Oatmeal Creme (Little Debbie)	1 pkg (1.33 oz)	170	135
Pecan (Little Debbie)	1 pkg (1.83 oz)	200	180
Raisin Creme (Little Debbie)	1 pkg (1.17 oz)	170	95
apple	1 (3 oz)	266	325
cherry	1 (3 oz)	266	325
lemon	1 (3 oz)	266	325

PIECRUST
(see also PIE)

FOOD	PORTION	CALORIES	SODIUM
FROZEN			
Pepperidge Farm			
Patty Shells	1	210	180
Puff Pastry Sheets	¼ sheet	260	290
HOME RECIPE			
9-inch crust	1	900	1100
MIX			
Betty Crocker			
Sticks	⅟₁₆ pkg	120	140
	⅟₁₆ pkg	120	140
Flako	⅛ of 9" pie	250	390
Pillsbury			
Mix	⅛ of 2-crust pie	270	420

FOOD	PORTION	CALORIES	SODIUM
Pillsbury *(cont.)*			
Stick	⅛ of 2-crust pie	270	420
as prep	2 crusts	1485	2602
READY-TO-USE			
Ready Crust			
Chocolate	1 (3" diam)	110	135
Chocolate	⅛ of 9" pie	100	120
Graham	1 (3" diam)	110	145
Graham	⅛ of 9" pie	100	130
REFRIGERATED			
Pillsbury All Ready	⅛ of 2-crust pie	240	200

PIEROGI

TAKE-OUT			
pierogi	¾ cup (4.4 oz)	307	369

PIG'S EARS

ears, frzn, simmered	1 ear (3.7 oz)	183	183

PIGEON PEAS

DRIED			
cooked	1 cup	204	9
cooked	½ cup	86	3

PIGNOLIA
   (*see* PINE NUTS)

PIKE

FRESH			
northern, cooked	½ fillet (5.4 oz)	176	76
northern, cooked	3 oz	96	42

FOOD	PORTION	CALORIES	SODIUM
northern, raw	3 oz	75	33
walleye, baked	3 oz	101	56
walleye fillet, baked	4.4 oz	147	81

PILLNUTS

pillnuts-canarytree dried	1 oz	204	1

PIMIENTOS

Dromedary	1 oz	10	5
canned	1 slice	0	0
canned	1 tbsp	3	2

PINE NUTS

pignolia, dried	1 oz	146	1
pignolia, dried	1 tbsp	51	0
pinyon, dried	1 oz	161	20

PINEAPPLE

CANNED			
All Cuts			
Juice Pack (Dole)	½ cup	70	10
Syrup Pack (Dole)	½ cup	90	10
Hawaiian Slice			
In Heavy Syrup (S&W)	½ cup	90	0
Juice Pack (S&W)	½ cup	70	10
Sliced, Unsweetened (S&W)	½ cup	60	10
chunks in heavy syrup	1 cup	199	3
chunks, juice pack	1 cup	150	4
crushed in heavy syrup	1 cup	199	3
slices in heavy syrup	1 slice	45	1
slices in light syrup	1 slice	30	1

FOOD	PORTION	CALORIES	SODIUM
slices, juice pack	1 slice	35	1
slices, water pack	1 slice	19	1
tidbits in heavy syrup	1 cup	199	3
tidbits in juice	1 cup	150	4
tidbits in water	1 cup	79	3
FRESH Dole	2 slices	90	10
diced	1 cup	77	1
sliced	1 slice	42	1
FROZEN chunks, sweetened	½ cup	104	2
JUICE Dole	6 oz	100	10
New Breakfast Juice	6 oz	100	5
Libby's Nectar	6 oz	110	30
S&W Unsweetened	6 oz	100	0
Tree Top	6 oz	100	0
canned	1 cup	139	2
frzn, as prep	1 cup	129	3
frzn, not prep	6 oz	387	6

PINK BEANS

CANNED Goya, Spanish Style	7.5 oz	140	800
DRIED cooked	1 cup	252	3

PINTO BEANS

CANNED Gebhardt	4 oz	100	600

FOOD	PORTION	CALORIES	SODIUM
Goya, Spanish Style	7.5 oz	140	860
Green Giant	½ cup	90	280
Picante	½ cup	100	580
Trappey's	½ cup	90	410
Hearty Texas	½ cup	110	440
Jalapinto	½ cup	90	480
pinto	1 cup	186	998
DRIED			
Arrowhead Red	2 oz	200	3
cooked	1 cup	235	3

PINYON
(*see* PINE NUTS)

PISTACHIOS

FOOD	PORTION	CALORIES	SODIUM
California Natural (Dole)	1 oz	90	250
Red Salted (Planters)	1 oz	170	250
dried	1 cup	739	7
dried	1 oz	164	2
dry roasted	1 oz	172	2
dry roasted, salted	1 cup	776	1040
dry roasted, salted	1 oz	172	260

PITANGA

FOOD	PORTION	CALORIES	SODIUM
fresh	1	2	0
fresh	1 cup	57	5

PIZZA

FOOD	PORTION	CALORIES	SODIUM
FROZEN			
Fox Deluxe			
Golden Topping	½ pizza	240	600

FOOD	PORTION	CALORIES	SODIUM
Fox Deluxe *(cont.)*			
Hamburger	½ pizza	260	700
Pepperoni	½ pizza	250	640
Sausage	½ pizza	260	630
Sausage & Pepperoni	½ pizza	260	640
Healthy Choice French Bread			
Cheese	1 (5.3 oz)	270	420
Deluxe	1 (6.25 oz)	330	490
Italian Turkey Sausage	1 (6.45 oz)	320	440
Pepperoni	1 (6.25 oz)	320	490
Jeno's 4-Pack			
Cheese	1 pizza	160	460
Combination	1 pizza	180	470
Hamburger	1 pizza	180	500
Pepperoni	1 pizza	170	460
Sausage	1 pizza	180	460
Jeno's Crisp 'n Tasty			
Canadian Bacon	½ pizza	250	880
Cheese	½ pizza	270	770
Hamburger	½ pizza	290	810
Pepperoni	½ pizza	280	760
Sausage	½ pizza	300	850
Sausage & Pepperoni	½ pizza	300	840
Jeno's Microwave Pizza Rolls			
Pepperoni & Cheese	6	240	440
Sausage & Cheese	6	250	440
Jeno's Pizza Rolls			
Cheese	6	240	350
Hamburger	6	240	280
Pepperoni & Cheese	6	230	390
Sausage & Pepperoni	6	230	380

FOOD	PORTION	CALORIES	SODIUM
Kid Cuisine			
Cheese	1 (6.85 oz)	380	390
Hamburger	6.85 oz	330	700
Mega Meal Cheese	1 (9.7 oz)	430	700
MicroMagic Deep Dish			
Combination	1 (6.5 oz)	605	1280
Pepperoni	1 (6.5 oz)	615	1300
Sausage	1 (6.5 oz)	590	1250
Mr. P's			
Combination	½ pizza	260	640
Golden Topping	½ pizza	240	600
Hamburger	½ pizza	260	700
Pepperoni	½ pizza	250	640
Sausage	½ pizza	260	630
Pappalo's French Bread			
Cheese	1 pizza	360	830
Combination	1 pizza	430	1120
Pepperoni	1 pizza	410	1130
Sausage	1 pizza	410	1000
Pappalo's Pan			
Combination	⅙ pizza	340	700
Hamburger	⅙ pizza	310	580
Pepperoni	⅙ pizza	330	710
Sausage	⅙ pizza	360	550
Pappalo's Thin Crust			
Combination	⅙ pizza	260	590
Hamburger	⅙ pizza	240	470
Pepperoni	⅙ pizza	270	600
Sausage	⅙ pizza	250	490
Pepperidge Farm Croissant Pastry			
Cheese	1	430	640
Deluxe	1	440	790
Pepperoni	1	420	690

FOOD	PORTION	CALORIES	SODIUM
Pillsbury Microwave			
Cheese	½ pizza	240	540
Combination	½ pizza	310	780
Pepperoni	½ pizza	300	790
Sausage	½ pizza	280	680
Pillsbury Microwave French Bread	1 pizza	370	680
Pepperoni	1 pizza	430	940
Sausage	1 pizza	410	860
Sausage & Pepperoni	1 pizza	450	950
Totino's Microwave			
Cheese	1 pizza	250	760
Pepperoni	1 pizza	280	880
Sausage	1 pizza	320	870
Sausage Pepperoni Combination	1 pizza	310	970
Totino's My Classic Deluxe			
Cheese	⅙ pizza	210	420
Combination	⅙ pizza	270	630
Pepperoni	⅙ pizza	260	630
Totino's Pan			
Pepperoni	⅙ pizza	330	730
Sausage	⅙ pizza	320	630
Sausage & Pepperoni Combination	⅙ pizza	340	720
Three Cheese	⅙ pizza	290	510
Totino's Party			
Bacon	½ pizza	370	1030
Canadian Bacon	½ pizza	310	1150
Cheese	½ pizza	340	1000
Combination	½ pizza	380	1230
Hamburger	½ pizza	370	1060
Mexican Style	½ pizza	380	970

FOOD	PORTION	CALORIES	SODIUM
Pepperoni	½ pizza	370	1310
Sausage	½ pizza	390	1180
Vegetable	½ pizza	300	910
Totino's Slices			
Cheese	1	170	350
Combination	1	200	630
Pepperoni	1	190	530
Sausage	1	200	540
Weight Watchers			
Cheese	1 (6.03 oz)	300	310
Pepperoni	1 (6.08 oz)	320	550
Sausage	1 (6.43 oz)	340	380
Weight Watchers Deluxe			
Combination	1 (7.32 oz)	320	370
French Bread	1 (5.94 oz)	260	480
SAUCE			
Ragu Pizza Quick Sauce			
Mushrooms	1.7 oz	35	330
Traditional	1.7 oz	35	330
w/ Cheese	1.7 oz	35	330
w/ Garlic & Basil	1.7 oz	35	330
w/ Pepperoni	1.7 oz	35	330
w/ Sausage	3 tbsp	35	330
TAKE-OUT			
cheese	⅛ of 12" pie	140	336
cheese	12" pie	1121	2680
cheese, meat & vegetables	⅛ of 12" pie	184	382
cheese, meat & vegetables	12" pie	1472	3054
pepperoni	⅛ of 12" pie	181	267
pepperoni	12" pie	1445	2133

FOOD	PORTION	CALORIES	SODIUM

PLANTAINS

| All Natural Plantain Chips (Top Banana) | 1 oz | 150 | 85 |

FRESH			
sliced, cooked	½ cup	89	4
uncooked	1	218	7

PLUMS

CANNED			
Halves			
Purple, Fancy, Unpeeled, in Extra Heavy Syrup (S&W)	½ cup	135	25
Unpeeled, Diet (S&W)	½ cup	52	0
Whole			
Purple, Fancy, Unpeeled, in Extra Heavy Syrup (S&W)	½ cup	135	25
Unpeeled, Diet (S&W)	½ cup	52	0
purple, in heavy syrup	1 cup	320	50
purple, in heavy syrup	3	119	26
purple, in light syrup	1 cup	158	50
purple, in light syrup	3	83	26
purple, juice pack	1 cup	146	3
purple, juice pack	3	55	1
purple, water pack	1 cup	102	2
purple, water pack	3	39	1
FRESH			
Dole	2	70	0
plum	1	36	0
sliced	1 cup	91	1
JUICE			
Kern's Nectar	6 oz	110	10

FOOD	PORTION	CALORIES	SODIUM

POI

poi	½ cup	134	14

POLLACK

FRESH

atlantic, baked	3 oz	100	94
atlantic fillet, baked	5.3 oz	178	166

FROZEN

Mrs. Paul's Light Fillets	1 fillet (4.5 oz)	240	530

POMEGRANATES

FRESH

pomegranates	1	104	5

POMPANO

florida, cooked	3 oz	179	65
florida, raw	3 oz	140	55

POPCORN
(*see also* CHIPS, PRETZELS, SNACKS)

Newman's Own	3⅓ cups	80	0
Newman's Own Microwave			
Butter	3 cups	140	150
Light, Butter	3 cups	90	100
Light, Natural	3 cups	90	100
Natural	3 cups	140	150
Natural No Salt	3 cups	140	0
Orville Redenbacher's Gourmet			
Hot Air	3 cups	40	0
Original	3 cups	80	0
White	3 cups	80	0

FOOD	PORTION	CALORIES	SODIUM
Orville Redenbacher's Microwave Gourmet	3 cups	100	200
Butter	3 cups	100	240
Butter Toffee	2½ cups	210	85
Caramel	2½ cups	240	90
Cheddar Cheese	3 cups	130	280
Frozen	3 cups	100	200
Frozen Butter	3 cups	100	240
Light	3 cups	70	115
Light Butter	3 cups	70	110
Salt Free	3 cups	100	0
Salt Free, Butter	3 cups	100	0
Sour Cream 'n Onion	3 cups	160	270
Pillsbury Microwave			
Butter	3 cups	210	410
Original	3 cups	210	410
Salt Free	3 cups	170	0
Pop Secret			
Butter Flavor	3 cups	100	170
Butter Flavor, Singles	6 cups	250	310
Natural Flavor	3 cups	100	170
Natural Flavor, Salt Free	3 cups	100	<5
Pop Secret Pop Quiz			
Butter Flavor	3 cups	100	170
Natural Flavor	3 cups	100	170
Pop Secret Light			
Butter Flavor	3 cups	70	115
Butter Flavor, Singles	6 cups	140	190
Natural Flavor	3 cups	70	160
Natural Flavor, Singles	6 cups	150	320
Ultra Slim-Fast Lite N' Tasty	½ oz	60	150

FOOD	PORTION	CALORIES	SODIUM
Weight Watchers Microwave	1 oz	100	5
Weight Watchers Ready-to-Eat Butter	.7 oz	90	100
White Cheddar Cheese	.7 oz	90	120
air-popped	1 cup	30	tr
popped w/ vegetable oil	1 cup	55	86
sugar syrup coated	1 cup	135	tr

POPPY SEEDS

poppy seeds	1 tsp	15	1

PORK

(*see also* BACON, BACON SUBSTITUTES, CANADIAN BACON, HAM, LUNCH-
EON MEATS/COLD CUTS, SAUSAGE)

The values for cooked pork may differ slightly from the values for
raw pork. When meat is cooked, some moisture and fat are lost,
changing the nutritive value slightly. As a rule of thumb, it can be
assumed that a 4-oz raw portion will equal a 3-oz cooked portion
of meat.

FRESH

blade chop, roasted	1 (3.1 oz)	321	54
center loin chop, broiled	1 (3.1 oz)	275	61
center loin, roasted	3 oz	259	54
loin w/ fat, roasted	3 oz	271	53
shoulder arm, picnic cured, lean only, roasted	3 oz	145	1046
shoulder blade, roll-cured, lean & fat	3 oz	304	1412
shoulder whole, roasted	3 oz	277	58
spareribs, braised	3 oz	338	79
tenderloin, lean only, roasted	3 oz	141	57

FOOD	PORTION	CALORIES	SODIUM

POSOLE
(*see* HOMINY)

POT PIE

FROZEN
Beef

(Swanson)	7 oz	370	730
Hungry Man (Swanson)	16 oz	610	1360

Chicken

(Swanson)	7 oz	380	760
Homestyle (Swanson)	8 oz	410	1030
Hungry Man (Swanson)	16 oz	630	1600

Turkey

(Swanson)	7 oz	380	720
Hungry Man (Swanson)	16 oz	650	1470

Vegetable Pie w/ Beef

(Banquet)	7 oz	510	870
(Morton)	7 oz	430	740

Vegetable Pie w/ Chicken

(Banquet)	7 oz	550	860
(Morton)	7 oz	420	740

Vegetable Pie w/ Turkey

(Banquet)	7 oz	510	860
(Morton)	7 oz	420	740

HOME RECIPE

beef, baked	⅓ of 9" pie (7.4 oz)	515	596
chicken	⅓ of 9" pie (8.1 oz)	545	594

POTATO
(*see also* CHIPS)

FOOD	PORTION	CALORIES	SODIUM
CANNED			
Hunt's Whole New	4 oz	70	230
S&W New Potatoes, Extra Small	½ cup	45	310
FRESH			
baked, skin only	1 skin (2 oz)	115	12
baked, w/ skin	1 (6½ oz)	220	16
baked, w/o skin	1 (5 oz)	145	8
baked, w/o skin	½ cup	57	3
boiled	½ cup	68	3
microwaved	1 (7 oz)	212	16
microwaved, w/o skin	½ cup	78	5
raw, w/o skin	1 (3.9 oz)	88	7
FROZEN			
Baked Potato			
Broccoli & Ham (Weight Watchers)	11.5 oz	280	520
Broccoli & Cheddar (Lean Cuisine)	10⅜ oz	290	590
Broccoli And Cheese (Weight Watchers)	1	270	570
Chicken Divan (Weight Watchers)	1	280	480
Homestyle Turkey (Weight Watchers)	1	250	510
w/ Broccoli & Cheese Sauce (Healthy Choice)	10 oz	240	510
Cheddar Browns (Ore Ida)	3 oz	90	330
Cheddared Potatoes (Budget Gourmet)	1 pkg	260	600
With Broccoli (Budget Gourmet)	1 pkg	150	410
Cottage Fries (Ore Ida)	3 oz	130	15
Crispers! (Ore Ida)	3 oz	220	490

FOOD	PORTION	CALORIES	SODIUM
Crispy Crowns! (Ore Ida)	3 oz	190	390
Crispy Crunchers (Ore Ida)	3 oz	180	410
Deep Fries			
Crinkle Cuts (Ore Ida)	3 oz	160	10
French Fries (Ore Ida)	3 oz	170	10
Dinner Fries, Country Style (Ore Ida)	3 oz	110	10
French Fries (MicroMagic)	1 pkg (3 oz)	290	30
Golden			
Crinkles (Ore Ida)	3 oz	120	10
Fries (Ore Ida)	3 oz	120	10
Patties (Ore Ida)	1 (2.5 oz)	130	210
Twirls (Ore Ida)	3 oz	160	15
Hash Browns			
Shredded (Ore Ida)	3 oz	70	15
Southern Style (Ore Ida)	3 oz	70	15
Lites, Crinkle Cuts (Ore Ida)	3 oz	90	10
Microwave			
Crinkle Cuts (Ore Ida)	3.5 oz	190	10
Hash Browns (Ore Ida)	2 oz	110	210
Tater Tots (Ore Ida)	4 oz	210	370
Nacho Potatoes (Budget Gourmet)	1 pkg	200	450
O'Brien Potatoes (Ore Ida)	3 oz	60	10
One Serve Potatoes			
& Broccoli In Cheese Sauce (Green Giant)	1 pkg	130	720
Au Gratin (Green Giant)	1 pkg	200	560
Pixie Crinkles (Ore Ida)	3 oz	140	15
Shoestrings (Ore Ida)	3 oz	150	15
Skinny Fries (MicroMagic)	1 pkg (3 oz)	350	40
Stuffed Potatoes			
w/ Cheddar Cheese (Oh Boy!)	1 (6 oz)	150	490

FOOD	PORTION	CALORIES	SODIUM
w/ Real Bacon (Oh Boy!)	1 (6 oz)	120	360
w/ Sour Cream & Chives (Oh Boy!)	1 (6 oz)	110	360
Tater Tots			
(Ore Ida)	3 oz	160	280
Bacon (Ore Ida)	3 oz	150	390
Onion (Ore Ida)	3 oz	150	370
Three Cheese Potatoes (Budget Gourmet)	1 pkg	230	470
Toaster Hash Browns (Ore Ida)	1 (1.75 oz)	100	230
Topped			
Broccoli & Cheese (Ore Ida)	1 (5.63 oz)	160	400
Vegetable Primavera (Ore Ida)	1 (6.13 oz)	160	390
Twice Baked			
Butter Flavor (Ore Ida)	1 (5 oz)	200	460
Cheddar Cheese (Ore Ida)	1 (5 oz)	210	570
Sour Cream & Chives (Ore Ida)	1 (5 oz)	190	430
Wedges, Home Style (Ore Ida)	3 oz	110	10
Zesties! (Ore Ida)	3 oz	160	300
french fries	10 strips	111	15
french fries, thick cut	10 strips	109	23
hashed brown	½ cup	170	27
potato puffs	½ cup	138	462
potato puffs, as prep	1 puff	16	52
HOME RECIPE			
au gratin	½ cup	160	528
hash brown	½ cup	163	19
mashed	½ cup	111	309
o'brien	1 cup	157	421
potato dumpling	3½ oz	334	1
potato pancakes	1 (2.7 oz)	495	388
scalloped	½ cup	105	409

FOOD	PORTION	CALORIES	SODIUM
MIX			
Au Gratin, as prep (Betty Crocker)	½ cup	140	580
Cheddar And Bacon Casserole (French's)	½ cup	130	390
Cheddar 'N Bacon, as prep (Betty Crocker)	½ cup	140	520
Cheesy, Scalloped, as prep (Betty Crocker)	½ cup	140	560
Creamy Italian Scalloped Potatoes (French's)	½ cup	120	430
Creamy Stroganoff Potatoes (French's)	½ cup	130	520
Crispy Top Scalloped Potatoes w/ Savory Onion (French's)	½ cup	140	390
Hash Browns (Betty Crocker)			
as prep	½ cup	160	460
as prep w/o salt	½ cup	160	100
Homestyle (Betty Crocker)			
American Cheese, as prep	½ cup	140	610
Broccoli Au Gratin, as prep	½ cup	130	540
Cheddar Cheese, as prep	½ cup	140	530
Cheesy, Scalloped, as prep	½ cup	140	590
Julienne, as prep (Betty Crocker)	½ cup	130	580
Mashed Potato Flakes (Hungry Jack)	½ cup	40	380
Potato Buds			
as prep (Betty Crocker)	½ cup	130	360
as prep w/o salt (Betty Crocker)	½ cup	130	90
Potatoes & Cheese (Kraft)			
2-Cheese	½ cup	130	540
Au Gratin	½ cup	130	570
Broccoli Au Gratin	½ cup	120	530

FOOD	PORTION	CALORIES	SODIUM
Scalloped	½ cup	140	500
Scalloped With Ham	½ cup	150	510
Sour Cream With Chives	½ cup	150	610
Real Cheese Scalloped Potatoes (French's)	½ cup	140	380
Real Sour Cream and Chives Potatoes (French's)	½ cup	150	550
Scalloped & Ham, as prep (Betty Crocker)	½ cup	160	620
as prep (Betty Crocker)	½ cup	140	570
Smokey Cheddar, as prep (Betty Crocker)	½ cup	140	680
Sour Cream 'N Chive, as prep (Betty Crocker)	½ cup	140	520
Spuds Mashed (French's)	½ cup	140	380
Tangy Au Gratin (French's)	½ cup	130	460
Twice Baked (Betty Crocker) Bacon And Cheddar, as prep	½ cup	210	600
Herbed Butter, as prep	½ cup	220	540
Mild Cheddar With Onion as prep	½ cup	190	640
Sour Cream & Chive, as prep	½ cup	200	570
au gratin, as prep	4½ oz	127	601
instant mashed flakes, as prep w/ whole milk & butter	½ cup	118	349
instant mashed flakes, not prep	½ cup	78	24
instant mashed granules, as prep w/ whole milk & butter	½ cup	114	270
instant mashed granules, not prep	½ cup	372	67
scalloped, as prep	4½ oz	127	467

FOOD	PORTION	CALORIES	SODIUM
SHELF STABLE			
Augratin Potatoes (Pantry Express)	½ cup	120	430
TAKE-OUT			
au gratin w/ cheese	½ cup	178	548
baked, topped w/ cheese sauce	1	475	381
& bacon	1	451	973
& broccoli	1	402	484
& chili	1	481	1570
baked, topped w/ sour cream & chives	1	394	182
french fried			
in beef tallow	1 lg	358	187
in beef tallow	1 reg	237	124
in vegetable oil	1 lg	355	187
in vegetable oil	1 reg	235	124
hash brown	½ cup	151	290
mashed w/ whole milk & margarine	⅓ cup	66	182
mustard potato salad	3.5 oz	120	393
potato salad	½ cup	179	661
potato salad	⅓ cup	108	312
potato salad w/ vegetables	3.5 oz	120	390
scalloped	½ cup	127	435
POTATO STARCH			
Manischewitz	1 cup	570	1
potato starch	3½ oz	335	8
POUT			
FRESH			
ocean, baked	3 oz	86	66

FOOD	PORTION	CALORIES	SODIUM
ocean fillet, baked	4.8 oz	139	107

PRESERVES
(*see* JAM/JELLY/PRESERVES)

PRETZELS
(*see also* CHIPS, POPCORN, SNACKS)

Estee Unsalted	7	50	0
J&J			
Soft	1 (2.25 oz)	170	140
Soft Bites	5 bites	110	95
Mister Salty			
Fat Free Sticks	1 oz	100	380
Fat Free Twists	1 oz	100	380
Twists	1 oz	110	580
Very Thin Sticks	1 oz	110	600
Mr. Phipps Chips	8	60	310
Lightly Salted	8	60	200
Sesame	8	60	250
Ultra Slim-Fast Lite N' Tasty	1 oz	100	460
Wege			
Sourdough	1 oz	102	548
Unsalted	1 oz	102	60
Whole Wheat	1 oz	109	25
sticks	10	10	48
twist	1 (½ oz)	65	258
twists thin	10 (2 oz)	240	966

PRICKLYPEAR

fresh	1	42	6

FOOD	PORTION	CALORIES	SODIUM

PRUNES

CANNED

in heavy syrup	1 cup	245	6
in heavy syrup	5	90	2

DRIED

cooked, w/ sugar	½ cup	147	2
cooked, w/o sugar	½ cup	113	2
dried	1 cup	385	6
dried	10	201	3

JUICE

S&W Unsweetened	6 oz	120	20
canned	1 cup	181	11

PUDDING
(*see also* CUSTARD)

HOME RECIPE

bread, w/ raisins	½ cup	180	185
corn	⅔ cup	181	92

MIX
Banana Cream

(Royal)	mix for 1 serving	80	110
Instant (Royal)	mix for 1 serving	90	390

Butterscotch

(My*T*Fine)	mix for 1 serving	90	190
(Royal)	mix for 1 serving	90	180
Instant (Royal)	mix for 1 serving	90	400
Cherry Vanilla Instant (Royal)	mix for 1 serving	90	300

FOOD	PORTION	CALORIES	SODIUM
Chocolate			
(Estee)	½ cup	70	75
(My*T*Fine)	mix for 1 serving	100	135
(Royal)	mix for 1 serving	90	90
Instant (Royal)	mix for 1 serving	110	450
Instant, as prep w/ skim milk (Weight Watchers)	½ cup	100	430
Sugar Free Instant (Royal)	mix for 1 serving	50	420
Chocolate Almond (My*T*Fine)	mix for 1 serving	100	135
Chocolate Almond Instant (Royal)	mix for 1 serving	120	440
Chocolate Chocolate Chip Instant (Royal)	mix for 1 serving	110	590
Chocolate Fudge (My*T*Fine)	mix for 1 serving	100	140
Chocolate Peanut Butter Instant (Royal)	mix for 1 serving	110	480
Creme Caramel Flan And Sauce, as prep (Knorr)	½ cup + 1 tbsp sauce	190	70
Dark 'n Sweet			
Chocolate (Royal)	mix for 1 serving	90	95
Instant (Royal)	mix for 1 serving	110	460
Lemon			
(My*T*Fine)	mix for 1 serving	90	170
Instant (Royal)	mix for 1 serving	90	320
Pistachio Instant (Royal)	mix for 1 serving	90	360

FOOD	PORTION	CALORIES	SODIUM
Strawberry Instant (Royal)	mix for 1 serving	100	330
Toasted Coconut Instant (Royal)	mix for 1 serving	100	450
Vanilla			
(Estee)	½ cup	70	75
(My*T*Fine)	mix for 1 serving	90	120
(Royal)	mix for 1 serving	80	160
Instant (Royal)	mix for 1 serving	90	325
Instant, as prep w/ skim milk (Weight Watchers)	½ cup	90	510
Vanilla Chocolate Chip Instant (Royal)	mix for 1 serving	90	350
Vanilla Tapioca (My*T*Fine)	mix for 1 serving	80	160
MIX W/ WHOLE MILK			
chocolate	½ cup	150	167
chocolate, instant	½ cup	155	440
rice	½ cup	155	140
tapioca	½ cup	145	152
vanilla	½ cup	145	178
vanilla, instant	½ cup	150	375
READY-TO-USE			
Banana (Snack Pack)	4.25 oz	145	180
Butterscotch			
(Snack Pack)	4.25 oz	170	210
(Swiss Miss)	4 oz	180	135
(Ultra Slim-Fast)	4 oz	100	230
Chocolate			
(Snack Pack)	4.25 oz	170	120

FOOD	PORTION	CALORIES	SODIUM
(Swiss Miss)	4 oz	180	160
(Ultra Slim-Fast)	4 oz	100	240
Chocolate Fudge (Snack Pack)	4.25 oz	165	125
(Swiss Miss)	4 oz	220	180
Light (Swiss Miss)	4 oz	100	120
Chocolate Light (Snack Pack)	4.25 oz	100	120
(Swiss Miss)	4 oz	100	120
Chocolate Marshmallow (Snack Pack)	4.25 oz	165	125
Chocolate Sundae (Swiss Miss)	4 oz	220	140
Lemon (Snack Pack)	4.25 oz	150	75
Tapioca (Snack Pack)	4.25 oz	150	125
(Swiss Miss)	4 oz	160	170
Light (Snack Pack)	4.25 oz	100	105
Vanilla (Snack Pack)	4.25 oz	170	150
(Swiss Miss)	4 oz	190	140
(Ultra Slim-Fast)	4 oz	100	230
Vanilla Chocolate Parfait, Light (Swiss Miss)	4 oz	100	110
Vanilla Light (Swiss Miss)	4 oz	100	105
Vanilla Parfait (Swiss Miss)	4 oz	180	150
Vanilla Sundae (Swiss Miss)	4 oz	200	180
TAKE-OUT rice w/ raisins	½ cup	246	270
tapicoa	½ cup	169	154

PUDDING POPS
(*see* ICE CREAM AND FROZEN DESSERT, PUDDING)

FOOD	PORTION	CALORIES	SODIUM

PUMMELO

FOOD	PORTION	CALORIES	SODIUM
fresh	1	228	7
sections	1 cup	71	2

PUMPKIN

FOOD	PORTION	CALORIES	SODIUM
CANNED			
pumpkin	½ cup	41	6
FRESH			
cooked, mashed	½ cup	24	6
flowers, cooked	½ cup	10	4
flowers, raw	1	0	0
leaves, cooked	½ cup	7	3
leaves, raw	½ cup	4	2
raw, cubed	½ cup	15	1
SEEDS			
dried	1 oz	154	5
roasted	1 cup	1184	40
roasted	1 oz	148	5
salted & roasted	1 cup	1184	1294
salted & roasted	1 oz	148	144
whole, roasted	1 cup	285	12
whole, roasted	1 oz	127	5
whole, salted & roasted	1 cup	285	268
whole, salted & roasted	1 oz	127	191

PURSLANE

FOOD	PORTION	CALORIES	SODIUM
cooked	1 cup	21	51
raw	1 cup	7	20

QUAHOGS
(see CLAMS)

FOOD	PORTION	CALORIES	SODIUM

QUAIL

FRESH
breast w/o skin, raw	1 (2 oz)	69	31
w/ skin, raw	1 quail (3.8 oz)	210	58
w/o skin, raw	1 quail (3.2 oz)	123	47

QUICHE

HOME RECIPE
lorraine	⅛ of 8″ pie	600	653

QUINCE

fresh	1	53	4

QUINOA

Seeds (Arrowhead)	2 oz	200	3

RABBIT

domestic, w/o bone, roasted	3 oz	167	40
wild, w/o bone, stewed	3 oz	147	38

RADICCHIO

raw, shredded	½ cup	5	4

RADISHES

DRIED
chinese	½ cup	157	161
daikon	½ cup	157	161

FRESH
Dole	7	20	35
chinese, raw	1 (12 oz)	62	71
chinese, raw, sliced	½ cup	8	9

FOOD	PORTION	CALORIES	SODIUM
chinese, sliced, cooked	½ cup	13	10
daikon, raw	1 (12 oz)	62	71
daikon, raw, sliced	½ cup	8	9
daikon, sliced, cooked	½ cup	13	10
red, raw	10	7	11
red, sliced	½ cup	10	14
white icicle, raw	1 (½ oz)	2	3
white icicle, raw, sliced	½ cup	7	8
SPROUTS			
raw	½ cup	8	1

RAISINS

Dole Golden	½ cup	260	25
Dole Seedless	½ cup	260	25
Sunbelt	1 bar (1 oz)	90	tr
golden, seedless	1 cup	437	17
seedless	1 cup	434	17

RASPBERRIES

CANNED			
in heavy syrup	½ cup	117	4
FRESH			
Dole	1 cup	45	0
raspberries	1 cup	61	0
raspberries	1 pint	154	0
FROZEN			
sweetened	1 cup	256	1
sweetened	1 pkg (10 oz)	291	1
JUICE			
Crystal Geyser Juice Squeeze, Mountain Raspberry	6 oz	70	15

FOOD	PORTION	CALORIES	SODIUM
Dole Pure & Light	6 oz	90	15
Smucker's	8 oz	120	10
Smucker's Juice Sparkler	10 oz	130	5

RED BEANS

CANNED
Green Giant	½ cup	90	340
Hunt's Small	4 oz	90	560
Van Camp's	1 cup	194	928

RELISH

Dill (Vlasic)	1 oz	2	415
Hamburger (Vlasic)	1 oz	40	255
Hog Dog (Vlasic)	1 oz	40	255
Hot Piccalilli (Vlasic)	1 oz	35	165
India (Vlasic)	1 oz	30	205
Sandwich Spread (Hellman's)	1 tbsp	55	170
Sweet (Vlasic)	1 oz	30	220
cranberry orange	½ cup	246	44
hamburger	1 tbsp	19	164
hamburger	½ cup	158	1338
hot dog	1 tbsp	14	164
hot dog	½ cup	111	1332
sweet	1 cup	159	990
sweet	1 tbsp	19	122

RHUBARB

fresh	½ cup	13	2
frzn	½ cup	60	1
frzn, as prep w/ sugar	½ cup	139	2

FOOD	PORTION	CALORIES	SODIUM

RICE
(*see also* BRAN, CEREAL, FLOUR, WILD RICE)

BROWN
Arrowhead

FOOD	PORTION	CALORIES	SODIUM
Basmati	2 oz	200	1
Brown Long	2 oz	200	1
Brown Medium	2 oz	200	1
Brown Short	2 oz	200	1
Arrowhead Quick			
Original	2 oz	200	0
Spanish Style	2 oz	150	150
Vegetable Herb	2 oz	150	50
Wild Rice & Herb	2 oz	140	150
S&W Quick			
Natural Long Grain	3.5 oz	110	0
Natural Long Grain, cooked	3.5 oz	119	0
long-grain, cooked	½ cup	109	5
medium-grain, cooked	½ cup	109	1
CANNED			
Van Camp's Spanish	1 cup	160	1270
DRY MIX			
Knorr Risotto			
Milanese With Saffron	½ cup	130	420
Tomato	½ cup	110	460
w/ Mushrooms	½ cup	110	430
w/ Onion	½ cup	110	390
With Peas And Corn	½ cup	110	470
La Choy Chinese Fried Rice	¾ cup	190	820
Lipton Golden Saute Fried Rice			
Beef	½ cup	124	516
Chicken	½ cup	129	509
Oriental	½ cup	127	675

FOOD	PORTION	CALORIES	SODIUM
Lipton Rice And Sauce			
Beef	½ cup	119	602
Cajun	½ cup	123	596
Cheddar Broccoli	½ cup	125	487
Chicken	½ cup	124	469
Chicken Broccoli	½ cup	129	495
Creamy Chicken	½ cup	142	417
Herbs & Butter	½ cup	123	446
Long Grain And Wild Rice, Original	½ cup	121	530
Mushroom	½ cup	123	497
Pilaf	½ cup	122	410
Skillet Style Spanish	½ cup	104	426
Spanish	½ cup	118	536
Lipton Rice, Asparaus With Hollandaise	½ cup	123	462
Nile Spice, Rozdali Vegetable Curry	½ cup	154	130
Rice-A-Roni			
Beef	½ cup	140	610
Beef & Mushroom	½ cup	150	740
Chicken	½ cup	150	560
Chicken & Broccoli	½ cup	150	710
Chicken & Mushroom	½ cup	180	840
Chicken & Vegetables	½ cup	140	790
Fried Rice	½ cup	110	700
Herb & Butter	½ cup	130	790
Long Grain & Wild, Chicken w/ Almonds	½ cup	140	690
Long Grain & Wild, Original	½ cup	130	660
Long Grain & Wild, Pilaf	½ cup	130	550
Pilaf	½ cup	150	620

FOOD	PORTION	CALORIES	SODIUM
Rice-A-Roni *(cont.)*			
Risotto	½ cup	200	1130
Spanish	½ cup	150	1090
Stroganoff	½ cup	200	810
Yellow Rice	½ cup	140	780
Ultra Slim-Fast			
Oriental Style	2.3 oz	240	900
Rice & Chicken Sauce	2.3 oz	240	1080
FROZEN			
Budget Gourmet			
Oriental Rice With Vegetables	1 pkg	240	420
Rice Mexicana	1 pkg	240	580
Rice Pilaf With Green Beans	1 pkg	240	520
Green Giant Garden Gourmet			
Asparagus Pilaf	1 pkg	190	610
Sherry Wild Rice	1 pkg	210	580
Green Giant One Serve			
Rice 'N Broccoli in Cheese Sauce	1 pkg	180	550
Rice, Peas And Mushrooms With Sauce	1 pkg	130	410
Green Giant Rice Originals			
Italian Rice & Spinach In Cheese Sauce	½ cup	140	400
Pilaf	½ cup	110	530
Rice Medley	½ cup	100	310
Rice 'N Broccoli In Cheese Sauce	½ cup	120	510
White And Wild	½ cup	130	540
TAKE-OUT			
pilaf	½ cup	84	362
spanish	¾ cup	363	1339

FOOD	PORTION	CALORIES	SODIUM
WHITE			
S&W Long Grain, cooked	3.5 oz	106	0
Superfino Arborio Rice	½ cup	100	5
glutinous, cooked	½ cup	116	6
long-grain, cooked	½ cup	131	2
long-grain, instant, cooked	½ cup	80	2
long-grain, parboiled, cooked	½ cup	100	3
medium-grain, cooked	½ cup	132	0
short-grain, cooked	½ cup	133	0
starch	3½ oz	343	61

ROCKFISH

FRESH			
pacific, cooked	1 fillet (5.2 oz)	180	114
pacific, cooked	3 oz	103	65
pacific, raw	3 oz	80	51

ROE

(*see* individual fish names)

ROLL

(*see also* BISCUIT, CROISSANT, ENGLISH MUFFIN, MUFFIN, SCONE)

FROZEN			
All Butter Cinnamon Roll			
w/ Icing (Sara Lee)	1	280	220
w/o Icing (Sara Lee)	1	230	220
Cinnamon Roll (Pepperidge Farm)	1 (2¼ oz)	220	190
Cinnamon Rolls (Weight Watchers)	1 (2.1 oz)	180	170
HOME RECIPE			
dinner	1 (1.2 oz)	120	98

FOOD	PORTION	CALORIES	SODIUM
MIX			
Hot Roll Mix			
(Dromedary)	2	239	410
(Pillsbury)	2	240	430
READY-TO-EAT			
Big Marty			
Poppy (Martin's)	1	170	320
Sesame (Martin's)	1	170	320
Brown 'N Serve			
Club (Pepperidge Farm)	1	100	190
French (Pepperidge Farm)	½ roll	180	380
Hearth (Pepperidge Farm)	1	50	100
Buns (Wonder)	1	70	160
Dinner			
(Pepperidge Farm)	1	60	95
Country Style Classic (Pepperidge Farm)	1	50	90
Finger			
Poppy Seed (Pepperidge Farm)	1	50	80
Sesame Seed (Pepperidge Farm)	1	60	85
Frankfurter			
Dijon (Pepperidge Farm)	1	160	230
Side Sliced (Pepperidge Farm)	1	140	270
Top Sliced (Pepperidge Farm)	1	140	270
w/ Poppy Seeds (Pepperidge Farm)	1	130	280
French Style (Pepperidge Farm)	1	100	230
Hamburger			
(Pepperidge Farm)	1	130	240
Light (Wonder)	1	80	210
Heat & Serve			
Butter Crescent (Pepperidge Farm)	1	110	150

FOOD	PORTION	CALORIES	SODIUM
Golden Twist (Pepperidge Farm)	1	110	150
Hoagie (Martin's)	1	240	430
Sesame (Martin's)	1	240	430
Soft (Pepperidge Farm)	1	210	320
Hotdog Light (Wonder)	1	80	210
Old Fashioned (Pepperidge Farm)	1	50	85
Parker House (Pepperidge Farm)	1	60	80
Party (Pepperidge Farm)	1	30	50
Potato Dinner (Martin's)	1	100	135
Long (Martin's)	1	140	200
Party (Martin's)	1	50	70
Sandwich (Martin's)	1	140	200
Sandwich (Pepperidge Farm)	1	160	260
Salad Roll (Matthew's)	1	110	190
Sandwich (Matthew's)	1	110	180
Onion w/ Poppy Seeds (Pepperidge Farm)	1	150	260
Salad (Pepperidge Farm)	1	110	150
Whole Wheat, 100% Stoneground (Martin's)	1	160	290
w/ Sesame Seeds (Pepperidge Farm)	1	140	230
Soft Family (Pepperidge Farm)	1	100	190
Sourdough French (Pepperidge Farm)	1	100	240
dinner	1 (1 oz)	85	155
frankfurter	1 (8/pkg)	115	241
hamburger	1 (8/pkg)	115	241

FOOD	PORTION	CALORIES	SODIUM
hard	1	155	313
submarine	1 (4.7 oz)	155	313
REFRIGERATED Pillsbury			
Best Quick Cinnamon Rolls w/ Icing	1	110	260
Butterflake	1	140	530
Crescent	1	100	230

ROSE HIP

fresh	3½ oz	91	146

ROSELLE

fresh	1 cup	28	3

ROSEMARY

dried	1 tsp	4	1

ROUGHY

orange, baked	3 oz	75	69

RUTABAGA

FRESH cooked, mashed	½ cup	41	22
raw, cubed	½ cup	25	14

SABLEFISH

baked	3 oz	213	61
fillet, baked	5.3 oz	378	108
SMOKED sablefish	1 oz	72	206
sablefish	3 oz	218	626

FOOD	PORTION	CALORIES	SODIUM
SAFFRON			
saffron	1 tsp	2	1
SAGE			
ground	1 tsp	2	tr
SALAD			
(see also PASTA SALAD)			
MIX			
Suddenly Salad			
Caesar, as prep	½ cup	170	450
Ranch And Bacon, as prep	½ cup	210	320
Ranch And Bacon, as prep, lowfat recipe	½ cup	160	350
TAKE-OUT			
chef, w/o dressing	1½ cup	386	279
tossed			
w/o dressing	1½ cup	32	53
w/o dressing	¾ cup	16	27
w/o dressing, w/ cheese & egg	1½ cup	102	119
w/o dressing, w/ chicken	1½ cup	105	209
w/o dressing, w/ pasta & seafood	1½ cup	380	1572
w/o dressing, w/ shrimp	1½ cup	107	487
waldorf	½ cup	79	49
SALAD DRESSING			
HOME RECIPE			
french	1 tbsp	88	92
vinegar & oil	1 tbsp	72	tr
READY-TO-USE			
Catalina	1 tbsp	15	120

FOOD	PORTION	CALORIES	SODIUM
Catalina French	1 tbsp	60	180
Estee			
Blue Cheese	1 tbsp	8	50
Dijon Creamy	1 tbsp	8	100
French	1 tbsp	4	10
Garlic Creamy	1 tbsp	2	10
Italian Creamy	1 tbsp	4	12
Red Wine Vinegar	1 tbsp	2	10
Thousand Island	1 tbsp	8	30
Healthy Sensation			
Blue Cheese	1 tbsp	19	144
French	1 tbsp	21	121
Honey Dijon	1 tbsp	26	142
Italian	1 tbsp	7	141
Ranch	1 tbsp	15	138
Thousand Island	1 tbsp	20	134
Kraft Bacon			
& Tomato	1 tbsp	70	130
& Tomato, Reduced Calorie	1 tbsp	30	150
Creamy	1 tbsp	30	150
Kraft Blue Cheese			
Chunky	1 tbsp	60	230
Chunky, Reduced Calorie	1 tbsp	30	240
Kraft Buttermilk			
Creamy	1 tbsp	80	120
Creamy, Reduced Calorie	1 tbsp	30	125
Kraft Coleslaw	1 tbsp	70	200
Kraft Creamy			
Garlic	1 tbsp	50	170
Italian With Real Sour Cream	1 tbsp	50	120

FOOD	PORTION	CALORIES	SODIUM
Kraft Cucumber			
Creamy	1 tbsp	70	190
Creamy, Reduced Calorie	1 tbsp	25	220
Kraft Free			
French, Nonfat	1 tbsp	26	120
Italian, Nonfat	1 tbsp	6	210
Ranch, Nonfat	1 tbsp	16	150
Thousand Island, Nonfat	1 tbsp	20	135
Kraft French Reduced Calorie	1 tbsp	20	120
Kraft French	1 tbsp	60	125
Kraft Golden Caesar	1 tbsp	70	180
Kraft House			
Italian	1 tbsp	60	115
Italian, Reduced Calorie	1 tbsp	30	115
Kraft Italian			
Creamy, Reduced Calorie	1 tbsp	25	120
Oil-Free	1 tbsp	4	220
Kraft Miracle French	1 tbsp	70	240
Kraft Oil & Vinegar	1 tbsp	70	210
Kraft Presto Italian	1 tbsp	70	150
Kraft Red Wine Vinegar And Oil	1 tbsp	60	200
Kraft Russian			
Creamy	1 tbsp	60	150
Reduced Calorie	1 tbsp	30	130
With Pure Honey	1 tbsp	60	130
Kraft Thousand Island	1 tbsp	60	150
& Bacon	1 tbsp	60	100
Reduced Calorie	1 tbsp	20	135
Kraft Zesty Italian	1 tbsp	50	260
Reduced Calorie	1 tbsp	20	230
Newman's Own			
Italian Light	1 tbsp	40	150

FOOD	PORTION	CALORIES	SODIUM
Newman's Own *(cont.)*			
Olive Oil & Vinegar	1 tbsp	80	80
Rancher's Choice	1 tbsp	90	140
Creamy	1 tbsp	30	150
Roka Blue Cheese	1 tbsp	60	170
Reduced Calorie	1 tbsp	15	280
S&W			
Blue Cheese, Low Calorie	1 tbsp	25	200
Cucumber, Creamy Low Calorie	1 tbsp	25	190
French, Low Calorie	1 tbsp	18	120
Italian, Creamy Low Calorie	1 tbsp	10	180
Italian, No-Oil	1 tbsp	2	290
Russian, Low Calorie	1 tbsp	25	120
Thousand Island, Low Calorie	1 tbsp	25	105
Seven Seas Buttermilk	1 tbsp	80	130
Ranch! Light	1 tbsp	50	135
Seven Seas French			
Creamy	1 tbsp	60	240
Light	1 tbsp	35	210
Seven Seas Herb & Spice	1 tbsp	60	170
Seven Seas Italian, Creamy	1 tbsp	70	240
Seven Seas Thousand Island			
Creamy	1 tbsp	50	150
Light	1 tbsp	30	160
Seven Seas Free			
Ranch, Nonfat	1 tbsp	16	120
Red Wine Vinegar, Nonfat	1 tbsp	6	190
Seven Seas Viva			
Free, Italian, Nonfat	1 tbsp	4	220
Herbs & Spices! Light	1 tbsp	30	200
Italian	1 tbsp	50	240

FOOD	PORTION	CALORIES	SODIUM
Italian! Light	1 tbsp	30	230
Ranch	1 tbsp	80	135
Ranch! Light	1 tbsp	50	125
Red Wine Vinegar & Oil	1 tbsp	70	290
Red Wine! Vinegar & Oil, Light	1 tbsp	45	190
Ultra Slim-Fast			
French	1 tbsp	20	150
Italian	1 tbsp	6	170
Walden Farms			
Bleu Cheese	1 tbsp	27	270
Creamy Italian With Parmesan	1 tbsp	35	210
French	1 tbsp	33	132
Italian	1 tbsp	9	300
Italian, No Sugar Added	1 tbsp	6	180
Ranch	1 tbsp	35	165
Thousand Island	1 tbsp	24	132
Weight Watchers			
Ceasar	1 pkg (¾ oz)	6	280
Ceasar	1 tbsp	4	200
Cucumber, Creamy	1 tbsp	18	85
Italian	1 pkg (¾ oz)	8	270
Italian	1 tbsp	6	200
Italian, Creamy	1 tbsp	12	85
Peppercorn, Creamy	1 tbsp	8	85
Ranch, Creamy	1 pkg (¾ oz)	35	130
Ranch, Creamy	1 tbsp	25	100
Russian	1 tbsp	50	80
Thousand Island	1 tbsp	50	80
Wishbone Blue Cheese			
Chunky	1 tbsp	73	148
Chunky Lite	1 tbsp	40	197

FOOD	PORTION	CALORIES	SODIUM
Wishbone Caesar With Olive Oil Lite	1 tbsp	28	172
Wishbone Dijon Vinaigrette			
Classic	1 tbsp	57	159
Classic Lite	1 tbsp	30	176
Wishbone French			
Deluxe	1 tbsp	57	83
Fat Free	1 tbsp	6	249
Lite	1 tbsp	30	67
Red	1 tbsp	64	170
Red, Lite	1 tbsp	17	155
Sweet 'N Spicy	1 tbsp	613	156
Sweet 'N Spicy, Lite	1 tbsp	17	134
Wishbone Italian	1 tbsp	45	281
Creamy	1 tbsp	54	149
Creamy, Lite	1 tbsp	26	148
Lite	1 tbsp	6	249
Robusto	1 tbsp	46	288
Wishbone Olive Oil			
Italian Classic	1 tbsp	33	190
Italian Classic, Lite	1 tbsp	20	155
Vinaigrette	1 tbsp	30	126
Vinaigrette, Lite	1 tbsp	16	133
Wishbone Ranch	1 tbsp	76	103
Lite	1 tbsp	42	148
Wishbone Red Wine			
Olive Oil Vinaigrette	1 tbsp	34	191
Olive Oil Vinaigrette, Lite	1 tbsp	20	151
Wishbone Russian	1 tbsp	54	173
Lite	1 tbsp	21	142
Wishbone Thousand Island	1 tbsp	66	168
Lite	1 tbsp	22	135

FOOD	PORTION	CALORIES	SODIUM
french	1 tbsp	67	214
french, reduced calorie	1 tbsp	22	128
italian	1 tbsp	69	116
italian, reduced calorie	1 tbsp	16	118
russian	1 tbsp	76	133
russian, reduced calorie	1 tbsp	23	141
sesame seed	1 tbsp	68	153
thousand island	1 tbsp	59	109
thousand island, reduced calorie	1 tbsp	24	153

SALMON

FOOD	PORTION	CALORIES	SODIUM
CANNED			
Bumble Bee			
Pink	2 oz	160	490
Pink, Skinless, Boneless	3.25 oz	120	420
Red Sockeye	2 oz	180	490
Deming's			
Alaska Keta	½ cup	140	450
Alaska Pink	½ cup	140	450
Alaska Red Sockeye	½ cup	170	450
Double "Q" Alaska Pink	½ cup	140	450
Humpty Dumpty Alaska Chum	½ cup	140	450
S&W Bluepack, Fancy, Diet	½ cup	188	45
S&W Red Fancy, Sockeye, Bluepack	½ cup	190	590
chum, w/ bone	1 can (13.9 oz)	521	1797
chum, w/ bone	3 oz	120	414
pink, w/ bone	1 can (15.9 oz)	631	2514
pink, w/ bone	3 oz	118	471
sockeye, w/ bone	1 can (12.9 oz)	566	1987
sockeye, w/ bone	3 oz	130	458

FOOD	PORTION	CALORIES	SODIUM
FRESH			
atlantic, baked	3 oz	155	48
chinook, baked	3 oz	196	51
chum, baked	3 oz	131	54
coho, cooked	½ fillet (5.4 oz)	286	91
coho, cooked	3 oz	157	50
coho, raw	3 oz	124	39
pink, baked	3 oz	127	73
sockeye, cooked	½ fillet (5.4 oz)	334	102
sockeye, cooked	3 oz	183	102
sockeye, raw	3 oz	143	40
SMOKED			
chinook	1 oz	33	220
chinook	3 oz	99	666
TAKE-OUT			
salmon cake	1 (3 oz)	241	602

SALSA

FOOD	PORTION	CALORIES	SODIUM
Chi Chi's			
Hot	1 oz	8	138
Medium	1 oz	8	130
Mild	1 oz	9	96
Ortega			
Hot Green Chili	1 tbsp	6	190
Medium Green Chili	1 tbsp	6	190
Mild Green Chili	1 tbsp	8	190
Rosarita			
Chunky Hot	3 tbsp	25	300
Chunky Medium	3 tbsp	25	350
Chunky Mild	3 tbsp	25	340
Rosarita Taco Salsa			
Chunky Medium	3 tbsp	25	310

FOOD	PORTION	CALORIES	SODIUM
Chunky Mild	3 tbsp	25	300

SALSIFY

FRESH
cooked, sliced	½ cup	46	11
raw, sliced	½ cup	55	13

SALT/SEASONED SALT
(*see also* SALT SUBSTITUTES)

salt	1 tsp	0	2132

SALT SUBSTITUTES

Estee Salt-It	⅛ tsp	0	0
Papa Dash			
Lite Lite Lite Salt	¼ tsp	1	87
Salt Lover's Blend	¼ tsp	tr	231

SAPODILLA

fresh	1	140	20
fresh, cut up	1 cup	199	29

SAPOTES

fresh	1	301	21

SARDINES

CANNED
Empress Skinless & Boneless
Olive Oil	1 can (3.8 oz)	420	530
Soy Oil	1 can (4.4 oz)	500	630
S&W Norwegian Brisling	1.5 oz	130	220
atlantic in oil, w/ bone	1 can (3.2 oz)	192	465
atlantic in oil, w/ bone	2	50	121

FOOD	PORTION	CALORIES	SODIUM
pacific in tomato sauce, w/ bone	1 can (13 oz)	658	1532
pacific in tomato sauce, w/ bone	1	68	157
FRESH			
raw	3½ oz	135	100

SAUCE
(see also GRAVY, PIZZA, SPAGHETTI SAUCE, TOMATO)

FOOD	PORTION	CALORIES	SODIUM
DRY			
Au Jus, as prep (Knorr)	2 oz	8	160
Bearnaise, as prep (Knorr)	2 oz	170	340
Classic Brown Gravy, as prep (Knorr)	2 oz	25	300
Demi-Glace, as prep (Knorr)	2 oz	30	310
Hollandaise, as prep (Knorr)	2 oz	170	310
Hunter, as prep (Knorr)	2 oz	25	340
Lyonnaise, as prep (Knorr)	2 oz	20	360
Mushroom, as prep (Knorr)	2 oz	60	240
Napoli, as prep (Knorr)	4 oz	100	960
Pepper, as prep (Knorr)	2 oz	20	380
bearnaise, as prep w/ milk & butter	1 cup	701	1265
cheese, as prep w/ milk	1 cup	307	1566
curry, as prep w/ milk	1 cup	270	1276
mushroom, as prep w/ milk	1 cup	228	1533
sour cream, as prep w/ milk	1 cup	509	1007
stroganoff	1 cup	271	1829
sweet & sour	1 cup	294	779
teriyaki	1 cup	131	4791
white, as prep w/ milk	1 cup	241	796

FOOD	PORTION	CALORIES	SODIUM
JARRED			
Bandito Diavalo Spicy (Newman's Own)	4 oz	70	530
Barbecue			
(Estee)	1 tbsp	18	5
(Kraft)	2 tbsp	45	460
Country Style (Hunt's)	1 tbsp	20	140
Garlic (Kraft)	2 tbsp	40	420
Hickory (Hunt's)	1 tbsp	20	160
Hickory Smoke (Kraft)	2 tbsp	45	440
Hickory Smoke, Onion Bits (Kraft)	2 tbsp	50	340
Homestyle (Hunt's)	1 tbsp	20	170
Hot (Kraft)	2 tbsp	45	520
Hot, Hickory Smoke (Kraft)	2 tbsp	45	360
Italian Seasoning (Kraft)	2 tbsp	50	280
Kansas City Style (Hunt's)	1 tbsp	20	85
Kansas City Style (Kraft)	2 tbsp	50	270
Mesquite Smoke (Kraft)	2 tbsp	45	410
New Orleans Style (Hunt's)	1 tbsp	20	150
Onion Bits (Kraft)	2 tbsp	50	340
Original (Hunt's)	1 tbsp	20	160
Select (Heinz)	1 oz	40	275
Select Hickory (Heinz)	1 oz	35	260
Southern Style (Hunt's)	1 tbsp	20	170
Texas Style (Hunt's)	1 tbsp	25	150
Barbecue Thick & Rich (Heinz)			
Cajun Style	1 oz	35	360
Chunky	1 oz	30	380
Hawaiian Style	1 oz	40	210
Hickory Smoke	1 oz	35	380

FOOD	PORTION	CALORIES	SODIUM
Barbecue Thick & Rich *(cont.)*			
Mesquite Smoke	1 oz	30	380
Mushroom	1 oz	30	460
Old Fashioned	1 oz	35	350
Onion	1 oz	30	420
Original	1 oz	35	390
Texas Hot	1 oz	30	390
Barbecue Thick'n Spicy (Kraft)			
Chunky	2 tbsp	60	420
Hickory Smoke	2 tbsp	50	430
Kansas City Style	2 tbsp	60	270
Mesquite Smoke	2 tbsp	50	430
Original	2 tbsp	50	430
With Honey	2 tbsp	60	340
Barbecue Western Style (Hunt's)	1 tbsp	20	170
Cajun Style (Golden Dipt)	1 oz	90	360
Chili 7 Spice Tabasco (McIlhenny)	4 oz	56	575
Cocktail (Sauceworks)	1 tbsp	14	170
Creole (Golden Dipt)	1 oz	20	190
Diable (Escoffier)	1 Tbsp	20	160
Dijonaisse (Golden Dipt)	1 oz	52	130
Duck Sauce Sweet & Sour (La Choy)	1 tbsp	25	40
Enchilada Sauce (Gebhardt)	3 tbsp	25	170
French, White (Golden Dipt)	1 oz	55	210
Ginger Teriyaki Marinade (Golden Dipt)	1 oz	120	920
Grilling And Broiling (Knorr)			
Chardonnay	1.6 oz	50	630
Spicey Plum	1.7 oz	60	790
Tequilla Lime	1.6 oz	50	690
Tuscan Herb	1.6 oz	50	600

FOOD	PORTION	CALORIES	SODIUM
Hot Dog			
(Just Rite)	2 oz	60	220
(Wolf Brand)	1.25 oz	44	199
Chili Sauce (Gebhardt)	2 tbsp	30	180
Hot Sauce (Gebhardt)	½ tsp	tr	55
Lemon Butter Dill (Golden Dipt)	1 oz	100	190
Lemon Herb Marinade (Golden Dipt)	1 oz	130	210
Manwich Mexican	2.5 oz	35	460
Microwave (Knorr)			
Hollandaise	1 oz	50	190
Mandarin Ginger	1.6 oz	50	690
Parmesano	1.6 oz	50	680
Vera Cruz	3.3 oz	70	580
Rib (Gold's)	1 oz	60	250
Seafood Cocktail (Golden Dipt)	1 tbsp	20	210
Extra Hot (Golden Dipt)	1 tbsp	20	210
Sloppy Joe (Manwich)	2.5 oz	40	390
Steak			
(Estee)	1 tbsp	14	35
(Lea & Perrins)	1 oz	40	220
(Mrs. Dash)	1 tbsp	17	10
Stir-Fry (Kikkoman)	1 tbsp	16	369
Sweet & Sour			
(Kikkoman)	1 tbsp	19	97
(La Choy)	1 tbsp	25	40
Sweet 'N Sour (Sauceworks)	1 tbsp	25	50
Tabasco (McIlhenny)	¼ tsp	tr	9
Tartar			
(Best Foods)	1 tbsp	70	190
(Golden Dipt)	1 tbsp	70	100

FOOD	PORTION	CALORIES	SODIUM
Tartar *(cont.)*			
(Hellman's)	1 tbsp	70	190
(Sauceworks)	1 tbsp	50	85
(Weight Watchers)	1 tbsp	35	80
Lite (Golden Dipt)	1 tbsp	50	40
Natural Lemon And Herb (Kraft)	1 tbsp	70	85
Teriyaki (Kikkoman)	1 tbsp	15	626
Worcestershire			
(Heinz)	1 tbsp	6	170
(Lea & Perrins)	1 tsp	5	55
White Wine (Lea & Perrins)	1 tsp	4	40
barbecue	1 cup	188	2038
teriyaki	1 oz	30	1380
teriyaki	1 tbsp	15	690

SAUERKRAUT

CANNED			
S&W	½ cup	25	850
SnowFloss Kraut	4 oz	28	780
SnowFloss Kraut Bavarian Style	4 oz	64	780
Vlasic Old Fashioned	1 oz	4	280
canned	½ cup	22	780
JUICE			
S&W	4 oz	14	1120

SAUSAGE

(*see also* HOT DOG, SAUSAGE DISHES)

Perdue			
Breakfast Links, Turkey, cooked	1 (1.3 oz)	40	106
Breakfast Patties, Turkey, cooked	1 (1.3 oz)	61	175

FOOD	PORTION	CALORIES	SODIUM
Hot Italian, Turkey, cooked	1 (2 oz)	94	348
Sweet Italian, Turkey, cooked	1 (2 oz)	94	348
blutwurst, uncooked	3½ oz	424	680
brotwurst, pork	1 oz	92	315
brotwurst, pork & beef	1 link (2.5 oz)	226	778
bratwurst, pork, cooked	1 link (3 oz)	256	473
country-style pork, cooked	1 link (½ oz)	48	168
country-style pork, cooked	1 patty (1 oz)	100	349
gelbwurst, uncooked	3½ oz	363	640
italian, pork, cooked	1 (2.4 oz)	216	618
italian, pork, cooked	1 (3 oz)	268	765
kielbasa, pork	1 oz	88	305
knockwurst, pork & beef	1 (2.4 oz)	209	687
knockwurst, pork & beef	1 oz	87	286
mettwurst, uncooked	3½ oz	483	1090
polish, pork	1 (8 oz)	739	1989
polish, pork	1 oz	92	248
pork & beef, cooked	1 link (½ oz)	52	105
pork & beef, cooked	1 patty (1 oz)	107	217
pork, cooked	1 link (½ oz)	48	168
pork, cooked	1 patty (1 oz)	100	349
smoked pork	1 link (2.4 oz)	265	1020
smoked pork	1 sm link (½ oz)	62	240
smoked pork & beef	1 link (2.4 oz)	229	151
smoked pork & beef	1 sm link (½ oz)	54	151
vienna, canned	1 (½ oz)	45	152
vienna, canned	7 (4 oz)	315	1077
weisswurst, uncooked	3½ oz	305	620
TAKE-OUT			
pork	1 link (.5 oz)	48	168

FOOD	PORTION	CALORIES	SODIUM
pork	1 patty (1 oz)	100	349

SAUSAGE DISHES

FROZEN
Ovenstuffs French Roll
| Italian Sausage | 1 (4.75 oz) | 390 | 910 |
| Pepperoni | 1 (4.75 oz) | 370 | 870 |

SAVORY

| ground | 1 tsp | 4 | tr |

SCALLOP

FRESH			
raw	3 oz	75	137
FROZEN			
Fried (Mrs. Paul's)	2 oz	160	320
HOME RECIPE			
breaded & fried	2 lg	67	144
TAKE-OUT			
breaded & fried	6 (5 oz)	386	919

SCONE

| HOME RECIPE | | | |
| apricot scone | 1 | 232 | 201 |

SCROD

| FROZEN | | | |
| Microwave Entree, Baked (Gorton's) | 1 pkg | 320 | 420 |

SCUP

| FRESH | | | |
| baked | 3 oz | 115 | 46 |

FOOD	PORTION	CALORIES	SODIUM

SEA BASS
(see BASS)

SEA TROUT
(see TROUT)

SEAWEED

FOOD	PORTION	CALORIES	SODIUM
DRIED			
agar	1 oz	87	29
FRESH			
agar	1 oz	tr	3
irishmoss	1 oz	14	19
kelp	1 oz	12	66
kombu	1 oz	12	66
laver	1 oz	10	14
nori	1 oz	10	14
spirulina	1 oz	7	28
tangle	1 oz	12	66
wakame	1 oz	13	249

SEMOLINA

FOOD	PORTION	CALORIES	SODIUM
dry	½ cup	303	1

SESAME

FOOD	PORTION	CALORIES	SODIUM
Seeds (Arrowhead)	1 oz	160	5
Sesame Butter (Erewhon)	2 tbsp	190	20
Sesame Tahini (Arrowhead)	1 oz	170	tr
(Erewhon)	2 tbsp	200	65
seeds	1 tsp	16	1
seeds, dried	1 cup	825	16

FOOD	PORTION	CALORIES	SODIUM
seeds, dried	1 tbsp	52	1
seeds, roasted & toasted	1 oz	161	3
sesame butter	1 tbsp	95	2
tahini, from roasted & toasted kernels	1 tbsp	89	17
tahini, from stone-ground kernels	1 tbsp	86	11
tahini, from unroasted kernels	1 tbsp	85	0

SESBANIA

flower	1	1	0
flowers	1 cup	5	3
flowers, cooked	1 cup	23	11

SHAD

american, baked	3 oz	214	56

SHALLOTS

DRIED			
dried	1 tbsp	3	1
FRESH			
raw, chopped	1 tbsp	7	1

SHARK

batter-dipped & fried	3 oz	194	103
raw	3 oz	111	67

SHEEPSHEAD FISH

cooked	1 fillet (6.5 oz)	234	136
cooked	3 oz	107	62
raw	3 oz	92	61

SHELLFISH
(*see* individual names, SHELLFISH SUBSTITUTES)

FOOD	PORTION	CALORIES	SODIUM

SHELLFISH SUBSTITUTES

FOOD	PORTION	CALORIES	SODIUM
crab, imitation	3 oz	87	715
scallop, imitation	3 oz	84	676
shrimp, imitation	3 oz	86	599
surimi	1 oz	28	40
surimi	3 oz	84	122

SHELLIE BEANS

FOOD	PORTION	CALORIES	SODIUM
CANNED			
shellie beans	½ cup	37	408

SHRIMP

FOOD	PORTION	CALORIES	SODIUM
canned	1 cup	154	216
canned	3 oz	102	143
FRESH			
cooked	3 oz	84	190
cooked	4 large	22	49
raw	3 oz	90	126
raw	4 large	30	42
FROZEN			
Butterfly Shrimp (Gorton's)	4 oz	160	540
Light Seafood Entrees, Shrimp And Clams With Linguini (Mrs. Paul's)	10 oz	240	750
Microwave Crunchy Shrimp (Gorton's)	5 oz	380	870
Entree, Shrimp Scampi (Gorton's)	1 pkg	390	470
Shrimp Crisps (Gorton's)	4 oz	280	740
TAKE-OUT			
breaded & fried	3 oz	206	292
breaded & fried	4 large	73	103

FOOD	PORTION	CALORIES	SODIUM
breaded & fried	6 to 8 (6 oz)	454	1447
jambalaya	¾ cup	188	83

SMELT

FOOD	PORTION	CALORIES	SODIUM
rainbow, cooked	3 oz	106	65
rainbow, raw	3 oz	83	51

SNACKS
(*see also* CHIPS, FRUIT SNACKS, NUTS MIXED, POPCORN, PRETZELS)

FOOD	PORTION	CALORIES	SODIUM
Apple Chips (Weight Watchers)	¾ oz	70	110
Bugles	1 oz	150	290
Nacho Cheese	1 oz	160	250
Ranch	1 oz	150	290
Carrot Lites (Health Valley)	½ oz	75	5
Cheddar Lites (Health Valley)	¼ oz	40	35
With Green Onion	¼ oz	40	35
Cheese Curls (Weight Watchers)	½ oz	70	45
Chex Snack Mix			
Barbecue	⅔ cup	130	480
Cool Sour Cream And Onion	⅔ cup	130	300
Golden Cheddar	⅔ cup	130	300
Traditional	⅔ cup	120	320
Doo Dads	1 oz	140	360
Easy Cheddar Nacho (Nabisco)	1 oz	80	340
Easy Cheese (Nabisco)			
American	1 oz	80	340
Cheddar	1 oz	80	360
Cheese 'n Bacon	1 oz	80	340
Sharp Cheddar	1 oz	80	360
Ultra Slim-Fast Lite N' Tasty Cheese Curls	1 oz	110	360
Wheat Snax (Estee)	1 oz	100	15

FOOD	PORTION	CALORIES	SODIUM

SNAIL

FRESH
cooked	3 oz	233	350
raw	3 oz	117	175

SNAP BEANS

CANNED
green	½ cup	13	170
green, low sodium	½ cup	13	1
italian	½ cup	13	170
italian, low sodium	½ cup	13	1
yellow	½ cup	13	170
yellow, low sodium	½ cup	13	1

FRESH
green, cooked	½ cup	22	2
green, raw	½ cup	17	3
green, raw	½ cup	17	3
yellow, cooked	½ cup	22	2
yellow, raw	½ cup	17	3

FROZEN
green, cooked	½ cup	18	9
italian, cooked	½ cup	18	9
yellow, cooked	½ cup	18	9

SNAPPER

FRESH
cooked	1 fillet (6 oz)	217	96
cooked	3 oz	109	48
raw	3 oz	85	54

FOOD	PORTION	CALORIES	SODIUM

SODA
(see also DRINK MIXER)

FOOD	PORTION	CALORIES	SODIUM
Crystal Geyser Mountain Spring Sparkler			
Black Cherry	6 oz	65	tr
Cranberry Raspberry	6 oz	65	tr
Kiwi Lemon	6 oz	65	tr
Peach	6 oz	65	tr
Vanilla Creme	6 oz	65	tr
Health Valley			
Ginger Ale	12 oz	153	30
Rootbeer Old Fashioned	12 oz	120	12
Sarsaparilla Rootbeer	12 oz	153	27
Wild Berry	12 oz	142	27
Manischewitz Seltzer, No Salt Added, No Calories	8 oz	0	9
Orangina	9 oz	150	200
club	12 oz	0	75
cola	12 oz	151	14
cream	12 oz	191	43
diet cola	12 oz	2	21
diet cola w/ nutrasweet	12 oz	2	21
diet cola w/ saccharin	12 oz	2	57
ginger ale	12 oz	124	25
grape	12 oz	161	57
lemon lime	12 oz	149	41
orange	12 oz	177	49
pepper-type	12 oz	151	38
quinine	12 oz	125	15
root beer	12 oz	152	49
tonic water	12 oz	125	15

FOOD	PORTION	CALORIES	SODIUM

SOLE

FRESH

lemon, raw	3½ oz	85	80
raw	3½ oz	90	100

FROZEN

Fishmarket Fresh (Gorton's)	5 oz	110	140
Light Fillets (Mrs. Paul's)	1 fillet	240	450
Microwave Entree			
In Lemon Butter (Gorton's)	1 pkg	380	560
In Wine Sauce (Gorton's)	1 pkg	180	770

SOUFFLE

HOME RECIPE

cheese	1 cup	308	899
grand marnier	1 cup	109	58
lemon, chilled	1 cup	176	108
raspberry, chilled	1 cup	173	108
spinach souffle	1 cup	218	763

SOUP

CANNED

Asparagus, Cream Of, as prep (Campbell)	8 oz	80	820
Bean And Ham (Healthy Choice)	½ can (7.5 oz)	220	480
Home Cookin' (Campbell)	10¾ oz	210	1000
Beef, as prep (Campbell)	8 oz	80	830
Bean Homestyle, as prep (Campbell)	8 oz	130	700
Bean With Bacon as prep (Campbell)	8 oz	140	840

FOOD	PORTION	CALORIES	SODIUM
Bean With Bacon *(cont.)*			
Healthy Request, as prep (Campbell)	8 oz	140	470
Beef Broth			
(College Inn)	½ can (7 oz)	16	960
(Health Valley)	7½ oz	10	420
(Swanson)	7¼ oz	18	750
as prep (Campbell)	8 oz	16	820
No Salt Added (Health Valley)	7½ oz	10	5
Beef Chunky, Ready-To-Serve (Campbell)	10¾ oz	200	1100
Beef Noodle			
as prep (Campbell)	8 oz	70	830
Homestyle, as prep (Campbell)	8 oz	80	810
Beef Stroganoff, Chunky, Ready-To-Serve (Campbell)	10¾ oz	320	1230
Beef With Vegetables And Pasta, Home Cookin' (Campbell)	10¾ oz	140	1060
Beefy Mushroom, as prep (Campbell)	8 oz	60	960
Black Bean			
(Goya)	7.5 oz	160	720
(Health Valley)	7½ oz	150	280
No Salt Added (Health Valley)	7½ oz	150	20
Borscht			
(Gold's)	8 oz	100	1280
Lo-Cal (Gold's)	8 oz	20	1160
Low Calorie (Manischewitz)	8 oz	20	725
With Beets (Manischewitz)	8 oz	80	660
Broccoli, Cream Of, as prep (Campbell)	8 oz	80	790
as prep w/ 2% milk (Campbell)	8 oz	140	850
Celery, Cream Of, as prep (Campbell)	8 oz	100	820

FOOD	PORTION	CALORIES	SODIUM
Cheddar Cheese, as prep (Campbell)	8 oz	110	810
Chicken & Stars, as prep (Campbell)	8 oz	60	870
Chicken Alphabet, as prep (Campbell)	8 oz	80	800
Chicken Barley, as prep (Campbell)	8 oz	70	850
Chicken Broth			
(College Inn)	½ can (7 oz)	35	990
(Health Valley)	7½ oz	35	410
(Swanson)	7¼ oz	30	900
as prep (Campbell)	8 oz	30	710
Healthy Request, Ready-To-Serve (Campbell)	8 oz	10	400
Low Sodium, Ready-To-Serve (Campbell)	10½ oz	30	85
Lower Salt (College Inn)	½ can (7 oz)	20	550
No Salt Added (Health Valley)	7½ oz	35	0
Chicken Broth & Noodles, as prep (Campbell)	8 oz	45	860
Chicken Corn Chowder, Chunky, Ready-To-Serve (Campbell)	10¾ oz	340	1200
Chicken, Cream Of, as prep (Campbell)	8 oz	110	810
Chicken Gumbo			
as prep (Campbell)	8 oz	60	900
With Sausage, Home Cookin' (Campbell)	10¾ oz	140	1090
Chicken Minestrone, Home Cookin' (Campbell)	10¾ oz	180	950
Chicken Mushroom, Creamy, as prep (Campbell)	8 oz	120	920
Chicken 'n Dumplings, as prep (Campbell)	8 oz	80	960

FOOD	PORTION	CALORIES	SODIUM
Chicken Noodle			
(Weight Watchers)	10.5 oz	80	1230
as prep (Campbell)	8 oz	60	900
Chunky, Ready-To-Serve (Campbell)	10¾ oz	200	1140
Healthy Request, as prep (Campbell)	8 oz	60	460
Homestyle, as prep (Campbell)	8 oz	70	880
Chicken Noodle-O's, as prep (Campbell)	8 oz	70	820
Chicken Nuggets w/ Vegetables & Noodles, Chunky (Campbell)	10¾ oz	190	1060
Chicken Rice, Home Cookin' (Campbell)	10¾ oz	150	1090
Chicken Vegetable			
as prep (Campbell)	8 oz	70	850
Chunky, Ready-To-Serve (Campbell)	9½ oz	170	1080
Chicken Beef, Low Sodium, Ready-To-Serve (Campbell)	10¾ oz	180	90
Chicken With Noodles			
Home Cookin' (Campbell)	10¾ oz	140	1150
Low Sodium, Ready-To-Serve (Campbell)	10¾ oz	170	90
Chicken w/ Rice			
(Healthy Choice)	½ can (7.5 oz)	140	510
as prep (Campbell)	8 oz	60	790
Chunky, Ready-To-Serve (Campbell)	9½ oz	140	1060
Healthy Request, as prep (Campbell)	8 oz	60	480
Chili Beef			
as prep (Campbell)	8 oz	140	840
Chunky, Ready-To-Serve (Campbell)	11 oz	290	1120

FOOD	PORTION	CALORIES	SODIUM
Chunky Beef Vegetable (Healthy Choice)	½ can (7.5 oz)	110	490
Chunky Chicken Noodle And Vegetable (Healthy Choice)	½ can (7.5 oz)	160	500
Chunky Chicken Vegetable (Health Valley)	7½ oz	125	290
Chunky Five Bean Vegetable (Health Valley)	7.5 oz	110	290
Chunky Five Bean Vegetable, No Salt Added (Health Valley)	7½ oz	110	60
Chunky Vegetable Chicken, No Salt Added (Health Valley)	7½ oz	125	60
Clam Chowder, Manhattan Style as prep (Campbell)	8 oz	70	820
Chunky, Ready-To-Serve (Campbell)	10¾ oz	160	1110
Clam Chowder, New England as prep (Campbell)	8 oz	80	870
as prep w/ whole milk (Campbell)	8 oz	150	930
Chunky, Ready-To-Serve (Campbell)	10¾ oz	290	1200
Consomme, as prep (Campbell)	8 oz	25	750
Country Vegetable (Healthy Choice)	½ can (7.5 oz)	120	540
Home Cookin' (Campbell)	10¾ oz	120	1070
Cream of Chicken, Healthy Request (Campbell)	8 oz	70	490
Cream of Mushroom, Healthy Request, as prep (Campbell)	8 oz	60	460
Creamy Chicken Mushroom, Chunky, Ready-To-Serve (Campbell)	10½ oz	270	1280
Creole Style, Chunky, Ready-To-Serve (Campbell)	10¾ oz	240	910

FOOD	PORTION	CALORIES	SODIUM
Curly Noodle With Chicken, as prep (Campbell)	8 oz	80	800
French Onion, as prep (Campbell)	8 oz	60	900
Green Pea, as prep (Campbell)	8 oz	160	820
Green Split Pea (Health Valley)	7½ oz	180	290
No Salt Added (Health Valley)	7½ oz	180	25
Ham 'n Butter Bean, Chunky, Ready-To-Serve (Campbell)	10¾ oz	280	1180
Hearty Beef (Healthy Choice)	½ can (7.5 oz)	120	580
Hearty Chicken (Healthy Choice)	½ can (7.5 oz)	150	530
Hearty Chicken Noodle, Healthy Request, Ready-To-Serve (Campbell)	8 oz	80	470
Hearty Chicken Rice, Healthy Request, Ready-To-Serve (Campbell)	8 oz	110	400
Hearty Chicken Vegetable, Healthy Request (Campbell)	8 oz	120	460
Hearty Lentil, Home Cookin' (Campbell)	10¾ oz	170	930
Hearty Minestrone, Healthy Request, Ready-To-Serve (Campbell)	8 oz	90	430
Hearty Vegetable Beef, Healthy Request, Ready-To-Serve (Campbell)	8 oz	120	490
Hearty Vegetable Healthy Request, Ready-To-Serve (Campbell)	8 oz	110	480
Lentil (Health Valley)	7½ oz	220	290
No Salt Added (Health Valley)	7½ oz	220	25
Manhattan Clam Chowder (Health Valley)	7½ oz	110	290

FOOD	PORTION	CALORIES	SODIUM
No Salt Added (Health Valley)	7½ oz	110	60
Mediterranean Vegetable, Chunky, Ready-To-Serve (Campbell)	9½ oz	170	1010
Minestrone			
(Health Valley)	7½ oz	130	290
(Healthy Choice)	½ can (7.5 oz)	160	520
as prep (Campbell)	8 oz	80	900
Chunky, Ready-To-Serve (Campbell)	9½ oz	160	870
Home Cookin' (Campbell)	10¾ oz	140	1220
No Salt Added (Health Valley)	7½ oz	130	90
Mushroom Barley			
(Health Valley)	7½ oz	100	290
No Salt Added (Health Valley)	7½ oz	100	20
Mushroom, Cream Of			
(Weight Watchers)	10.5 oz	90	1250
as prep (Campbell)	8 oz	100	820
Low Sodium, Ready-To-Serve (Campbell)	10½ oz	210	55
Mushroom, Golden, as prep (Campbell)	8 oz	70	870
Nacho Cheese			
as prep (Campbell)	8 oz	110	740
as prep w/ milk (Campbell)	8 oz	180	800
Natural Goodness, Clear Chicken Broth (Swanson)	7¼ oz	20	580
New England Clam Chowder, as prep w/ whole milk (Gorton's)	¼ can	140	740
Noodles & Ground Beef, as prep (Campbell)	8 oz	90	820
Old Fashioned Bean w/ Ham, Chunky, Ready-To-Serve (Campbell)	11 oz	290	1110

FOOD	PORTION	CALORIES	SODIUM
Old Fashioned Chicken, Chunky, Ready-To-Serve (Campbell)	10¾ oz	180	1220
Old Fashioned Chicken Noodle (Healthy Choice)	½ can (7.5 oz)	90	520
Old Fashioned Vegetable Beef, Chunky, Ready-To-Serve (Campbell)	10¾ oz	190	1100
Onion Cream Of			
as prep (Campbell)	8 oz	100	830
as prep w/ whole milk & water (Campbell)	8 oz	140	860
Oyster Stew			
as prep (Campbell)	8 oz	70	840
as prep w/ whole milk (Campbell)	8 oz	140	890
Pepper Pot, as prep (Campbell)	8 oz	90	970
Pepper Steak, Chunky, Ready-To-Serve (Campbell)	10¾ oz	180	1050
Potato, Cream Of			
as prep (Campbell)	8 oz	80	870
as prep w/ whole milk & water (Campbell)	8 oz	120	900
Potato Leek			
(Health Valley)	7½ oz	130	290
No Salt Added (Health Valley)	7½ oz	130	20
Schav			
(Gold's)	8 oz	25	1380
(Manischewitz)	1 cup	11	4
Scotch Broth, as prep (Campbell)	8 oz	80	870
Shrimp, Cream Of			
as prep (Campbell)	8 oz	90	810
as prep w/ whole milk (Campbell)	8 oz	160	860
Sirloin Burger, Chunky, Ready-To-Serve (Campbell)	10¾ oz	220	1240

FOOD	PORTION	CALORIES	SODIUM
Split Pea			
And Ham (Healthy Choice)	½ can (7.5 oz)	170	460
Low Sodium, Ready-To-Serve (Campbell)	10¾ oz	230	30
With Bacon, as prep (Campbell)	8 oz	160	780
w/ Ham, Chunky, Ready-To-Serve (Campbell)	10¾ oz	230	1080
Ham, Home Cookin' (Campbell)	10¾ oz	230	1310
Steak And Potato, Chunky, Ready-To-Serve (Campbell)	10¾ oz	200	1140
Teddy Bear, as prep (Campbell)	8 oz	70	790
Tomato			
(Health Valley)	7½ oz	130	290
as prep (Campbell)	8 oz	90	680
as prep, w/ 2% milk (Campbell)	8 oz	150	740
Tomato Bisque, as prep (Campbell)	8 oz	120	820
Tomato Garden			
(Healthy Choice)	½ can (7.5 oz)	130	510
Home Cookin' (Campbell)	10¾ oz	150	930
Tomato Healthy Request			
as prep (Campbell)	8 oz	90	430
as prep w/ skim milk (Campbell)	8 oz	130	490
Tomato, Homestyle, Cream Of			
as prep (Campbell)	8 oz	110	810
as prep w/ whole milk (Campbell)	8 oz	180	860
Tomato, No Salt Added (Health Valley)	7½ oz	130	40
Tomato, Rice, Old Fashioned, as prep (Campbell)	8 oz	110	730

FOOD	PORTION	CALORIES	SODIUM
Tomato With Tomato Pieces, Low Sodium, Ready-To-Serve (Campbell)	10½ oz	190	45
Tomato, Zesty, as prep (Campbell)	8 oz	100	760
Turkey Noodle, as prep (Campbell)	8 oz	70	880
Turkey Vegetable, as prep (Campbell)	8 oz	70	710
Turkey Vegetable, Chunky, Ready-To-Serve (Campbell)	9⅜ oz	150	1060
Vegetable			
(Health Valley)	7.5 oz	110	300
as prep (Campbell)	8 oz	90	830
Chunky, Ready-To-Serve (Campbell)	10¾ oz	160	1100
Healthy Request, as prep (Campbell)	8 oz	90	500
Homestyle, as prep (Campbell)	8 oz	60	880
No Salt Added (Health Valley)	7½ oz	110	40
Old Fashioned, as prep (Campbell)	8 oz	60	880
Vegetable Beef (Healthy Choice)	½ can (7.5 oz)	130	530
Vegetable Beef, as prep (Campbell)	8 oz	70	780
Vegetable Beef, Healthy Request, as prep (Campbell)	8 oz	70	490
Vegetable Beef, Home Cookin' (Campbell)	10¾ oz	140	1160
Vegetarian Vegetable, as prep (Campbell)	8 oz	80	790
Won Ton, as prep (Campbell)	8 oz	40	850
asparagus, cream of, as prep w/ milk	1 cup	161	1041

FOOD	PORTION	CALORIES	SODIUM
asparagus, cream of, as prep w/ water	1 cup	87	981
beef broth, ready-to-serve	1 can (14 oz)	27	1294
beef broth, ready-to-serve	1 cup	16	782
beef noodle, as prep w/ water	1 cup	84	952
black bean, as prep w/ water	1 cup	116	1198
black bean, turtle soup	1 cup	218	922
celery, cream of, as prep w/ milk	1 cup	165	1010
celery, cream of, as prep w/ water	1 cup	90	949
celery, cream of, not prep	1 can (10¾ oz)	219	2308
cheese, as prep w/ milk	1 cup	230	1020
cheese, as prep w/ water	1 cup	155	959
cheese, not prep	1 can (11 oz)	377	2331
chicken broth, as prep w/ water	1 cup	39	776
chicken, cream of, as prep w/ milk	1 cup	191	1046
chicken, cream of, as prep w/ water	1 cup	116	986
chicken gumbo, as prep w/ water	1 cup	56	955
chicken noodle, as prep w/ water	1 cup	75	1107
chicken rice, as prep w/ water	1 cup	251	814
clam chowder, Manhattan, as prep w/ water	1 cup	77	1029
clam chowder, New England, as prep w/ milk	1 cup	163	992
clam chowder, New England, as prep w/ water	1 cup	95	914
consomme w/ gelatin, as prep w/ water	1 cup	29	637
consomme w/ gelatin, not prep	1 can (10½ oz)	71	1550
escarole, ready-to-serve	1 cup	27	3865

FOOD	PORTION	CALORIES	SODIUM
french onion, as prep w/ water	1 cup	57	1053
gazpacho, ready-to-serve	1 cup	57	1183
minestrone, as prep w/ water	1 cup	83	911
mushroom, cream of, as prep w/ milk	1 cup	203	1076
mushroom, cream of, as prep w/ water	1 cup	129	1031
oyster stew, as prep w/ milk	1 cup	134	1040
oyster stew, as prep w/ water	1 cup	59	980
pepperpot, as prep w/ water	1 cup	103	970
potato, cream of, as prep w/ milk	1 cup	148	1060
potato, cream of, as prep w/ water	1 cup	73	1000
scotch broth, as prep w/ water	1 cup	80	1012
split pea w/ ham, as prep w/ water	1 cup	189	1008
tomato, as prep w/ milk	1 cup	160	932
tomato, as prep w/ water	1 cup	86	872
vegetarian vegetable, as prep w/ water	1 cup	72	823
vichyssoise	1 cup	148	1060
DRY			
Asparagus, as prep (Knorr)	8 oz	80	770
Bean With Bacon 'n Ham, Microwave (Campbell)	7½ oz	230	830
Beef, as prep (Ramen Noodle)	8 oz	190	1010
Beef Bouillon, as prep (Knorr)	8 oz	15	1220
Beef Broth, Instant, (Weight Watchers)	1 pkg	8	910
Beef, Instant, Oriental Noodle (Lipton)	8 oz	177	912
Beef, Low Fat, as prep (Ramen Noodle)	8 oz	160	890

FOOD	PORTION	CALORIES	SODIUM
Beef Mushroom (Lipton)	8 oz	38	763
Beef Noodle (Campbell's Cup)	1 (1.35 oz)	130	1270
(Ultra Slim-Fast)	6 oz	45	700
Beef With Vegetables as prep (Cup-A-Ramen)	8 oz	270	1530
Low Fat, as prep (Cup-A-Ramen)	8 oz	220	1600
Beefy Onion (Lipton)	8 oz	27	635
Cauliflower, as prep (Knorr)	8 oz	100	750
Chick 'n Pasta, as prep (Knorr)	8 oz	90	850
Chicken, as prep (Ramen Noodle)	8 oz	190	970
Chicken Bouillon, as prep (Knorr)	8 oz	16	1200
Chicken Broth (Cup-A-Soup)	6 oz	19	605
Instant (Weight Watchers)	1 pkg	8	900
Chicken, Instant, Oriental Noodle (Lipton)	8 oz	180	785
Chicken Leek (Ultra Slim-Fast)	6 oz	50	1070
Chicken Low Fat, as prep (Ramen Noodle)	8 oz	160	940
Chicken Noodle (Campbell's Cup)	1 (1.35 oz)	140	1340
(Lipton)	8 oz	82	702
(Ultra Slim-Fast)	6 oz	45	970
(Weight Watchers)	7.5 oz	90	450
as prep (Campbell)	8 oz	100	710
as prep (Knorr)	8 oz	100	710
Hearty (Lipton)	8 oz	81	766
Microwave (Campbell)	7½ oz	100	870
w/ White Meat, as prep (Campbell's Cup)	6 oz	90	770

FOOD	PORTION	CALORIES	SODIUM
Chicken Vegetable (Cup-a-Soup)	6 oz	47	566
Chicken With Rice, Microwave (Campbell)	7½ oz	100	820
Chicken w/ Vegetables as prep (Cup-a-Ramen)	8 oz	270	1470
Low Fat, as prep (Cup-a-Ramen)	8 oz	220	1500
Chili Beef, Microwave (Campbell)	7½ oz	190	870
Chunky Beef Stew (Weight Watchers)	7.5 oz	120	450
Country Barley, as prep (Knorr)	8 oz	120	940
Country Vegetable (Lipton)	8 oz	80	803
Creamy Broccoli (Ultra Slim-Fast)	6 oz	75	800
Creamy Broccoli And Cheese (Cup-a-Soup)	6 oz	70	595
Creamy Chicken w/ White Meat, as prep (Campbell's Cup)	6 oz	90	1020
Creamy Tomato (Ultra Slim-Fast)	6 oz	60	800
Fine Herb, as prep (Knorr)	8 oz	130	990
Fish Bouillon, as prep (Knorr)	8 oz	10	1130
French Onion, as prep (Knorr)	8 oz	50	970
Giggle Noodle (Lipton)	8 oz	72	708
Green Pea (Cup-A-Soup)	6 oz	113	553
Hearty Chicken And Noodles (Cup-A-Soup)	6 oz	110	587
Hearty Creamy Chicken, Lots-A-Noodles (Cup-A-Soup)	7 oz	179	639
Hearty Minestrone, as prep (Knorr)	10 oz	130	940
Hearty Noodle, as prep (Campbell)	8 oz	90	840
Hearty Noodle With Vegetable (Lipton)	8 oz	75	687

FOOD	PORTION	CALORIES	SODIUM
Hearty Noodles With Vegetables (Campbell's Cup)	1 (1.7 oz)	180	1320
Hearty Noodles With Vegetables (Lipton)	8 oz	75	687
Hearty Vegetable (Ultra Slim-Fast)	6 oz	50	750
Leek, as prep (Knorr)	8 oz	110	800
Lobster Bisque (Golden Dipt)	¼ pkg	30	560
Manhattan Clam Chowder (Golden Dipt)	¼ pkg	80	700
Minestrone, as prep (Manischewitz)	6 oz	50	160
Mushroom			
as prep (Knorr)	8 oz	100	870
Cream Of (Cup-A-Soup)	6 oz	71	756
New England Clam Chowder (Golden Dipt)	¼ pkg	24	680
(Weight Watchers)	7.5 oz	90	450
Noodle			
as prep (Campbell)	8 oz	110	700
With Chicken Broth (Campbell's Cup)	1 (1.35 oz)	130	1360
With Chicken Broth, as prep (Campbell's Cup)	6 oz	90	910
Onion			
(Cup-A-Soup)	6 oz	27	665
(Lipton)	8 oz	20	632
(Ultra Slim-Fast)	6 oz	45	930
as prep (Campbell)	8 oz	30	700
Golden (Lipton)	8 oz	62	716
Onion Mushroom (Lipton)	8 oz	41	684
Oriental			
as prep (Ramen Noodle)	8 oz	190	930
Hot And Sour, as prep (Knorr)	8 oz	80	690

FOOD	PORTION	CALORIES	SODIUM
Oriental *(cont.)*			
Low Fat, as prep (Ramen Noodle)	8 oz	150	940
With Vegetables, as prep (Cup-A-Ramen)	8 oz	270	1210
With Vegetables, Low Fat, as prep (Cup-A-Ramen)	8 oz	220	1400
Oxtail Hearty Beef, as prep (Knorr)	8 oz	70	1120
Pork			
as prep (Ramen Noodle)	8 oz	200	860
Low Fat, as prep (Ramen Noodle)	8 oz	150	1140
Potato			
Leek (Ultra Slim-Fast)	6 oz	80	780
Leek, as prep (Nile Spice)	10 oz	160	450
Potato Romano, as prep (Nile Spice)	10 oz	150	450
Potato Tomato, as prep (Nile Spice)	10 oz	160	440
Ring-O-Noodle (Lipton)	8 oz	67	708
Seafood Chowder (Golden Dipt)	¼ pkg	70	730
Shrimp Bisque (Golden Dipt)	¼ pkg	30	570
Shrimp With Vegetables, Low Fat, as prep (Cup-a-Ramen)	8 oz	230	1290
Shrimp With Vegetables, as prep (Cup-a-Ramen)	8 oz	280	1190
Split Pea, as prep (Manischewitz)	6 oz	45	320
Spring Vegetable With Herbs, as prep (Knorr)	8 oz	30	710
Tomato			
(Cup-A-Soup)	6 oz	103	524
Basil, as prep (Knorr)	8 oz	90	940
Tortellini In Brodo, as prep (Knorr)	8 oz	60	820

FOOD	PORTION	CALORIES	SODIUM
Vegetable (Lipton)	8 oz	37	640
as prep (Campbell)	8 oz	40	710
as prep (Knorr)	8 oz	35	840
as prep (Manischewitz)	6 oz	50	65
Vegetable Beef (Weight Watchers)	7.5 oz	90	450
Vegetable Beef, Microwave (Campbell)	7½ oz	100	830
Vegetarian Vegetable, Bouillon, as prep (Knorr)	8 oz	16	990
asparagus, cream of, as prep w/ water	1 cup	59	801
beef broth	1 pkg (.2 oz)	14	1019
beef broth, as prep w/ water	1 cup	19	1368
beef broth, cube	1 cub (3.6 g)	6	864
beef broth, cube, as prep w/ water	1 cup	8	1152
celery, cream of, as prep w/ water	1 cup	63	839
chicken broth	1 pkg (.2 oz)	16	1116
as prep w/ water	1 cup	21	1484
cube	1 cube (4.8 g)	9	1152
cube, as prep w/ water	1 cup	13	792
chicken, cream of, as prep w/ water	1 cup	107	1184
chicken noodle, as prep w/ water	1 cup	53	1284
french onion, not prep	1 pkg (1.4 oz)	115	3493
leek, as prep w/ water	1 cup	71	966
onion, as prep w/ water	1 cup	28	848
tomato, as prep w/ water	1 cup	102	943
FROZEN Asparagus, Cream Of (Kettle Ready)	6 oz	62	415

FOOD	PORTION	CALORIES	SODIUM
Barley & Mushroom (Jaclyn's)	7.5 oz	90	234
Black Bean With Ham (Kettle Ready)	6 oz	154	567
Boston Clam Chowder (Kettle Ready)	6 oz	131	420
Broccoli, Cream Of (Kettle Ready)	6 oz	94	487
Cauliflower, Cream Of (Kettle Ready)	6 oz	93	432
Cheddar Broccoli, Cream Of (Kettle Ready)	6 oz	137	595
Chicken, Cream Of (Kettle Ready)	6 oz	98	676
Chicken Gumbo (Kettle Ready)	6 oz	94	380
Chicken Noodle (Kettle Ready)	6 oz	94	599
Chili (Kettle Ready)	6 oz	161	425
Corn & Broccoli Chowder (Kettle Ready)	6 oz	102	451
Creamy Cheddar (Kettle Ready)	6 oz	158	625
French Onion (Kettle Ready)	6 oz	42	508
Garden Vegetable (Kettle Ready)	6 oz	85	460
Hearty Beef Vegetable (Kettle Ready)	6 oz	85	353
Minestrone (Kettle Ready)	6 oz	104	352
Manhattan Clam Chowder (Kettle Ready)	6 oz	69	564
Mushroom, Cream Of (Kettle Ready)	6 oz	85	422
New England Clam Chowder (Kettle Ready)	6 oz	116	336
Potato, Cream Of (Kettle Ready)	6 oz	121	404
Savory Bean With Ham (Kettle Ready)	6 oz	113	404
Split Pea (Jaclyn's)	7.5 oz	180	183

FOOD	PORTION	CALORIES	SODIUM
With Ham (Kettle Ready)	6 oz	155	351
Tomato Florentine (Kettle Ready)	6 oz	106	389
Tortellini In Tomato (Kettle Ready)	6 oz	122	548
Vegetable (Jaclyn's)	7.5 oz	90	195
HOME RECIPE			
black bean turtle soup	1 cup	241	6
corn & cheese chowder	¾ cup	215	386
greek	¾ cup	63	386
SHELF STABLE			
Chunky Beef Vegetable (Healthy Choice)	7.5 oz cup	110	490
Chunky Chicken Noodle & Vegetable (Healthy Choice)	7.5 oz cup	160	500
TAKE-OUT			
gazpacho	1 cup	46	63

SOUR CREAM
(*see also* SOUR CREAM SUBSTITUTES)

FOOD	PORTION	CALORIES	SODIUM
Breakstone	1 tbsp	30	5
Light Choice Cultured Half&Half	1 tbsp	25	10
Cabot	1 oz	60	15
Light	1 oz	33	72
Knudsen			
Hampshire	1 oz	60	10
Light N'Lively Light	1 oz	40	20
Land O'Lakes			
Light	2 tbsp	40	35
Light With Chives	2 tbsp	40	150
Sealtest	1 tbsp	30	5
Light Cultured Half&Half	1 tbsp	25	10

FOOD	PORTION	CALORIES	SODIUM
Weight Watchers Light Sour	2 tbsp	35	40
sour cream	1 cup	493	123
sour cream	1 tbsp	26	6

SOUR CREAM SUBSTITUTES

nondairy	1 cup	479	235
nondairy	1 oz	59	29

SOURSOP

fresh	1	416	87
fresh, cut up	1 cup	150	31

SOY
(*see also* TOFU)

Soo Moo Beverage (Health Valley)	1 cup	120	55
Soy Sauce			
(Kikkoman)	1 tbsp	12	938
(La Choy)	½ tsp	2	230
Lite (Kikkoman)	1 tbsp	13	564
Lite (La Choy)	½ tsp	1	110
Soybean Flakes (Arrowhead)	2 oz	250	2
Soybeans (Arrowhead)	2 oz	230	2
milk	1 cup	79	30
soy sauce	1 tbsp	7	1024
shoyu	1 tbsp	9	1029
tamari	1 tbsp	11	1005
soybean sprouts			
raw	½ cup	43	5
steamed	½ cup	38	5
stir fried	1 cup	125	14
soybeans			
cooked	1 cup	298	1

FOOD	PORTION	CALORIES	SODIUM
dry roasted	½ cup	387	2
roasted	½ cup	405	140
roasted & toasted	1 cup	490	4
roasted & toasted	1 oz	129	1
salted, roasted & toasted	1 cup	490	176
slated, roasted & toasted	1 oz	129	54

SPAGHETTI
(*see* PASTA, PASTA DINNERS, PASTA SALAD, SPAGHETTI SAUCE)

SPAGHETTI SAUCE
(*see also* PIZZA, TOMATO)

FOOD	PORTION	CALORIES	SODIUM
JARRED			
Estee	4 oz	60	30
Hunt's			
Chunky	4 oz	50	470
Homestyle	4 oz	60	530
Homestyle With Meat	4 oz	60	570
Homestyle With Mushrooms	4 oz	50	530
Traditional	4 oz	70	530
With Meat	4 oz	70	570
With Mushrooms	4 oz	70	560
Newman's Own	4 oz	70	630
Sockarooni	4 oz	70	630
With Mushrooms	4 oz	70	630
Prego			
Marinara	4 oz	100	620
Meat Flavored	4 oz	140	660
Mushroom	4 oz	130	630
Onion And Garlic	4 oz	110	510
Regular	4 oz	130	630

FOOD	PORTION	CALORIES	SODIUM
Prego *(cont.)*			
Three Cheese	4 oz	100	410
Tomato & Basil	4 oz	100	370
Prego Chunky			
Sausage & Green Peppers	4 oz	160	500
Prego Extra Chunky			
Garden Combination	4 oz	80	420
Mushroom And Green Pepper	4 oz	100	410
Mushroom And Onion	4 oz	100	490
Mushroom And Tomato	4 oz	110	500
Mushroom With Extra Spice	4 oz	100	450
Tomato And Onion	4 oz	110	490
Ragu			
Italian Cooking Sauce	4 oz	70	540
Joe	3.5 oz	50	650
Ragu Chunky Gardenstyle			
Extra Tomatoes, Garlic & Onions	4 oz	70	440
Green & Red Peppers	4 oz	70	440
Italian Garden Combination	4 oz	70	440
Mushrooms & Onions	4 oz	70	440
Ragu Homestyle			
w/ Meat	4 oz	110	510
w/ Mushrooms	4 oz	110	530
w/ Tomato & Herbs	4 oz	110	510
Ragu Old World Style			
Marinara	4 oz	80	740
Pizza	1.6 oz	25	200
Plain	4 oz	80	740
w/ Meat	4 oz	80	740
w/ Mushrooms	4 oz	80	740
Ragu Thick & Hearty			
Plain	4 oz	100	460

FOOD	PORTION	CALORIES	SODIUM
w/ Meat	4 oz	120	460
w/ Mushrooms	4 oz	100	460
Weight Watchers w/ Meat	⅓ cup	45	310
With Mushrooms	⅓ cup	35	300
marinara sauce	1 cup	171	1572
spaghetti sauce	1 cup	272	1236

SPARERIBS
(see PORK)

SPICES
(see HERBS/SPICES, individual names)

SPINACH

CANNED			
S&W Northwest Premium	½ cup	25	395
spinach	½ cup	25	29
FRESH			
Dole	3 oz	9	107
cooked	½ cup	21	63
new zealand, chopped, cooked	½ cup	11	97
new zealand, raw	½ cup	4	36
raw, chopped	1 pkg (10 oz)	46	160
raw, chopped	½ cup	6	22
FROZEN			
Budget Gourmet Au Gratin	1 pkg	160	620
Green Giant	½ cup	25	100
Creamed	½ cup	70	480
Cut Leaf In Butter Sauce	½ cup	40	380
Harvest Fresh	½ cup	25	170
cooked	½ cup	27	82

FOOD	PORTION	CALORIES	SODIUM
JUICE			
spinach juice	3½ oz	7	73

SPOT

FRESH			
baked	3 oz	134	32

SQUASH
(see also ZUCCHINI*)*

CANNED			
crookneck, sliced	½ cup	14	5
FRESH			
acorn, cooked, mashed	½ cup	41	3
acorn, cubed, baked	½ cup	57	4
butternut, baked	½ cup	41	4
crookneck, sliced, cooked	½ cup	18	1
crookneck, raw, sliced	½ cup	12	1
hubbard, baked	½ cup	51	8
hubbard, cooked, mashed	½ cup	35	6
scallop, raw, sliced	½ cup	12	1
scallop, sliced, cooked	½ cup	14	1
spaghetti, cooked	½ cup	23	14
FROZEN			
butternut, cooked, mashed	½ cup	47	2
crookneck, sliced, cooked	½ cup	24	6
SEEDS			
dried	1 cup	747	24
dried	1 oz	154	5
roasted	1 cup	1184	40
roasted	1 oz	148	5
salted & roasted	1 cup	1184	1294

FOOD	PORTION	CALORIES	SODIUM
salted & roasted	1 oz	148	5
whole, roasted	1 cup	285	12
whole, roasted	1 oz	127	5
whole, salted, roasted	1 cup	285	368
whole, salted, roasted	1 oz	127	191

SQUID

FRESH			
fried	3 oz	149	260
raw	3 oz	78	37

SQUIRREL

roasted	3 oz	147	102

STRAWBERRIES

CANNED			
in heavy syrup	½ cup	117	5
FRESH			
Dole	8	50	0
strawberries	1 cup	45	2
strawberries	1 pint	97	4
FROZEN			
sweetened, sliced	1 cup	245	8
sweetened, sliced	1 pkg (10 oz)	273	9
unsweetened	1 cup	52	3
whole, sweetened	1 cup	200	3
whole, sweetened	1 pkg (10 oz)	223	3
JUICE			
Kern's Nectar	6 oz	110	0
Libby's			
Nectar	6 oz	110	0

FOOD	PORTION	CALORIES	SODIUM
Libby's *(cont.)*			
Ripe Nectar	8 oz	150	5
Smucker's	8 oz	130	10
Wylers Drink Mix, Unsweetened, Strawberry Split	8 oz	2	28

STUFFING/DRESSING

FOOD	PORTION	CALORIES	SODIUM
HOME RECIPE			
bread, as prep w/ water & fat	½ cup	251	627
bread, as prep w/ water, egg & fat	½ cup	107	319
sausage	½ cup	292	258
MIX			
Betty Crocker			
Chicken	½ cup	180	620
Traditional Herb	½ cup	180	640
Golden Grain Bread Stuffing			
Chicken	½ cup	180	730
Corn Bread	½ cup	180	870
Herb & Butter	½ cup	180	810
With Wild Rice	½ cup	180	710
Pepperidge Farm			
Corn Bread	1 oz	110	320
Country Style	1 oz	100	400
Cube	1 oz	110	400
Distinctive Apple Raisin	1 oz	110	410
Distinctive Classic Chicken	1 oz	110	410
Distinctive Country Garden Herb	1 oz	120	300
Distinctive Vegetable & Almond	1 oz	110	250
Distinctive Wild Rice & Mushroom	1 oz	130	310

FOOD	PORTION	CALORIES	SODIUM
Herb Seasoned	1 oz	110	380
bread, dry	1 cup	500	1254

SUCKER

white, baked	3 oz	101	44

SUGAR
(*see also* FRUCTOSE, SUGAR SUBSTITUTES, SYRUP)

brown	1 cup	820	97
powdered, sifted	1 cup	385	2
white	1 cup	770	5
white	1 packet (6 g)	25	tr
white	1 tbsp	45	tr

SUGAR SUBSTITUTES
(*see also* FRUCTOSE)

Equal	1 pkg	4	0
Estee Swiss			
Sweet Packet	6 pkg	4	0
Sweet Tablet	1	0	0
S&W Liquid Table Sweetener	⅛ tsp	0	0
Sprinkle Sweet	1 tsp	2	1
SugarTwin	1 pkg	3	5
SugarTwin	1 tsp	2	3
SugarTwin, Brown	1 tsp	2	3
Sweet One	1 pkg	4	0
Sweet*10	⅛ tsp	0	2
Weight Watchers Sweet'ner	1 pkg	4	20

SUGAR-APPLE

fresh	1	146	15
fresh, cut up	1 cup	236	24

FOOD	PORTION	CALORIES	SODIUM

SUNDAE TOPPINGS
(see ICE CREAM TOPPINGS)

SUNFISH

FOOD	PORTION	CALORIES	SODIUM
pumpkinseed, baked	3 oz	97	87

SUNFLOWER SEEDS

FOOD	PORTION	CALORIES	SODIUM
Sunflower Butter (Erewhon)	2 tbsp	200	20
Sunflower Nuts, Dry Roasted, Unsalted (Planters)	1 oz	170	0
Sunflower Seeds			
(Arrowhead)	1 oz	160	3
(Planters)	1 oz	160	30
dried	1 cup	821	4
dried	1 oz	162	1
dry roasted	1 cup	745	4
dry roasted	1 oz	165	1
dry roasted, salted	1 cup	745	975
dry roasted, salted	1 oz	165	195
oil roasted	1 cup	830	4
oil roasted, salted	1 cup	830	804
oil roasted, salted	1 oz	175	201
sunflower butter	1 tbsp	93	82
sunflower butter, w/o salt	1 tbsp	93	1
toasted	1 cup	826	4
toasted	1 oz	176	1
toasted, salted	1 cup	826	817
toasted, salted	1 oz	176	204

FOOD	PORTION	CALORIES	SODIUM

SWAMP CABBAGE

FRESH			
chopped, cooked	½ cup	10	60
raw, chopped	1 cup	11	63

SWEET POTATO
(see also YAM)

CANNED			
in syrup	½ cup	106	38
pieces	1 cup	183	107
FRESH			
baked, w/ skin	1 (3½ oz)	118	12
leaves, cooked	½ cup	11	4
mashed	½ cup	172	21
FROZEN			
Candied			
Sweet Potatoes (Mrs. Paul's)	4 oz	170	40
Sweets 'N Apples (Mrs. Paul's)	4 oz	160	60
cooked	½ cup	88	7
HOME RECIPE			
candied	3½ oz	144	73

SWEETBREADS

beef, braised	3 oz	230	51
lamb, braised	3 oz	199	44

SWISS CHARD

FRESH			
cooked	½ cup	18	158
raw, chopped	½ cup	3	38

FOOD	PORTION	CALORIES	SODIUM

SWORDFISH

FOOD	PORTION	CALORIES	SODIUM
cooked	3 oz	132	98
raw	3 oz	103	76

SYRUP
(*see also* ICE CREAM TOPPINGS, PANCAKE/WAFFLE SYRUP)

FOOD	PORTION	CALORIES	SODIUM
Blueberry			
(Estee)	1 tbsp	8	25
(Whistling Wings)	1 oz	45	1
Diet (S&W)	1 tbsp	4	25
Corn Syrup			
Dark (Karo)	1 cup	975	610
Dark (Karo)	1 tbsp	60	40
Light (Karo)	1 cup	960	480
Light (Karo)	1 tbsp	60	30
Fruit Syrup, All Flavors (Smucker's)	2 tbsp	100	<10
Maple Flavored, Diet (S&W)	1 tbsp	4	25
Raspberry (Whistling Wings)	1 oz	60	2
Strawberry, Diet (S&W)	1 tbsp	4	25
corn	2 tbsp	122	19
raspberry	3½ oz	267	2

TAHINI
(*see* SESAME)

TAMARIND

FOOD	PORTION	CALORIES	SODIUM
fresh	1	5	1
fresh, cut up	1 cup	287	33

FOOD	PORTION	CALORIES	SODIUM

TANGERINE

CANNED

| in light syrup | ½ cup | 76 | 8 |
| juice pack | ½ cup | 46 | 7 |

FRESH

Dole	2	70	2
sections	1 cup	86	3
tangerine	1	37	1

JUICE

Dole Pure & Light	6 oz	100	20
canned, sweetened	1 cup	125	2
fresh	1 cup	106	2
frzn, sweetened, as prep	1 cup	110	2
frzn, sweetened, not prep	6 oz	344	7

TAPIOCA

| pearl, dry | ⅓ cup | 174 | 0 |
| starch | 3½ oz | 344 | 4 |

TARO

chips	½ cup	57	44
chips	10	110	85
leaves, cooked	½ cup	18	2
raw, sliced	½ cup	56	6
shoots, sliced, cooked	½ cup	10	1
sliced, cooked	½ cup	94	10
tahitian, sliced, cooked	½ cup	30	37

TARRAGON

| ground | 1 tsp | 5 | 1 |

FOOD	PORTION	CALORIES	SODIUM

TEA/HERBAL TEA

REGULAR
Lipton Iced Tea

Lemon w/ Vitamin C	6 oz	58	6
Mix, Lemon	6 oz	55	1
Sugar Free	8 oz	1	6
Sugar Free, Peach	8 oz	5	1
Sugar Free, Raspberry	8 oz	5	1
With Nutrasweet	8 oz	3	1
With Nutrasweet, Decaffeinated	8 oz	3	1
Lipton Instant	6 oz	0	0
Lemon	8 oz	3	1
Raspberry	8 oz	3	1
Decaffeinated	6 oz	0	0
Nestea			
100% Instant Tea, as prep	8 oz	2	0
Decaffeinated 100% Instant, as prep	8 oz	0	0
Iced Tea Mix With Sugar And Lemon, as prep	8 oz	70	0
Lemon	8 oz	6	0
Tea Bag, as prep	6 oz	0	0
Nestea Ice Teasers			
Citrus	8 oz	6	0
Lemon	8 oz	6	0
Orange	8 oz	6	0
Tropical	8 oz	6	0
Wild Cherry	8 oz	6	0
Nestea Ready-to-Drink			
Iced Tea With Sugar and Lemon	8 oz	70	0
Sugarfree Iced Tea w/ Lemon	8 oz	2	0

FOOD	PORTION	CALORIES	SODIUM
Nestea Sugarfree			
Decaffeinated Iced Tea Mix	2 tsp	6	0
Iced Tea Mix	8 oz	4	0
brewed tea	6 oz	2	5
Instant			
artificially sweetened, lemon flavored, as prep w/ water	8 oz	5	24
unsweetened, as prep w/ water	8 oz	2	8
unsweetened, lemon flavor, as prep w/ water	8 oz	4	14

TEFF

Seeds (Arrowhead)	2 oz	200	6

TEMPEH

tempeh	½ cup	165	5

THYME

ground	1 tsp	4	1

TILEFISH

FRESH			
cooked	½ fillet (5.3 oz)	220	88
cooked	3 oz	125	50
raw	3 oz	81	45

TOFU

Azumaya			
Blue Label	3.5 oz	46	2
Green Label	3.5 oz	68	2
Name Age Fried	3.5 oz	144	2
Red Label	3.5 oz	68	3

FOOD	PORTION	CALORIES	SODIUM
Jaclyn's, Grilled			
in Black Bean Sauce	10.75 oz	270	170
In Peanut Sauce	10.75 oz	260	145
Mori-Nu Silken			
Extra-Firm	½ box (5¼ oz)	90	95
Firm	½ box (5¼ oz)	90	50
Soft	½ box (5¼ oz)	80	10
Spring Creek			
Baked Barbecue	2 oz	88	234
Baked Cajun	2 oz	87	228
Baked Teriyaki	2 oz	84	393
Great Balls Of Tofu!	2 (3 oz)	107	485
Nigari, Firm	4 oz	140	30
Spring Creek Tofu Salads			
Missing Egg	2 oz	49	167
!Onion Dip	2 oz	46	155
!Taco Dip	2 oz	46	175
firm	½ cup	183	17
firm	¼ block (3 oz)	118	11
fresh, fried	1 piece (½ oz)	35	2
fuyu, salted & fermented	1 block (⅓ oz)	13	316
koyadofu, dried, frzn	1 piece (½ oz)	82	1
okara	½ cup	47	6
regular	½ cup	94	9
regular	¼ block (4 oz)	88	8
YOGURT			
Stir Fruity			
Black Cherry	6 oz	141	51
Blueberry	6 oz	140	43
Lemon Chiffon	6 oz	152	43
Mixed Berry	6 oz	149	34
Orange	6 oz	143	51

FOOD	PORTION	CALORIES	SODIUM
Peach	6 oz	160	34
Piña Colada	6 oz	162	43
Raspberry	6 oz	155	34
Spiced Apple	6 oz	167	43
Strawberry	6 oz	140	51
Tropical Fruit	6 oz	170	43

TOFUTTI
(*see* ICE CREAM AND FROZEN DESSERT)

TOMATILLO
fresh	1 (1.2 oz)	11	0
fresh, chopped	½ cup	21	1

TOMATO
(*see also* PIZZA, SPAGHETTI SAUCE)

CANNED			
Health Valley			
Sauce	1 cup	70	460
Sauce, Low Sodium	1 cup	70	35
Hunt's			
Crushed Angela Mia	4 oz	35	260
Crushed Italian	4 oz	40	460
Italian Pear Shaped	4 oz	20	320
Peeled, Choice-Cut	4 oz	20	460
Puree	4 oz	45	150
Paste	2 oz	45	135
Paste Italian Style	2 oz	50	430
Paste No Salt Added	2 oz	45	25
Paste With Garlic	2 oz	50	440
Sauce	4 oz	30	650
Sauce Herb	4 oz	70	470

FOOD	PORTION	CALORIES	SODIUM
Hunt's *(cont.)*			
Sauce Italian	4 oz	60	460
Sauce Meatloaf Fixin's	4 oz	20	580
Sauce No Salt Added	4 oz	35	20
Sauce Special	4 oz	35	280
Sauce With Bits	4 oz	30	620
Sauce With Garlic	4 oz	70	480
Sauce With Mushrooms	4 oz	25	710
Stewed	4 oz	35	400
Stewed Italian	4 oz	40	370
Stewed No Salt Added	4 oz	35	20
Whole	4 oz	20	330
Whole Italian	4 oz	25	420
Whole No Salt Added	4 oz	20	15
S&W			
Aspic Supreme	½ cup	60	860
Diced In Rich Puree	½ cup	35	290
Italian, Stewed, Sliced	½ cup	35	355
Italian Style w/ Basil	½ cup	25	220
Mexican Style, Stewed	½ cup	40	360
Paste	6 oz	150	100
Peeled, Ready Cut	½ cup	25	220
Puree	½ cup	60	35
Sauce	½ cup	40	620
Sauce Chunky	½ cup	45	615
Stewed Sliced	½ cup	35	355
Stewed 50% Salt Reduced	½ cup	35	180
Whole Diet	½ cup	25	20
Whole Peeled	½ cup	25	220
paste	½ cup	110	86

FOOD	PORTION	CALORIES	SODIUM
puree	1 cup	102	532
puree, w/o salt	1 cup	102	49
red, whole	½ cup	24	195
sauce	½ cup	37	738
sauce w/ mushrooms	½ cup	42	552
sauce w/ onion	½ cup	52	672
stewed	½ cup	34	325
w/ green chiles	½ cup	18	481
wedges in tomato juice	½ cup	34	285
DRIED			
sun dried	1 cup	140	1131
sun dried	1 piece	5	42
sun dried, in oil	1 cup	235	293
sun dried, in oil	1 piece	6	8
FRESH			
cooked	½ cup	32	13
green	1	30	16
red	1 (4½ oz)	26	11
red, chopped	1 cup	35	16
JUICE			
Campbell	6 oz	40	540
Hunt's	6 oz	30	520
No Salt Added	6 oz	35	25
Libby's	6 oz	35	450
S&W California	5½ oz	35	550
S&W California	6 oz	35	600
S&W Diet	½ cup	35	20
beef broth & tomato	5½ oz	61	220
clam & tomato	1 can (5½ oz)	77	664
tomato juice	½ cup	21	441

FOOD	PORTION	CALORIES	SODIUM
tomato juice	6 oz	32	658
TAKE-OUT stewed	1 cup	80	460

TONGUE

beef, simmered	3 oz	241	51
lamb, braised	3 oz	234	57
pork, braised	3 oz	230	93

TOPPINGS
(*see* ICE CREAM TOPPINGS, WHIPPED TOPPINGS)

TREE FERN

chopped, cooked	½ cup	28	3

TRITICALE
(*see also* FLOUR)

dry	½ cup	323	5

TROUT

FRESH baked	3 oz	162	57
rainbow, cooked	3 oz	129	29
sea trout, baked	3 oz	113	63

TRUFFLES

fresh	3½ oz	25	77

TUNA
(*see also* TUNA DISHES)

CANNED Bumble Bee Chunk Light In Oil	2 oz	160	310

FOOD	PORTION	CALORIES	SODIUM
Chunk Light In Water	2 oz	60	310
Solid White In Oil	2 oz	130	310
Solid White In Water	2 oz	70	310
Empress			
Chunk Light	2 oz	60	310
Chunk Light Tongol	2 oz	50	55
Solid White	2 oz	70	310
S&W			
Chunk Light Fancy In Oil	2 oz	140	450
Chunk Light Fancy In Water	2 oz	60	500
Fancy White Albacore in Oil	2 oz	160	450
light, in oil	1 can (6 oz)	399	606
light, in oil	3 oz	169	301
light, in water	1 can (5.8 oz)	192	558
light, in water	3 oz	99	287
white, in oil	1 can (6.2 oz)	331	704
white, in oil	3 oz	158	336
white, in water	1 can (6 oz)	234	673
white, in water	3 oz	116	333
FRESH			
bluefin, cooked	3 oz	157	43
bluefin, raw	3 oz	122	33
skipjack, baked	3 oz	112	40
yellowfin, baked	3 oz	118	40

TUNA DISHES

FROZEN			
Microwave Tuna Sandwich (Mrs. Paul's)	1	200	590
MIX			
Tuna Helper			
Au Gratin, as prep	⅕ pkg (6 oz)	280	980

FOOD	PORTION	CALORIES	SODIUM
Tuna Helper *(cont.)*			
Buttery Rice, as prep	⅕ pkg (6 oz)	280	1040
Creamy Mushroom, as prep	⅕ pkg (7 oz)	220	740
Creamy Noodles, as prep	⅕ pkg (8 oz)	300	960
Cheesy Noodles, as prep	⅕ pkg (7.75 oz)	240	980
Fettucine Alfredo, as prep	⅕ pkg (7 oz)	300	1000
Romanoff, as prep	⅕ pkg (8 oz)	290	820
Tetrazzini, as prep	⅕ pkg (6 oz)	240	780
Tuna Pot Pie, as prep	⅙ pkg (5.1 oz)	420	890
Tuna Salad, as prep	⅕ pkg (5.5 oz)	420	870
Tuna Mix-ins Garden Herb	.2 oz	25	5
TAKE-OUT			
tuna salad	1 cup	383	824
tuna salad	3 oz	159	342
tuna salad, submarine sandwich w/ lettuce & oil	1	584	1294

TURBOT

FOOD	PORTION	CALORIES	SODIUM
FRESH			
european, baked	3 oz	104	163

TURKEY

(*see also* DINNER, HOT DOG, TURKEY DISHES)

FOOD	PORTION	CALORIES	SODIUM
CANNED			
White (Swanson)	2½ oz	80	260
w/ broth	1 can (5 oz)	231	663
w/ broth	½ can (2.5 oz)	116	332
FRESH			
Breast			
Cutlets, Thin-Sliced, Skinless & Boneless (Perdue)	1 oz	28	13

FOOD	PORTION	CALORIES	SODIUM
Fillets, Skinless & Boneless, Fit 'n Easy, cooked (Perdue)	1 oz	28	13
Hotel Style, Prime w/ Skin, cooked (Perdue)	1 oz	43	12
Skinless, Boneless, Fit 'n Easy, cooked (Perdue)	1 oz	28	13
Tenderloins, Skinless & Boneless, cooked (Perdue)	1 oz	29	12
w/ Skin, Fresh Young, cooked (Perdue)	1 oz	44	14
Drumsticks w/ Skin, Fresh Young, cooked (Perdue)	1 oz	36	19
Ground Breast Meat, cooked (Perdue)	1 oz	28	13
Ground, cooked (Perdue)	1 oz	35	17
Thighs Skinless & Boneless, Fit 'n Fresh, cooked (Perdue)	1 oz	36	15
w/ Skin, Fresh Young, cooked (Perdue)	1 oz	48	20
Whole Dark Meat w/ skin, cooked (Perdue)	1 oz	48	18
White Meat, Fresh Young w/ skin, cooked (Perdue)	1 oz	44	13
Wings Drummettes w/ Skin, Fresh Young, cooked (Perdue)	1 oz	43	18
Portions w/ Skin, Fresh Young, cooked (Perdue)	1 oz	51	18
w/ Skin, Fresh Young, cooked (Perdue)	1 oz	45	20
back, w/ skin, roasted	½ back (9 oz)	637	191
breast, w/ skin, roasted	4 oz	212	70
dark meat, w/ skin, roasted	3.6 oz	230	79
dark meat, w/o skin, roasted	1 cup (5 oz)	262	110

FOOD	PORTION	CALORIES	SODIUM
dark meat, w/o skin, roasted	3 oz	170	72
ground, cooked	3 oz	188	68
leg, w/ skin, roasted	1 (1.2 lb)	1133	420
leg, w/ skin, roasted	2.5 oz	147	55
light meat, w/ skin, roasted	4.7 oz	268	85
light meat, w/ skin, roasted	from ½ turkey (2.3 lb)	2069	658
light meat, w/o skin, roasted	4 oz	183	75
neck, simmered	1 (5.3 oz)	274	84
skin, roasted	1 oz	141	17
skin, roasted	from ½ turkey (9 oz)	1096	132
w/ skin, neck & giblets, roasted	½ turkey (8.8 lb)	4123	1358
w/ skin, roasted	½ turkey (4 lb)	3857	1269
w/ skin, roasted	8.4 oz	498	164
w/o skin, roasted	1 cup (5 oz)	238	99
w/o skin, roasted	7.3 oz	354	147
wing, w/ skin, roasted	1 (6.5 oz)	426	114
FROZEN			
roast, boneless, seasoned light & dark meat, roasted	1 pkg (1.7 lb)	1213	5320
READY-TO-USE			
Carl Buddig	1 oz	50	400
Turkey Ham	1 oz	40	430
Hansel & Gretel			
Doubledecker Turkey-Corned Beef	1 oz	30	195
Doubledecker Turkey-Ham	1 oz	30	185
Gourmet Breast	1 oz	28	170
Gourmet Smoked Breast	1 oz	31	170
Honey Breast	1 oz	28	170

FOOD	PORTION	CALORIES	SODIUM
Lessalt Cooked Breast	1 oz	25	140
Oven Cooked Breast	1 oz	26	180
Perdue Done It! Nuggets	1 (.67 oz)	54	112
Weight Watchers Deli Thin Smoked Breast	5 slices (⅓ oz)	10	80
Oven Roasted Breast	2 slices (¾ oz)	25	200
Oven Roasted Turkey Ham	2 slices (¾ oz)	25	210
Roasted And Smoked Breast	2 slices (¾ oz)	25	170
bologna	1 oz	57	249
breast	1 slice (¾ oz)	23	301
diced, light & dark, seasoned	1 oz	39	241
diced, light & dark, seasoned	½ lb	313	1928
ham, thigh meat	1 pkg (8 oz)	291	2260
ham, thigh meat	2 oz	73	565
pastrami	1 pkg (8 oz)	320	2372
pastrami	2 oz	80	698
patties, battered & fried	1 (2.3 oz)	181	512
patties, battered & fried	1 (3.3 oz)	266	752
patties, breaded & fried	1 (2.3 oz)	181	512
patties, breaded & fried	1 (3.3 oz)	266	752
poultry salad sandwich spread	1 oz	238	107
poultry salad sandwich spread	1 tbsp	109	49
prebasted breast w/ skin, roasted	1 breast (3.8 lb)	2175	6868
prebasted breast w/ skin, roasted	½ breast (1.9 lb)	1087	3434
prebasted thigh w/ skin, roasted	1 thigh (11 oz)	494	1371
roll, light & dark meat	1 oz	42	166
roll, light meat	1 oz	42	139
salami, cooked	1 pkg (8 oz)	446	2278
salami, cooked	2 oz	111	569
turkey loaf, breast meat	1 pkg (6 oz)	187	2433

FOOD	PORTION	CALORIES	SODIUM
turkey loaf, breast meat	2 slices (1.5 oz)	47	608
turkey sticks, battered & fried	1 stick (2.3 oz)	178	536
turkey sticks, breaded & fried	1 stick (2.3 oz)	178	536

TURKEY DISHES
(*see also* DINNER)

FROZEN			
Ovenstuffs Turkey Turnover	1 (4.75 oz)	350	700
gravy & turkey	1 cup (8.4 oz)	160	1328
gravy & turkey	1 pkg (5 oz)	95	786

TURMERIC

ground	1 tsp	8	1

TURNIPS

CANNED			
greens	½ cup	17	325
FRESH			
cooked, mashed	½ cup	21	58
greens, chopped, cooked	½ cup	15	21
greens, raw, chopped	½ cup	7	11
raw, cubed	½ cup	18	44
FROZEN			
greens, cooked	½ cup	24	12

TUSK FISH

raw	3½ oz	79	113

VANILLA

Vanilla Milk Chips (Hershey)	¼ cup	240	65

FOOD	PORTION	CALORIES	SODIUM

VEAL
(*see also* BEEF, DINNER, VEAL DISHES)

FRESH

cutlet, lean only, braised	3 oz	172	57
cutlet, lean only, fried	3 oz	156	65
ground, broiled	3 oz	146	70
loin chop, w/ bone, lean & fat, braised	1 chop (2.8 oz)	227	64
loin chop, w/ bone, lean only, braised	1 chop (2.4 oz)	155	58
shoulder, w/ bone, lean only, braised	3 oz	169	83
sirloin, w/ bone, lean & fat, roasted	3 oz	171	71
sirloin, w/ bone, lean only, roasted	3 oz	143	72

TAKE-OUT

parmigiana	4.2 oz	279	545

VEGETABLES MIXED
(*see also* individual vegetables)

CANNED

Chop Suey Vegetables (La Choy)	½ cup	10	320
Garden Medley (Green Giant)	½ cup	40	290
Garden Salad Marinated (S&W)	½ cup	60	670
Mixed Vegetables, Old Fashion Harvest Time (S&W)	½ cup	35	380
Peas & Carrots Water Pack (S&W)	½ cup	35	5
Succotash Country Style (S&W)	½ cup	80	250
Sweet Peas & Diced Carrots (S&W)	½ cup	50	310
w/ Tiny Pearl Onions (S&W)	½ cup	60	490

FOOD	PORTION	CALORIES	SODIUM
mixed vegetables	½ cup	39	122
peas & carrots	½ cup	48	332
peas & carrots, low sodium	½ cup	48	332
peas & onions	½ cup	30	265
succotash	½ cup	102	325
FROZEN			
American Mixtures			
California (Green Giant)	½ cup	25	40
Heartland (Green Giant)	½ cup	25	35
New England (Green Giant)	½ cup	70	75
San Francisco (Green Giant)	½ cup	25	35
Sante Fe (Green Giant)	½ cup	70	0
Seattle (Green Giant)	½ cup	25	35
Breaded Medley (Ore Ida)	3 oz	160	490
Broccoli, Cauliflower And Carrots			
In Butter Sauce (Green Giant)	½ cup	30	240
in Cheese Sauce (Green Giant)	½ cup	60	490
Harvest Fresh Mixed Vegetables (Green Giant)	½ cup	40	125
Mandarin Vegetables (Budget Gourmet)	1 pkg	160	440
Mixed Fancy (La Choy)	½ cup	12	30
Mixed Vegetables			
(Green Giant)	½ cup	40	40
In Butter Sauce (Green Giant)	½ cup	60	300
New England Recipe Vegetables (Budget Gourmet)	1 pkg	230	390
One Serve			
Broccoli, Carrots & Rotini In Cheese Sauce (Green Giant)	1 pkg	120	520
Broccoli, Cauliflower And Carrots (Green Giant)	1 pkg	25	45

FOOD	PORTION	CALORIES	SODIUM
Peas			
& Cauliflower In Cream Sauce (Budget Gourmet)	1 pkg	150	550
And Waterchestnuts Oriental (Budget Gourmet)	1 pkg	110	410
Spring Vegetables In Cheese Sauce (Budget Gourmet)	1 pkg	150	440
Stew Vegetables (Ore Ida)	3 oz	50	35
Valley Combinations, Broccoli & Cauliflower (Green Giant)	½ cup	60	340
mixed vegetables, cooked	½ cup	54	32
peas & carrots, cooked	½ cup	38	55
succotash, cooked	½ cup	79	38
HOME RECIPE			
succotash	½ cup	111	16
JUICE			
Smucker's Vegetable Juice Hearty	8 oz	58	714
Hot & Spicy	8 oz	58	650
V8	6 oz	35	560
V8, No Salt Added	6 oz	35	45
V8, Spicy Hot	6 oz	35	650
vegetable juice cocktail	½ cup	22	442
vegetable juice cocktail	6 oz	34	664
SHELF STABLE			
Corn, Green Beans, Carrots, Pasta In Tomato Sauce (Pantry Express)	½ cup	80	330
Green Beans, Potatoes And Mushrooms In A Seasoned Sauce (Pantry Express)	½ cup	50	430
Mixed Vegetables (Pantry Express)	½ cup	35	300

FOOD	PORTION	CALORIES	SODIUM

VENISON

roasted	3 oz	134	46

VINEGAR

Apple Cider (White House)	2 tbsp	2	0
Red Wine			
(Regina)	1 oz	4	0
(White House)	2 tbsp	4	5
cider	1 tbsp	tr	tr

WAFFLES

FROZEN			
Apple Cinnamon			
(Aunt Jemima)	2.5 oz	176	616
(Eggo)	1	130	250
Belgian			
(Weight Watchers)	1 (1.5 oz)	120	220
And Sausage (Great Starts)	2.85 oz	280	420
Strawberries And Sausage (Great Starts)	3½ oz	210	240
Blueberry			
(Aunt Jemima)	2.5 oz	175	684
(Eggo)	1	130	250
Batter, as prep (Aunt Jemima)	3.6 oz	204	688
Buttermilk			
(Aunt Jemima)	2.5 oz	179	615
(Eggo)	1	130	40
Homestyle (Eggo)	1	130	250
Minis (Eggo)	4	90	190
Multi Bran (Nutri-Grain)	1	120	220
Multi-Grain, Belgian (Weight Watchers)	1 (1.5 oz)	120	200

FOOD	PORTION	CALORIES	SODIUM
Nut And Honey (Eggo)	1	130	60
Oat Bran (Common Sense)	1	110	220
Fruit And Nut (Common Sense)	1	120	220
Original (Aunt Jemima)	2.5 oz	173	591
Plain (Nutri-Grain)	1	120	250
Raisin And Bran (Nutri-Grain)	1	120	250
Special K (Kellogg's)	1	80	120
Strawberry (Eggo)	1	130	50
Waffle (Kid Cuisine)	3.6 oz	160	340
With Bacon (Great Starts)	2.2 oz	230	710
Wholegrain Wheat/Oat Bran (Aunt Jemima)	2.5 oz	154	676
HOME RECIPE waffle	7" diam	245	445
MIX as prep w/ egg & milk	1 waffle (2.6 oz)	205	515

WALNUTS

FOOD	PORTION	CALORIES	SODIUM
Black (Planters)	1 oz	180	0
English Halves (Planters)	1 oz	190	0
black, dried	1 oz	172	0
black, dried, chopped	1 cup	759	2
english, dried	1 oz	182	3
english, dried, chopped	1 cup	770	12

WATER CHESTNUTS

FOOD	PORTION	CALORIES	SODIUM
CANNED Empress Sliced	2 oz	14	10

FOOD	PORTION	CALORIES	SODIUM
Empress *(cont.)*			
Whole	2 oz	14	10
La Choy			
Sliced	¼ cup	18	3
Whole	4	14	2
chinese, sliced	½ cup	35	6
FRESH			
sliced	½ cup	66	9

WATERCRESS
(*see also* CRESS)

raw, chopped	½ cup	2	7

WATERMELON

cut up	1 cup	50	3
wedge	1⁄16	152	10
SEEDS			
dried	1 cup	602	28
dried	1 oz	158	28

WAX BEANS

CANNED			
Golden Cut, Premium (S&W)	½ cup	20	385

WHALE

raw	3.5 oz	134	100

WHEAT
(*see also* BRAN, BULGUR, CEREAL, COUSCOUS, FLOUR, WHEAT GERM)

Hard Red			
Spring (Arrowhead)	2 oz	190	tr
Winter (Arrowhead)	2 oz	190	tr

FOOD	PORTION	CALORIES	SODIUM
Soft Red (Arrowhead)	2 oz	190	tr
Vital Wheat Gluten (Arrowhead)	2 oz	200	tr
Wheat Flakes (Arrowhead)	2 oz	210	1
sprouted	⅓ cup	71	6
starch	3½ oz	348	2

WHEAT GERM

Arrowhead Raw	2 oz	210	1
Kretschmer	¼ cup	103	2
Honey Crunch	¼ cup	105	2
plain, toasted	1 cup	431	4
plain, toasted	¼ cup	108	1
plain, untoasted	¼ cup	104	4
w/ brown sugar & honey, toasted	1 cup	426	3
w/ brown sugar & honey, toasted	1 oz	107	1

WHELK
(*see* SNAIL)

WHIPPED TOPPINGS
(*see also* CREAM)

Estee Whipped Topping, as prep	1 tbsp	4	0
Kraft			
Real Cream Topping	¼ cup	30	5
Whipped Topping	¼ cup	35	10
cream, pressurized	1 cup	154	78
cream, pressurized	1 tbsp	8	4
nondairy, frzn	1 tbsp	13	1
nondairy, powdered, as prep w/ whole milk	1 cup	151	53
nondairy, powdered, as prep w/ whole milk	1 tbsp	8	3

FOOD	PORTION	CALORIES	SODIUM
nondairy, pressurized	1 cup	184	43
nondairy, pressurized	1 tbsp	11	2

WHITE BEANS

CANNED			
Goya Spanish Style	7.5 oz	130	990
white beans	1 cup	306	13
DRIED			
regular, cooked	1 cup	249	11
small, cooked	1 cup	253	4

WHITEFISH

FRESH			
baked	3 oz	146	56
SMOKED			
whitefish	1 oz	39	285
whitefish	3 oz	92	866

WHITING

FRESH			
cooked	3 oz	98	113
raw	3 oz	77	61

WILD RICE

cooked	½	83	3

WINE

red	3½ oz	74	6
rose	3½ oz	73	5
sweet, dessert	2 oz	90	5
white	3½ oz	70	5

FOOD	PORTION	CALORIES	SODIUM
WINGED BEANS			
DRIED			
cooked	1 cup	252	22
WOLFFISH			
FRESH			
atlantic, baked	3 oz	105	93
YAM			
(see also SWEET POTATO)			
CANNED			
S&W			
Candied	½ cup	180	355
Southern, Whole, In Extra Heavy Syrup	½ cup	139	27
FRESH			
mountain yam, hawaii, cooked	½ cup	59	9
yam, cubed, cooked	½ cup	79	6
YAMBEAN			
cooked	¾ cup	38	4
YARDLONG BEANS			
DRIED			
cooked	1 cup	202	9
YEAST			
Fleischmann's			
Active Dry	1 pkg (¼ oz)	20	10
Fresh Active	1 pkg (.6 oz)	15	5
Household Yeast	½ oz	15	5
RapidRise	1 pkg (¼ oz)	20	10

FOOD	PORTION	CALORIES	SODIUM
baker's dry, active	1 pkg (7 g)	20	4
brewer's dry	1 tbsp	25	10

YELLOW BEANS

DRIED			
cooked	1 cup	254	8

YELLOWTAIL

FRESH			
baked	3 oz	159	42

YOGURT
(*see also* YOGURT FROZEN)

All Flavors (Cabot)	8 oz	220	120
All Flavors Ultimate 90 (Weight Watchers)	1 cup	90	120
Apple Crisp Lowfat (New Country)	6 oz	150	85
Apple Original (Yoplait)	6 oz	190	110
Apples 'N Spice Nonfat Lite (Colombo)	8 oz	190	140
B! Lowfat, French Style (Colombo)	6 oz	140	105
Banana			
Custard Style (Yoplait)	6 oz	190	95
Fruit On Bottom (Dannon)	8 oz	240	120
Banana Strawberry			
Classic (Colombo)	8 oz	250	140
Nonfat Lite (Colombo)	8 oz	190	140
Nonfat Lite, Swiss Style (Colombo)	4.4 oz	100	70
Black Cherry			
100 Calorie With Aspartame (Light N'Lively)	8 oz	100	100

FOOD	PORTION	CALORIES	SODIUM
Classic (Colombo)	8 oz	230	140
Lowfat (Breyers)	8 oz	260	120
Lowfat (Light N'Lively)	8 oz	230	125
With Aspartame (Knudsen Cal 70)	8 oz	70	75
Blueberry			
(Dannon)	8 oz	200	160
100 Calorie With Aspartame (Light N'Lively)	8 oz	90	110
Classic (Colombo)	8 oz	230	140
Custard Style (Yoplait)	6 oz	190	95
Fat Free (Yoplait)	6 oz	150	95
Fruit On Bottom (Dannon)	4.4 oz	130	65
Fruit On Bottom (Dannon)	8 oz	240	120
Light (Yoplait)	4 oz	60	75
Light (Yoplait)	6 oz	80	80
Lowfat (Breyers)	8 oz	250	120
Lowfat (Light N'Lively)	4.4 oz	130	70
Lowfat (Light N'Lively)	8 oz	240	130
Nonfat (Dannon)	6 oz	140	105
Nonfat Light (Dannon)	4.4 oz	60	70
Nonfat Light (Dannon)	8 oz	100	130
Nonfat Lite (Colombo)	8 oz	190	140
Nonfat Lite, Swiss Style (Colombo)	4.4 oz	100	70
Original (Yoplait)	4 oz	120	75
Original (Yoplait)	6 oz	190	110
Supreme Lowfat (New Country)	6 oz	150	90
With Aspartame (Knudsen Cal 70)	8 oz	70	80
With Aspartame (Light N'Lively Free)	8 oz	50	60

FOOD	PORTION	CALORIES	SODIUM
Boysenberry			
Fruit On Bottom (Dannon)	8 oz	240	120
Lowfat (Knudsen)	8 oz	240	135
Original (Yoplait)	6 oz	190	110
Cherry			
Custard Style (Yoplait)	6 oz	180	95
Fat Free (Yoplait)	6 oz	150	95
Fruit On Bottom (Dannon)	4.4 oz	130	65
Fruit On Bottom (Dannon)	8 oz	240	120
Light (Yoplait)	4 oz	60	75
Light (Yoplait)	6 oz	80	80
Lowfat (Knudsen)	8 oz	240	135
Lowfat (Light N'Lively)	4.4 oz	140	70
Nonfat Lite (Colombo)	8 oz	190	140
Original (Yoplait)	6 oz	190	110
Supreme Lowfat (New Country)	6 oz	150	90
Cherry Vanilla, Nonfat Light (Dannon)	8 oz	100	130
Coffee			
Lowfat (Dannon)	8 oz	200	120
Nonfat Lite (Colombo)	8 oz	190	140
Dutch Apple, Fruit on Bottom (Dannon)	8 oz	240	120
Exotic Fruit, Fruit on Bottom (Dannon)	8 oz	240	120
French Vanilla			
Classic (Colombo)	8 oz	215	140
Lowfat (New Country)	6 oz	150	90
Fruit Cocktail, Nonfat Lite (Colombo)	8 oz	190	140
Fruit Crunch, Lowfat (New Country)	6 oz	150	90

FOOD	PORTION	CALORIES	SODIUM
Grape, Lowfat (Light N'Lively)	4.4 oz	130	70
Hawaiian Salad, Lowfat (New Country)	6 oz	150	90
Lemon			
100 Calorie With Aspartame (Light N'Lively)	8 oz	100	150
Custard Style (Yoplait)	6 oz	190	95
Lowfat (Dannon)	8 oz	200	120
Lowfat (Knudsen)	8 oz	240	135
Nonfat Lite (Colombo)	8 oz	190	140
Original (Yoplait)	6 oz	190	110
Supreme Lowfat (New Country)	6 oz	150	90
With Aspartame (Knudsen Cal 70)	8 oz	70	125
Lime, Lowfat (Knudsen)	8 oz	240	135
Mixed Berries			
Fruit On Bottom (Dannon)	4.4 oz	130	65
Fruit On Bottom (Dannon)	8 oz	240	120
Lowfat (Dannon)	8 oz	240	120
Lowfat (New Country)	6 oz	150	85
Mixed Berry			
Custard Style (Yoplait)	6 oz	180	95
Fat Free (Yoplait)	6 oz	150	95
Lowfat (Breyers)	8 oz	250	120
Original (Yoplait)	6 oz	190	110
Orange			
Original (Yoplait)	6 oz	190	110
Supreme Lowfat (New Country)	6 oz	150	90
Peach			
100 Calorie With Aspartame (Light N'Lively)	8 oz	100	115

FOOD	PORTION	CALORIES	SODIUM
Peach *(cont.)*			
Fat Free (Yoplait)	6 oz	150	95
Fruit Mousette (Colombo)	3.5 oz	80	55
Fruit On Bottom (Dannon)	8 oz	240	120
Light (Yoplait)	4 oz	60	75
Light (Yoplait)	6 oz	80	80
Lowfat (Breyers)	8 oz	250	120
Lowfat (Knudsen)	8 oz	240	135
Lowfat (Light N'Lively)	4.4 oz	130	65
Lowfat (Light N'Lively)	8 oz	240	120
Lowfat Blended With Fruit (Dannon)	4 oz	110	55
Lowfat Blended With Fruit (Dannon)	4.4 oz	130	80
Nonfat (Dannon)	6 oz	140	105
Nonfat Light (Dannon)	8 oz	100	130
Nonfat Lite (Colombo)	8 oz	190	140
Nonfat Lite, Swiss Style (Colombo)	4.4 oz	100	70
Original (Yoplait)	4 oz	120	75
Original (Yoplait)	6 oz	190	110
With Aspartame (Knudsen Cal 70)	8 oz	70	95
Peach Melba Classic (Colombo)	8 oz	230	140
Peaches 'n Cream, Lowfat (New Country)	6 oz	150	90
Piña Colada			
Fruit On Bottom (Dannon)	8 oz	240	120
Original (Yoplait)	6 oz	190	110
Pineapple			
Lowfat (Breyers)	8 oz	250	120
Lowfat (Light N'Lively)	4.4 oz	130	65

FOOD	PORTION	CALORIES	SODIUM
Lowfat (Light N'Lively)	8 oz	230	120
Original (Yoplait)	6 oz	190	110
With Aspartame (Knudsen Cal 70)	8 oz	70	125
Plain			
(Cabot)	8 oz	140	160
(Knudsen)	8 oz	200	170
Classic (Colombo)	8 oz	150	160
Extra Mild, Sweetened (Colombo)	8 oz	200	140
Lowfat (Breyers)	8 oz	140	170
Lowfat (Dannon)	8 oz	140	125
Lowfat (Knudsen)	8 oz	160	180
Nonfat (Colombo)	8 oz	110	160
Nonfat (Dannon)	8 oz	110	140
Nonfat (Weight Watchers)	1 cup	90	135
Nonfat (Yoplait)	8 oz	120	160
Original (Yoplait)	6 oz	130	140
Raspberry			
Classic (Colombo)	8 oz	230	140
Custard Style (Yoplait)	6 oz	190	95
Fat Free (Yoplait)	6 oz	150	95
Fruit Mousette (Colombo)	3.5 oz	80	55
Fruit On Bottom (Dannon)	4.4 oz	120	65
Fruit On Bottom (Dannon)	8 oz	240	120
Light (Yoplait)	4 oz	60	75
Light (Yoplait)	6 oz	80	80
Lowfat (Knudsen)	8 oz	240	135
Lowfat Blended With Fruit (Dannon)	4 oz	110	55
Lowfat Blended With Fruit (Dannon)	4.4 oz	130	80

FOOD	PORTION	CALORIES	SODIUM
Raspberry *(cont.)*			
Nonfat (Dannon)	6 oz	140	105
Nonfat (Dannon)	8 oz	200	160
Nonfat Light (Dannon)	8 oz	100	130
Nonfat Lite (Colombo)	8 oz	190	140
Nonfat Lite, Swiss Style (Colombo)	4.4 oz	100	70
Original (Yoplait)	4 oz	120	75
Original (Yoplait)	6 oz	190	110
Supreme Lowfat (New Country)	6 oz	150	90
Red Raspberry			
100 Calorie With Aspartame (Light N'Lively)	8 oz	90	105
Lowfat (Breyers)	8 oz	250	120
Lowfat (Light N'Lively)	4.4 oz	130	70
Lowfat (Light N'Lively)	8 oz	230	130
With Aspartame (Knudsen Cal 70)	8 oz	70	80
With Aspartame (Light N'Lively Free)	8 oz	50	60
Strawberry			
100 Calorie With Aspartame (Light N'Lively)	8 oz	90	105
Classic (Colombo)	8 oz	230	140
Custard Style (Yoplait)	4 oz	130	60
Custard Style (Yoplait)	6 oz	190	95
Fat Free (Yoplait)	6 oz	150	95
Fruit Basket With Aspartame (Knudsen Cal 70)	8 oz	70	90
Fruit Cup Lowfat (Light N'Lively)	4.4 oz	130	65
Fruit Cup Lowfat (Light N'Lively)	8 oz	240	120

FOOD	PORTION	CALORIES	SODIUM
Fruit Cup Lowfat (New Country)	6 oz	150	85
Fruit Cup Nonfat Light (Dannon)	8 oz	100	130
Fruit Cup With Aspartame (Light N'Lively Free)	8 oz	50	55
Fruit Mousette (Colombo)	3.5 oz	80	55
Fruit On Bottom (Dannon)	4.4 oz	130	65
Fruit On Bottom (Dannon)	8 oz	240	120
Light (Yoplait)	4 oz	60	75
Light (Yoplait)	6 oz	80	110
Lowfat (Breyers)	8 oz	250	120
Lowfat (Dannon)	8 oz	200	160
Lowfat (Knudsen)	8 oz	250	135
Lowfat (Light N'Lively)	4.4 oz	130	70
Lowfat (Light N'Lively)	8 oz	240	130
Lowfat Blended With Fruit (Dannon)	4 oz	110	55
Lowfat Blended With Fruit (Dannon)	4.4 oz	130	80
Nonfat (Dannon)	6 oz	140	105
Nonfat Light (Dannon)	4.4 oz	60	70
Nonfat Light (Dannon)	8 oz	100	130
Nonfat Lite (Colombo)	8 oz	190	140
Nonfat Lite, Swiss Style (Colombo)	4.4 oz	100	70
Original (Yoplait)	4 oz	120	75
Original (Yoplait)	6 oz	190	110
Supreme Lowfat (New Country)	6 oz	150	90
With Aspartame (Knudsen Cal 70)	8 oz	70	85

FOOD	PORTION	CALORIES	SODIUM
Strawberry *(cont.)*			
With Aspartame (Light N'Lively Free)	8 oz	50	60
Strawberry Banana			
100 Calorie With Aspartame (Light N'Lively)	8 oz	90	100
Custard Style (Yoplait)	4 oz	130	60
Custard Style (Yoplait)	6 oz	190	95
Fat Free (Yoplait)	6 oz	150	95
Fruit On Bottom (Dannon)	4.4 oz	130	65
Light (Yoplait)	4 oz	60	75
Light (Yoplait)	6 oz	80	80
Lowfat (Breyers)	8 oz	250	120
Lowfat (Dannon)	8 oz	200	160
Lowfat (Knudsen)	8 oz	250	135
Lowfat (Light N'Lively)	4.4 oz	140	65
Lowfat (Light N'Lively)	8 oz	260	120
Lowfat (New Country)	6 oz	150	85
Lowfat Blended With Fruit (Dannon)	4 oz	110	55
Lowfat Blended With Fruit (Dannon)	4.4 oz	130	80
Nonfat Light (Dannon)	8 oz	100	130
Original (Yoplait)	6 oz	190	110
With Aspartame (Knudsen Cal 70)	8 oz	70	80
w/ Aspartame (Light N'Lively Free)	8 oz	50	60
Strawberry Rhubarb Original (Yoplait)	6 oz	190	110
Vanilla			
Bean, Lowfat (Breyers)	8 oz	230	150
Custard Style (Yoplait)	4 oz	130	70

FOOD	PORTION	CALORIES	SODIUM
Custard Style (Yoplait)	6 oz	180	110
Lowfat (Dannon)	8 oz	200	120
Lowfat (Knudsen)	8 oz	240	135
Nonfat (Yoplait)	8 oz	180	140
Nonfat Light (Dannon)	8 oz	100	130
Nonfat Lite (Colombo)	8 oz	160	140
Nonfat Lite, Swiss Style (Colombo)	4.4 oz	100	110
Original (Yoplait)	6 oz	180	120
With Aspartame (Knudsen Cal 70)	8 oz	70	90
coffee, lowfat	8 oz	194	149
fruit, lowfat	4 oz	113	60
fruit, lowfat	8 oz	225	121
plain	8 oz	139	105
plain, lowfat	8 oz	144	159
plain, no fat	8 oz	127	174
vanilla lowfat	8 oz	194	149

YOGURT FROZEN
(see also TOFU YOGURT)

FOOD	PORTION	CALORIES	SODIUM
All Flavors (Just 10)	1 oz	10	14
Banana Strawberry (Edy's)	3 oz	80	40
Black Cherry (Sealtest Free)	½ cup	110	50
Blueberry			
(Edy's)	3 oz	80	40
(Elan)	4 oz	130	50
Softy (Dannon)	4 oz	110	65
Butter Pecan Softy (Dannon)	4 oz	110	65
Cappuccino Softy (Dannon)	4 oz	110	65
Caramel Almond Praline (Elan)	4 oz	150	90

FOOD	PORTION	CALORIES	SODIUM
Cheesecake Softy (Dannon)	4 oz	110	65
Cherry			
(Ben & Jerry's)	4 oz	160	150
(Edy's)	3 oz	80	40
Chocolate			
(Ben & Jerry's)	4 oz	121	69
(Edy's)	3 oz	80	40
(Elan)	4 oz	130	50
(Haagen-Dazs)	3 oz	130	30
(Sealtest Free)	½ cup	110	55
Bee-Lite	4 oz	100	55
Fi-Bar	1	190	160
Kissed With Honey	3.5 oz	100	50
Kissed With Honey, Nonfat	3.5 oz	85	60
Nonfat Softy (Dannon)	4 oz	110	65
Shake (Weight Watchers)	7.5 oz	220	140
Softy (Dannon)	4 oz	140	65
Yogurt Bar (Dole)	1	70	50
Chocolate Almond (Elan)	4 oz	160	50
Chocolate Chip (Edy's)	3 oz	100	55
Citrus Heights (Edy's)	3 oz	80	40
Coffee (Elan)	4 oz	130	60
Cookies 'N' Cream (Edy's)	3 oz	100	55
Decaffeinated Coffee (Elan)	4 oz	130	60
Dutch Chocolate Desserve	4 oz	80	62
Golden Vanilla Nonfat Softy (Dannon)	4 oz	100	65
Lemon Meringue Softy (Dannon)	4 oz	110	65
Marble Fudge (Edy's)	3 oz	100	55
Peach			
(Ben & Jerry's)	4 oz	133	113

FOOD	PORTION	CALORIES	SODIUM
(Elan)	4 oz	130	50
(Haagen-Dazs)	3 oz	120	30
(Sealtest Free)	½ cup	100	35
Softy (Dannon)	4 oz	110	65
Peanut Butter Softy (Dannon)	4 oz	130	70
Perfectly Peach (Edy's)	3 oz	80	40
Piña Colada Softy (Dannon)	4 oz	110	65
Plain Softy (Dannon)	4 oz	90	60
Raspberry			
(Ben & Jerry's)	4 oz	133	116
(Edy's)	3 oz	80	40
Softy (Dannon)	4 oz	110	65
Raspberry Vanilla Swirl (Edy's)	3 oz	80	45
Red Raspberry			
(Sealtest Free)	½ cup	100	40
Nonfat Softy (Dannon)	4 oz	100	60
Rum Raisin (Elan)	4 oz	135	55
Nonfat Softy (Dannon)	4 oz	100	65
Strawberry			
(Borden)	½ cup	100	50
(Edy's)	3 oz	80	40
(Elan)	4 oz	125	50
(Haagen-Dazs)	3 oz	120	30
(Meadow Gold)	½ cup	100	50
(Sealtest Free)	½ cup	100	35
Bar (Dole)	1	70	25
Fi-Bar	1	190	150
Nonfat (Dannon)	6 oz	140	105
Nonfat Softy (Dannon)	4 oz	100	60
Softy (Dannon)	4 oz	110	65

FOOD	PORTION	CALORIES	SODIUM
Strawberry Banana			
Softy (Dannon)	4 oz	110	65
Yogurt Bar (Dole)	1	60	15
Sweet Cream (Ben & Jerry's)	4 oz	130	140
Vanilla			
(Edy's)	3 oz	80	50
(Elan)	4 oz	130	60
(Haagen-Dazs)	3 oz	130	40
(Sealtest Free)	½ cup	100	45
Bee-Lite	4 oz	110	55
Deserve	4 oz	70	57
Fi-Bar	1	190	150
Kissed With Honey	3.5 oz	100	75
Kissed With Honey Nonfat	3.5 oz	85	50
Softy (Dannon)	4 oz	110	65
Vanilla Almond Crunch (Haagen-Dazs)	3 oz	150	65

ZUCCHINI

CANNED			
Italian Style (S&W)	½ cup	45	467
italian style	½ cup	33	427
FRESH			
baby, raw	1 (½ oz)	3	0
raw, sliced	½ cup	9	2
sliced, cooked	½ cup	14	2
FROZEN			
Breaded Zucchini (Ore Ida)	3 oz	150	340
cooked	½ cup	19	2

PART II
Restaurant, Take-Out and Fast-Food Chains

FOOD	PORTION	CALORIES	SODIUM
ARBY'S			
BEVERAGES			
7-Up	12 oz	144	34
Coca-Cola Classic	12 oz	141	15
Coffee	8 oz	3	3
Diet Coke	12 oz	1	30
Diet 7-Up	12 oz	4	22
Hot Chocolate	8 oz	110	120
Iced Tea	16 oz	6	12
Milk Lo Fat 2%	8 oz	121	122
Nehi Orange	12 oz	190	21
Orange Juice	6 oz	82	2
Pepsi-Cola	12 oz	159	10
R.C. Cola	12 oz	173	1
Diet Rite	12 oz	1	10
Root Beer	12 oz	173	16
Upper Ten	12 oz	169	40
BREAKFAST SELECTIONS			
Biscuit			
Bacon	1	318	904
Ham	1	323	1169
Plain	1	280	730
Sausage	1	460	1000
Blueberry Muffin	1	200	269
Cinnamon Nut Danish	1	340	230
Croissant			
Bacon/Egg	1	389	582
Ham/Cheese	1	345	939
Mushroom/Cheese	1	493	935
Plain	1	260	300

FOOD	PORTION	CALORIES	SODIUM
Croissant *(cont.)*			
Sausage/Egg	1	519	632
Maple Syrup	1½ oz	120	52
Platter			
Bacon	1	860	1051
Egg	1	460	491
Ham	1	518	1177
Sausage	1	640	861
Toastix	1 serving	420	440
DESSERTS			
Cheese Cake	1 serving	306	220
Chocolate Chip Cookie	1	130	95
Chocolate Shake	12 oz	451	410
Jamocha Shake	11.5 oz	368	262
Polar Swirl			
Butterfinger	1	457	318
Heath	1	543	346
Oreo	1	482	521
P'nut Butter Cup	1	517	385
Snickers	1	511	351
Turnover			
Apple	1	303	178
Blueberry	1	320	240
Cherry	1	280	200
Vanilla Shake	11 oz	330	686
MAIN MENU SELECTIONS			
Arby's Sauce	½ oz	15	113
Au Jus	4 oz	7	750
Bac N'Cheddar Deluxe Sandwich	1	532	422
Baked Potato			
Broccoli 'N Cheddar	1	417	1455

FOOD	PORTION	CALORIES	SODIUM
Deluxe	1	621	1520
Mushroom & Cheese	1	515	1445
Plain	1	240	1333
With Butter/Margarine And Sour Cream	1	463	203
Beef N'Cheddar Sandwich	1	451	955
Cheddar Fries	1 serving (5 oz)	399	443
Chicken Breast Sandwich	1	489	1019
Chicken Cordon Bleu Sandwich	1	658	1824
Chicken Fajita Pita	1	272	887
Curly Fries	1 serving (3.5 oz)	337	167
Fish Fillet Sandwich	1	537	994
French Dip	1	345	678
French Dip 'n Swiss	1	425	1078
French Fries	1 serving	246	114
Grilled Chicken Barbecue Sandwich	1	378	1059
Deluxe Sandwich	1	426	877
Ham 'N Cheese Sandwich	1	330	1350
Horsey Sauce	½ oz	55	105
Ketchup	½ oz	16	143
Light Ham Deluxe	1	255	1037
Light Roast Beef Deluxe	1	294	826
Light Roast Chicken Deluxe	1	263	620
Light Roast Turkey Deluxe	1	260	1172
Mayonnaise, Cholesterol Free	½ oz	90	75
Mustard	½ oz	11	160
Philly Beef N' Swiss Sandwich	1	498	1194
Potato Cakes	1 serving	204	397

FOOD	PORTION	CALORIES	SODIUM
Roast Beef Sandwich			
Giant	1	530	908
Junior	1	218	345
Regular	1	353	588
Super	1	529	798
Roast Chicken Club Sandwich	1	513	1423
Roast Chicken Deluxe Sandwich	1	373	913
Roast Chicken Salad	1	184	441
Sub Deluxe	1	482	1530
Sugar Substitute	⅓ oz	4	5
Turkey Deluxe Sandwich	1	399	1047
SALADS AND DRESSINGS			
Blue Cheese Dressing	2 oz	295	489
Buttermilk Ranch Dressing	2 oz	349	471
Cashew Chicken Salad	1	590	1140
Chef Salad	1	210	7207
Croutons	½ oz	59	155
Garden Salad	1	149	99
Honey French Dressing	2 oz	322	486
Italian Dressing Light	2 oz	23	1110
Thousand Island Dressing	2 oz	298	493
Weight Watchers			
Creamy French	1 oz	48	170
Creamy Italian	1 oz	29	280
SOUPS			
Beef With Vegetables & Barley	8 oz	96	996
Boston Clam Chowder	8 oz	207	1157
Cream of Broccoli	8 oz	180	1133
French Onion	8 oz	67	1248
Lumberjack Mixed Vegetable	8 oz	89	1075

FOOD	PORTION	CALORIES	SODIUM
Old Fashioned Chicken Noodle	8 oz	99	929
Pilgrim's Corn Chowder	5 oz	193	1157
Split Pea With Ham	8 oz	200	1029
Tomato Florentine	8 oz	244	910
Wisconsin Cheese	8 oz	287	1129

AU BON PAIN

BREAD AND ROLLS
FOOD	PORTION	CALORIES	SODIUM
3 Seed Raisin Roll	1	250	480
Alpine Roll	1	220	810
Baguette Loaf	1	810	1830
Cheese Loaf	1	1670	4140
Country Seed Roll	1	220	460
Four Grain Loaf	1	1420	3050
French Roll	1	320	710
Hearth Roll	1	250	510
Hearth Sandwich Roll	1	370	600
Onion Herb Loaf	1	1430	2390
Parisienne Loaf	1	1490	3380
Petit Pain Roll	1	220	490
Pumpernickel Roll	1	210	1005
Sandwich Croissant	1	300	240
Soft Roll	1	310	410
Vegetable Roll	1	230	410

COOKIES
FOOD	PORTION	CALORIES	SODIUM
Chocolate Chip	1	280	70
Chocolate Chunk Pecan	1	290	200
Oatmeal Raisin	1	250	230
Peanut Butter	1	290	250
White Chocolate Chunk Pecan	1	300	200

FOOD	PORTION	CALORIES	SODIUM
CROISSANTS			
Almond	1	420	250
Apple	1	250	150
Blueberry Cheese	1	380	280
Chocolate	1	400	220
Chocolate Hazelnut	1	480	220
Cinnamon Raisin	1	390	240
Coconut Pecan	1	440	290
Ham & Cheese	1	370	280
Plain	1	220	240
Raspberry Cheese	1	400	280
Spinach & Cheese	1	290	310
Strawberry Cheese	1	400	280
Sweet Cheese	1	420	310
Turkey & Cheddar	1	410	680
Turkey & Havarti	1	410	630
MUFFINS			
Blueberry	1	390	410
Bran	1	390	940
Carrot	1	450	610
Corn	1	460	510
Cranberry Walnut	1	350	730
Oat Bran Apple	1	400	590
Pumpkin	1	410	500
Whole Grain	1	440	310
SALADS			
Chicken			
Cracked Pepper	1	100	360
Grilled	1	110	330
Tarragon	1	310	332

FOOD	PORTION	CALORIES	SODIUM
Garden			
Large	1	40	20
Small	1	20	10
Shrimp	1	102	193
Tuna	1	350	480
SANDWICH FILLINGS			
Boursin	1 serving	290	390
Brie	1 serving	300	510
Chicken			
Cracked Pepper	1 serving	120	680
Grilled	1 serving	130	610
Tarragon	1 serving	270	304
Country Ham	1 serving	150	970
Roast Beef	1 serving	180	310
Smoked Turkey	1 serving	100	950
Swiss	1 serving	330	230
Tuna Salad	1 serving	310	450
SOUPS			
Beef Barley	1 bowl	125	933
Beef Barley	1 cup	80	600
Chicken Noodle	1 bowl	125	933
Chicken Noodle	1 cup	80	600
Clam Chowder	1 bowl	390	1130
Clam Chowder	1 cup	270	790
Cream Of Broccoli	1 bowl	380	1280
Cream Of Broccoli	1 cup	250	840
Garden Vegetarian	1 bowl	70	1630
Garden Vegetarian	1 cup	50	1120
Minestrone	1 bowl	190	1090
Minestrone	1 cup	120	720

FOOD	PORTION	CALORIES	SODIUM
Split Pea	1 bowl	380	1500
Split Pea	1 cup	250	1000
Tomato Florentine	1 bowl	120	1420
Tomato Florentine	1 cup	90	990
Vegetarian Chili	1 bowl	280	1050
Vegetarian Chili	1 cup	180	660

BASKIN-ROBBINS

FOOD	PORTION	CALORIES	SODIUM
Chocolate Raspberry Truffle	1 scoop	310	115
Chocolate Vanilla Twist Fat Free	½ cup	100	0
Chocolate w/ Caramel Ribbon Bar Light	1	150	75
Daiquiri Ice	1 scoop	140	15
Jamoca Swiss Almond Sugar Free	½ cup	90	100
Just Peachy Fat Free	½ cup	100	0
Praline Dream Light	½ cup	130	85
Praline 'n Cream Ice Cream Bar	1	310	145
Rainbow Sherbet	1 scoop	160	85
Strawberry Frozen Yogurt Low Fat	½ cup	120	40
Frozen Yogurt Nonfat	½ cup	110	40
Strawberry Royal Light	½ cup	110	120
Strawberry Sugar Free	½ cup	80	70
Sugar Cone	1	60	45
Vanilla Ice Cream	1 scoop	240	115
Very Berry Strawberry Ice Cream	1 scoop	220	95
Waffle Cone	1	140	5
World Class Chocolate Ice Cream	1 scoop	280	145

FOOD	PORTION	CALORIES	SODIUM

BURGER KING

BEVERAGES
Shake

Chocolate	1 med	326	198
Vanilla	1 med	334	213

BREAKFAST SELECTIONS

Breakfast Buddy	1	255	492
Breakfast Croissan'wich			
w/ Bacon	1	353	780
w/ Ham	1	351	1373
w/ Sausage	1	534	985

MAIN MENU SELECTIONS

Bacon Double Cheeseburger	1	530	860
BK Broiler	1	280	770
Cheeseburger	1	300	660
Chicken Sandwich	1	620	1430
Chicken Tenders	6 pieces	236	541
Double Whopper With Cheese	1	890	1250
French Fries	1 med	372	238
Hamburger	1	260	500
Ocean Catch Fish Fillet Sandwich	1	450	760
Onion Rings	1 serving	339	628
Whopper Jr.	1	300	500
With Cheese	1	350	650
Whopper Sandwich	1	570	870
With Cheese	1	660	1190

SALADS AND DRESSINGS

Bleu Cheese Dressing	2 oz	300	512
Chef Salad	1	178	568
Chunky Chicken Salad	1	142	443

FOOD	PORTION	CALORIES	SODIUM
French Dressing	2 oz	290	400
Garden Salad	1	95	125
Italian Dressing Light	2 oz	30	710
Ranch Dressing	2 oz	350	316
Side Salad	1	25	27
Thousand Island Dressing	2 oz	290	403

CARL'S JR.

FOOD	PORTION	CALORIES	SODIUM
BAKERY SELECTIONS			
Chocolate Chip Cookies	2.5 oz	330	170
Cinnamon Roll	1	460	230
Danish	1	520	230
Fudge Brownie	1	430	210
Fudge Moussecake	1 slice	400	85
Muffin			
Blueberry	1	340	300
Bran	1	310	370
Raspberry Cheesecake	1 slice	310	200
BEVERAGES			
Iced Tea	1 reg	2	0
Milk 2%	10 oz	180	180
Orange Juice	1 sm	90	2
Shake	1 reg	330	230
Soda	1 reg	240	35
Diet	1 reg	2	15
BREAKFAST SELECTIONS			
Bacon	2 strips	45	40
Breakfast Burrito	1	430	740
English Muffin w/ Margarine	1	190	280
French Toast Dips w/o Syrup	1 serving	490	620

FOOD	PORTION	CALORIES	SODIUM
Hash Brown Nuggets	1 serving	270	410
Hot Cakes w/ Margarine, w/o Syrup	1 serving	510	950
Sausage	1 patty	190	520
Scrambled Eggs	1 serving	120	105
Sunrise Sandwich	1	300	550
MAIN MENU SELECTIONS			
All Star			
Chili Dog	1	720	1530
Hot Dog	1	540	1130
American Cheese	½ oz	60	290
Carl's Catch Fish Sandwich	1	560	1220
Cheeseburger			
Double Western Bacon	1	1030	1810
Western Bacon	1	730	1490
Chicken Club Charbroiler	1	570	1160
Chicken Sandwich Charbroiler BBQ	1	310	34
Chicken Sante Fe Sandwich	1	540	1180
Country Fried Steak Sandwich	1	720	1420
CrissCut Fries	1 serving	330	890
French Fries	1 reg	420	200
Guacamole	1 oz	50	100
Hamburger	1	220	590
Famous Star	1	610	890
Old Time Star	1	460	810
Super Star	1	820	1210
Jr. Crisp Burrito	1	140	200
Onion Rings	1 serving	520	960
Potato			
Bacon & Cheese	1	730	1670

FOOD	PORTION	CALORIES	SODIUM
Potato *(cont.)*			
Broccoli & Cheese	1	590	830
Fiesta	1	720	1470
Lite	1	250	60
Sour Cream & Chives	1	470	180
w/ Cheese	1	690	1160
Roast Beef Club	1	620	1950
Roast Beef Deluxe Sandwich	1	540	1340
Salsa	1 oz	8	210
Swiss Cheese	½ oz	60	220
Taco Sauce	1 oz	8	160
Zucchini	1 serving	390	1040
SALADS AND DRESSINGS			
1000 Island Dressing	1 oz	110	200
Blue Cheese Dressing	1 oz	150	250
French Reduced Calorie Dressing	1 oz	40	290
House Dressing	1 oz	110	170
Italian Dressing	1 oz	120	210
Salad-To-Go Chicken	1	200	300
Salad-To-Go Garden	1 sm	50	75

CARVEL

Lo-Yo Vanilla Frozen Yogurt	1 oz	34	13

CHICK-FIL-A

BEVERAGES			
Iced Tea, Unsweetened	9 oz	3	0
Lemonade	10 oz	124	tr
DESSERTS			
Fudge Brownie w/ Nuts	1	369	213

FOOD	PORTION	CALORIES	SODIUM
Icedream	4.5 oz	134	51
Lemon Pie	1 slice	329	300
MAIN MENU SELECTIONS			
Carrot-Raisin Salad	1 serving	116	8
Chargrilled Chicken	3.6 oz	128	698
Chargrilled Chicken Deluxe Sandwich	1	266	1125
Chargrilled Chicken Garden Salad	10.4 oz	126	567
Chargrilled Chicken Sandwich	1	258	1121
Chick-fil-A Chicken	1 piece (3.6 oz)	219	801
Chick-fil-A Chicken Deluxe Sandwich	1	368	1178
Chick-fil-A			
Nuggets	12 pack	430	1989
Nuggets	8 pack	287	1326
Chick-fil-A Sandwich	1	360	1174
Chick-n-Q Sandwich	1	206	660
Chicken Salad			
Cup	3.4 oz	309	543
Plate	1 (11.8 oz)	579	980
Chicken Salad Sandwich w/ Wheat Bread	1	449	888
Cole Slaw	1 serving	175	158
Grilled 'n Lites	1 skewer	97	280
Hearty Breast of Chicken Soup	8.5 oz	152	530
Nuggets	8	287	1326
Potato Salad	1 serving	198	337
Tossed Salad	4.5 oz	21	19
With Honey French Dressing	6 oz	246	519
With Lite Italian Dressing	6 oz	46	354
With Ranch Dressing	6 oz	177	206

FOOD	PORTION	CALORIES	SODIUM
Tossed Salad *(cont.)*			
With Thousand Island Dressing	6 oz	231	389
Waffle Potato Fries	1 reg	270	45

DAIRY QUEEN/BRAZIER

FOOD SELECTION			
¼ lb Super Dog	1	590	1360
BBQ Beef Sandwich	1	225	700
Baked Chicken Fillet Sandwich w/ Cheese	1	480	980
Breaded Chicken Fillet Sandwich	1	430	760
DQ Homestyle Ultimate Burger	1	700	1110
Double Hamburger	1	460	630
w/ Cheese	1	570	1070
Fish Fillet Sandwich	1	370	630
w/ Cheese	1	420	850
French Dressing, Reduced Calorie	2 oz	90	450
French Fries	1 lg	390	200
French Fries	1 reg	300	160
French Fries	1 sm	210	115
Garden Salad	1	200	240
Grilled Chicken Fillet Sandwich	1	300	800
Hot Dog	1	280	700
w/ Cheese	1	330	920
w/ Chili	1	320	720
Lettuce	½ oz	2	1
Onion Rings	1 reg	240	135
Side Salad	1	25	15
Single Hamburger	1	310	580
w/ Cheese	1	365	800

FOOD	PORTION	CALORIES	SODIUM
Thousand Island Dressing	2 oz	225	570
Tomato	½ oz	3	1
ICE CREAM			
Banana Split	1	510	250
Blizzard Strawberry	1 reg	740	230
Blizzard Strawberry	1 sm	500	160
Breeze Strawberry	1 reg	590	170
Breeze Strawberry	1 sm	400	115
Buster Bar	1	450	220
Cone			
Chocolate	1 lg	350	170
Chocolate	1 reg	230	115
Dipped Chocolate	1 reg	330	100
Vanilla	1 lg	340	140
Vanilla	1 reg	230	95
Vanilla	1 sm	140	60
Yogurt	1 lg	260	115
Yogurt	1 reg	180	80
Cup			
Yogurt	1 lg	230	100
Yogurt	1 reg	170	70
DQ Frozen Cake Slice, Undecorated	1	380	210
DQ Sandwich	1	140	135
Dilly Bar	1	210	50
Heath			
Blizzard	1 reg	820	410
Blizzard	1 sm	560	280
Breeze	1 reg	680	360
Breeze	1 sm	450	230
Hot Fudge Brownie Delight	1	710	340

FOOD	PORTION	CALORIES	SODIUM
Malt Vanilla	1 reg	610	230
Mr. Misty	1 reg	250	0
Nutty Double Fudge	1	580	170
Peanut Buster Parfait	1	710	410
QC Big Scoop			
Chocolate	1	310	100
Vanilla	1	300	100
Shake			
Chocolate	1 reg	540	290
Vanilla	1 lg	600	260
Vanilla	1 reg	520	230
Sundae			
Chocolate	1 reg	300	140
Waffle Cone, Strawberry	1	350	220
Yogurt, Strawberry	1 reg	200	80

D'ANGELO SANDWICH SHOPS

DESSERTS
Frozen Yogurt

Banana	5 oz	125	60
Banana w/ Cone	5 oz	215	60
Peach	5 oz	130	55
Peach w/ Cone	5 oz	220	60

SALADS

Beef	1 serving (3¼ oz)	350	890
Chicken	1 serving (3¼ oz)	325	980
Tuna	1 serving (2 oz)	305	805
Turkey	1 serving (3¼ oz)	375	660

FOOD	PORTION	CALORIES	SODIUM
SANDWICHES			
D'Lite Pocket			
Chicken Stir Fry	1	340	1025
Roast Beef	1	325	730
Steak	1	415	500
Steak & Mushroom	1	420	620
Steak & Pepper	1	420	500
Turkey	1	350	500
Vegetarian	1	350	995
D'Lite Small Sub			
Roast Beef	1	365	750
Turkey	1	390	520

DELTACO

FOOD	PORTION	CALORIES	SODIUM
BEVERAGES			
Coke Classic	1 lg	287	35
Coke Classic	1 med	198	24
Coke Classic	1 sm	144	17
Coke Classic, Best Value	1	395	48
Diet Coke	1 lg	2	39
Diet Coke	1 med	1	27
Diet Coke	1 sm	1	20
Diet Coke, Best Value	1	2	53
Iced Tea	1 lg	6	26
Iced Tea	1 med	4	18
Iced Tea	1 sm	3	13
Iced Tea, Best Value	1	8	36
Milk	1	126	152
Mr Pibb	1 lg	283	47
Mr Pibb	1 med	195	32

FOOD	PORTION	CALORIES	SODIUM
Mr Pibb	1 sm	142	23
Mr Pibb, Best Value	1	390	64
Orange Juice	1	83	19
Shake			
Chocolate	1	549	302
Orange	1	609	234
Strawberry	1	486	222
Sprite	1 lg	287	71
Sprite	1 med	198	49
Sprite	1 sm	144	35
Sprite, Best Value	1	395	97
CHILDREN'S MENU SELECTIONS			
Kid's Meal			
Hamburger	1	617	799
Taco	1	532	373
DESSERTS			
M & M's Toppers	1	256	112
Oreos Toppers	1	257	188
Snickers Toppers	1	254	128
MAIN MENU SELECTIONS			
American Cheese	1 slice	53	203
Beans And Cheese	1	122	892
Burrito			
Big Del	1	453	1047
Breakfast	1	256	409
Chicken	1	264	771
Combination	1	413	1035
Del Beef	1	440	878
Deluxe Chicken Fajita	1	435	944
Deluxe Del Beef	1	286	890

FOOD	PORTION	CALORIES	SODIUM
Egg And Cheese	1	443	792
Egg And Cheese With Beans	1	470	1035
Egg And Cheese With Beef	1	529	929
Green	1	229	714
Green Regular	1	330	1149
Macho Beef	1	893	1969
Macho Combo	1	774	2180
Red	1	235	656
Red Regular	1	324	1033
Steak And Egg	1	500	1068
Cheeseburger	1	284	852
Chicken Salad	1	254	476
Deluxe	1	716	1419
Del Burger	1	385	1065
Del Cheeseburger	1	439	1268
Double Del Cheeseburger	1	618	1638
French Fries			
Large	1	566	318
Regular	1	404	227
Small	1	242	136
Guacamole	1 oz	60	130
Hamburger	1	231	649
Hot Sauce	1 pkg	2	38
Nacho Cheese Sauce, Side Order	1 serving	100	401
Nachos	1	390	504
Super Deluxe	1	684	1469
Quesadilla	1	257	455
Chicken	1	544	1147
Large	1	483	871
Salsa	2 oz	14	308

FOOD	PORTION	CALORIES	SODIUM
Salsa Dressing	1 oz	33	85
Sour Cream	1 oz	60	15
Taco	1	140	99
Chicken	1	186	276
Chicken, Soft	1	197	401
Deluxe	1	166	107
Deluxe Chicken Fajita	1	211	492
Deluxe, Soft	1	177	231
Regular	1	224	195
Soft	1	146	223
Taco			
Salad	1	235	268
Salad Deluxe	1	741	1280
Tostada	1	140	333

DUNKIN' DONUTS
(see also DOUGHNUTS)

FOOD	PORTION	CALORIES	SODIUM
CROISSANTS			
Almond	1	420	280
Chocolate	1	440	220
Plain	1	310	240
DOUGHNUTS			
Apple Filled w/ Cinnamon Sugar	1	250	190
Bavarian Filled w/ Chocolate Frosting	1	240	260
Blueberry Filled	1	210	240
Chocolate Frosted Yeast Ring	1	200	190
Glazed			
Buttermilk Ring	1	290	370
Chocolate Ring	1	324	383
Coffee Roll	1	280	310

FOOD	PORTION	CALORIES	SODIUM
French Cruller	1	140	130
Whole Wheat Ring	1	330	380
Yeast Ring	1	200	230
Jelly Filled	1	220	230
Lemon Filled	1	260	280
Plain Cake Ring	1	270	330
MISCELLANEOUS Chocolate Chunk Cookie	1	200	110
w/ Nuts	1	210	100
Oatmeal Pecan Raisin Cookie	1	200	100
MUFFINS Apple N'Spice	1	300	360
Banana Nut	1	310	410
Blueberry	1	280	340
Bran w/ Raisins	1	310	560
Corn	1	340	560
Cranberry Nut	1	290	360
Oat Bran	1	330	450

EL POLLO LOCO

FOOD	PORTION	CALORIES	SODIUM
Beans	3.5 oz	110	450
Chicken	2 pieces	310	460
Coleslaw	2.8 oz	80	160
Combo Meal	1	720	890
Corn	3.3 oz	110	110
Dolewhip	4.5 oz	90	18
Potato Salad	4.3 oz	140	500
Rice	2.5 oz	100	250
Salsa	1.8 oz	10	90

FOOD	PORTION	CALORIES	SODIUM
Tortillas			
Corn	3.3 oz	210	70
Flour	3.3 oz	280	450

GODFATHER'S PIZZA

Golden Crust			
Cheese	1/10 lg	261	314
Cheese	1/6 sm	213	258
Cheese	1/8 med	229	272
Combo	1/10 lg	322	602
Combo	1/6 sm	273	542
Combo	1/8 med	283	526
Original Crust			
Cheese	1/10 lg	271	329
Cheese	1/4 mini	138	159
Cheese	1/6 sm	239	289
Cheese	1/8 med	242	285
Combo	1/10 lg	332	617
Combo	1/4 mini	164	287
Combo	1/6 sm	299	573
Combo	1/8 med	318	569

HAAGEN-DAZS

Banana Nonfat Soft Yogurt	1 oz	25	15
Blueberry Sorbet & Cream	4 oz	190	35
Butter Pecan	4 oz	390	100
Caramel Almond Crunch Bar	1	240	65
Caramel Nut Sundae	4 oz	310	100
Chocolate	4 oz	270	50
Chocolate Chocolate Chip	4 oz	290	40
Chocolate Chocolate Mint	4 oz	300	50

FOOD	PORTION	CALORIES	SODIUM
Chocolate Dark Chocolate Bar	1	390	60
Chocolate Frozen Yogurt	3 oz	130	30
Chocolate Nonfat Soft Yogurt	1 oz	30	20
Chocolate Soft Yogurt	1 oz	30	15
Coffee	4 oz	270	55
Coffee Soft Yogurt	1	28	13
Deep Chocolate	4 oz	290	70
Deep Chocolate Fudge	4 oz	290	90
Fudge Pop Bar	1	210	50
Honey Vanilla	4 oz	250	55
Keylime Sorbet & Cream	4 oz	190	30
Lemon Sorbet	4 oz	140	5
Macadamia Brittle	4 oz	280	60
Orange & Cream Pop	1	130	25
Orange Sorbet	4 oz	113	7
Orange Sorbet & Cream	4 oz	190	35
Peach Frozen Yogurt	3 oz	120	30
Peanut Butter Crunch Bar	1	270	55
Raspberry Soft Yogurt	1 oz	30	15
Raspberry Sorbet	4 oz	93	7
Raspberry Sorbet & Cream	4 oz	180	35
Rum Raisin	4 oz	250	45
Strawberry	4 oz	250	40
Frozen Yogurt	3 oz	120	30
Nonfat Soft Yogurt	1 oz	25	10
Vanilla	4 oz	260	55
Vanilla Almond Crunch Frozen Yogurt	3 oz	150	65
Vanilla Crunch Bar	1	220	55
Vanilla Frozen Yogurt	3 oz	130	40

FOOD	PORTION	CALORIES	SODIUM
Vanilla Fudge	4 oz	270	100
Vanilla Milk Chocolate Almond Bar	1	370	55
Vanilla Milk Chocolate Bar	1	360	55
Vanilla Milk Chocolate Brittle Bar	1	370	160
Vanilla Peanut Butter Swirl	4 oz	280	120
Vanilla Soft Yogurt	1 oz	28	13
Vanilla Swiss Almond	4 oz	290	55

HARDEE'S

BEVERAGES			
Shake			
Chocolate	12 oz	460	340
Strawberry	12 oz	440	300
Vanilla	12 oz	400	320
BREAKFAST SELECTIONS			
Bacon & Egg Biscuit	1	410	990
Bacon Biscuit	1	360	950
Bacon, Egg & Cheese Biscuit	1	460	1220
Big Country Breakfast			
Bacon	1	660	1540
Country Ham	1	670	2870
Ham	1	620	1780
Sausage	1	850	1980
Biscuit 'N' Gravy	1	440	1250
Canadian Rise 'N' Shine Biscuit	1	470	1550
Chicken Biscuit	1	430	1330
Cinnamon 'N' Raisin	1	320	510
Country Ham & Egg Biscuit	1	400	1600
Country Ham Biscuit	1	350	1550
Ham & Egg Biscuit	1	370	1050

FOOD	PORTION	CALORIES	SODIUM
Ham Biscuit	1	320	1000
Ham, Egg & Cheese Biscuit	1	420	1270
Hash Rounds	1 serving	230	560
Margarine/Butter Blend	1 tsp	35	40
Rise 'N' Shine Biscuit	1	320	740
Sausage & Egg Biscuit	1	490	1150
Sausage Biscuit	1	440	1100
Steak & Egg Biscuit	1	550	1370
Steak Biscuit	1	500	1320
Syrup	1.5 oz	120	25
Three Pancakes	1 serving	280	890
w/ 1 Sausage Pattie	1 serving	430	1290
w/ 2 Bacon Strips	1 serving	350	1110
DESSERTS			
Apple Turnover	1	270	250
Big Cookie	1	250	240
Cool Twist Cone			
Chocolate	1	200	65
Vanilla/Chocolate	1	190	80
Cool Twist Sundae			
Caramel	1	330	290
Hot Fudge	1	320	270
Strawberry	1	260	115
MAIN MENU SELECTIONS			
Bacon Cheeseburger	1	610	1030
Big Deluxe Burger	1	500	760
Big Fry	1 serving	500	180
Big Roast Beef	1	300	880
Big Twin	1	450	580
Cheeseburger	1	320	710

FOOD	PORTION	CALORIES	SODIUM
Chef Salad	1	240	930
Chicken Fillet	1	370	1060
Chicken 'N' Pasta Salad	1	414	380
Chicken			
Stix	6 pieces	210	680
Stix	9 pieces	310	1020
Crispy Curls	1 serving	300	840
Fisherman's Fillet	1	500	1030
French Fries	1 lg	360	135
French Fries	1 reg	230	85
Garden Salad	1	210	270
Grilled Chicken Sandwich	1	310	890
Hamburger	1	270	490
Hot Dog, All Beef	1	300	710
Hot Ham 'N' Cheese	1	330	1420
Mushroom 'N' Swiss Burger	1	490	940
Quarter-Pound Cheeseburger	1	500	1060
Regular Roast Beef	1	260	730
Side Salad	1	20	15
Turkey Club	1	390	1280

JACK IN THE BOX

BEVERAGES			
Coca-Cola Classic	12 oz	144	14
Coffee, Black	8 oz	2	26
Diet Coke	12 oz	1	26
Dr Pepper	12 oz	144	18
Iced Tea	12 oz	3	5
Lowfat Milk 2%	8 oz	122	122

FOOD	PORTION	CALORIES	SODIUM
Milk Shake			
Chocolate	11 oz	330	270
Strawberry	11 oz	320	240
Vanilla	11 oz	320	230
Orange Juice	6 oz	80	0
Ramblin' Root Beer	12 oz	176	20
Sprite	12 oz	144	46
BREAKFAST SELECTIONS			
Breakfast Jack	1	307	871
Country Crock Spread	1 pat	25	40
Grape Jelly	1 pkg	38	3
Hash Brown	1	156	312
Pancake Platter	1	612	888
Pancake Syrup	1 pkg	121	6
Sausage Crescent	1	584	1012
Scrambled Egg			
Platter	1	559	1060
Pocket	1	431	1060
Sourdough Breakfast Sandwich	1	381	1120
Supreme Crescent	1	547	1053
DESSERTS			
Cheesecake	1	309	208
Double Fudge Cake	1 slice	288	259
Hot Apple Turnover	1	354	479
MAIN MENU SELECTIONS			
BBQ Sauce	1 oz	44	300
Bacon Bacon Cheeseburger	1	705	1240
Cheeseburger	1	315	746
Chicken And Mushroom Sandwich	1	438	1340
Chicken Fajita Pita	1	292	703

FOOD	PORTION	CALORIES	SODIUM
Chicken			
Strips	4 pieces	285	695
Strips	6 pieces	451	1100
Chicken Supreme	1	641	1470
Double Cheeseburger	1	467	842
Egg Rolls	3 pieces	437	957
Egg Rolls	5 pieces	753	1640
Fish Supreme	1	510	1040
French Fries	1 jumbo	396	219
French Fries	1 reg	351	194
French Fries	1 sm	219	121
Grilled Chicken Fillet	1	431	1070
Grilled Sourdough Burger	1	712	1140
Guacamole	1 oz	55	130
Ham And Turkey Melt	1	592	1120
Hamburger	1	267	556
Jumbo Jack	1	584	733
With Cheese	1	677	1090
Old Fashioned Patty Melt	1	713	1360
Onion Rings	1 serving	380	451
Pastrami Melt	1	556	1340
Salsa	1 oz	8	27
Seasoned Curly French Fries	1 serving	358	1030
Sesame Breadsticks	1	70	110
Super Taco	1	281	718
Sweet & Sour Sauce	1 oz	40	160
Taco	1	187	414
Taquitos	7 pieces	511	681
Tortilla Chips	1 oz	139	134
Ultimate Cheeseburger	1	942	1176

FOOD	PORTION	CALORIES	SODIUM
SALADS AND DRESSINGS			
Bleu Cheese	1 pkg	262	918
Buttermilk House	1 pkg	362	694
Chef Salad	1	325	900
Italian Low Calorie	1 pkg	25	810
Side Salad	1	51	11
Taco Salad	1	503	1600
Thousand Island	1 pkg	312	700

KENTUCKY FRIED CHICKEN

CHICKEN DISHES			
Chicken Littles Sandwich	1	169	331
Colonel's Chicken Sandwich	1	482	1060
Extra Crispy			
Center Breast	1	342	790
Drumstick	1	204	324
Thigh	1	406	688
Wing	1	254	422
Kentucky Nuggets	1	46	140
Original			
Center Breast	1	283	735
Drumstick	1	146	275
Side Breast	1	267	735
Wing	1	178	372
SIDE DISHES			
Buttermilk Biscuit	1	235	655
Cole Slaw	1 serving	119	197
Corn-on-the-Cob	1 ear	176	21
French Fries	1 reg	244	139
Mashed Potatoes & Gravy	1 serving	71	339

FOOD	PORTION	CALORIES	SODIUM
Sauce			
Barbecue	1 oz	35	450
Honey	½ oz	49	*15*
Mustard	1 oz	36	346
Sweet & Sour	1 oz	58	148

LONG JOHN SILVER'S

CHILDREN'S MENU SELECTIONS

Chicken Planks, 2 Pieces & Fryes	7.8 oz	510	1060
Fish & Fryes, 1 Piece	6.9 oz	450	650
Fish Chicken & Fryes	8.9 oz	580	1140

DESSERTS

Apple Pie	1 slice	320	420
Cherry Pie	1 slice	360	200
Chocolate Chip Cookie	1	230	35
Lemon Pie	1 slice	340	130
Oatmeal Raisin Cookie	1	160	150
Walnut Brownie	1	440	150

MAIN MENU SELECTIONS
Batter Dipped Fish

1 Piece	3.1 oz	210	570
2 Pieces	6.2 oz	410	1130
Chicken	17.3 oz	620	2060
Chicken Planks			
1 Piece	2 oz	130	490
2 Pieces	4 oz	270	980
3 Pieces	5.9 oz	400	1470
Chicken Planks 2 Pieces & Fryes	6.9 oz	440	1040
Chicken Planks 3 Pieces w/ Fryes & Slaw	14.1 oz	860	1840

FOOD	PORTION	CALORIES	SODIUM
Chicken Planks 4 Pieces w/ Fryes & Slaw	16 oz	990	2330
Clams w/ Fryes & Slaw	12.7 oz	910	1390
Cole Slaw	3.4 oz	140	260
Corn Cobbette	1 piece	140	0
Fish & Chicken w/ Fryes & Slaw	15.2 oz	930	1920
Fish & Fryes, 2 Pieces	9.2 oz	580	1190
& Fryes, 3 Pieces	14 oz	930	1800
Fish & More, 2 Pieces	14 oz	860	1500
Fish & More, 3 Pieces w/ Fryes & Slaw	17.5 oz	1070	2070
Fish Light Portion w/ Lemon Crumb, 2 Pieces	10.3 oz	320	900
Fish Light Portion w/ Paprika, 2 Pieces	10 oz	300	650
Fish w/ Lemon Crumb, 3 Pieces	18.4 oz	640	1810
Fish w/ Paprika, 3 Pieces	18.2 oz	610	1560
Fish w/ Scampi Sauce, 3 Pieces	18.6 oz	660	1710
Fryes	1 reg	170	55
Green Beans	4 oz	113	480
Homestyle Fish 1 Piece	1.6 oz	125	200
2 Pieces	3.3 oz	250	400
3 Pieces	5 oz	380	610
Hushpuppies	1	70	25
Long John's Homestyle Fish 3 Pieces w/ Fryes & Slaw	13.1 oz	830	980
Ocean Chef Salad	8.2 oz	234	860
Rice Pilaf	5 oz	142	570
Sandwich Baked Chicken	6.4 oz	310	920
Sandwich Batter Dipped Chicken, 2 Pieces	6.5 oz	440	1280

FOOD	PORTION	CALORIES	SODIUM
Sandwich Batter Dipped Fish, 1 Piece	5.6 oz	380	860
Seafood Chowder w/ Cod	7 oz	140	590
Seafood Gumbo w/ Cod	7 oz	120	740
Seafood Salad	9.8 oz	230	580
Shrimp Scampi	10.6 oz	610	2050
SALAD DRESSINGS AND SAUCES			
Catsup	⅓ oz	12	135
Creamy Italian Dressing	1 oz	30	280
Dijon Herb Sauce	.88 oz	90	220
Honey Mustard Sauce	.88 oz	45	125
Malt Vinegar	.4 oz	2	20
Ranch Dressing	1 oz	90	230
Sea Salad Dressing	1 oz	90	160
Seafood Sauce	.88 oz	35	380
Sweet'n Sour Sauce	.88 oz	40	95
Tartar Sauce	.88 oz	70	70

MACHEEZMO MOUSE

CHILDREN'S MENU SELECTIONS			
Kid's Plate	7 oz	279	328
With Chicken	9 oz	349	358
MAIN MENU SELECTIONS			
Bean/Cheese			
Enchilada	12 oz	405	450
Enchilada Dinner	22 oz	670	710
Beans	6 oz	214	120
Boss Sauce	1 oz	30	140
Cheese	1 oz	81	180

FOOD	PORTION	CALORIES	SODIUM
Cheese Quesadilla	5 oz	337	535
Chicken	3 oz	105	45
Chicken Burrito	13 oz	543	653
Chicken Burrito Dinner	23 oz	808	913
Chicken Enchilada	10 oz	332	400
Chicken Enchilada Dinner	20 oz	597	660
Chicken Majita	18 oz	704	784
Chicken Quesadilla	9 oz	407	575
Chicken Salad Large	17 oz	612	750
Chicken Salad Small	10 oz	324	390
Chicken Tacos	6 oz	294	255
Chicken Tacos Dinner	16 oz	559	515
Chicken w/ Green Salad	13 oz	377	502
Chili	3 oz	135	300
Chili Tacos	6 oz	314	425
Chili Tacos Dinner	16 oz	579	685
Chips	3 oz	394	30
Combo Burrito	14 oz	598	838
Dinner	24 oz	863	1098
Enchilada Sauce	1 oz	6	65
Famouse #5	14 oz	583	637
Guacamole	2 oz	201	220
Mex Cheese	1 oz	100	280
Mixed Greens	4 oz	tr	20
Nacho Grande	8 oz	704	625
Rice	6 oz	274	300
Salad w/ Marinated Veggies Large	8 oz	54	130
Small	5 oz	32	85
Sour Cream Blend	1 oz	27	20

FOOD	PORTION	CALORIES	SODIUM
Tortilla			
Corn	2 oz	128	10
Flour	2 oz	160	140
Mini Corn	3 oz	160	13
Whole Wheat	2 oz	160	130
Vegetables	4 oz	43	80
Vegetarian			
Burrito	14 oz	601	748
Burrito Dinner	24 oz	866	1008
Vegetarian Plate	15 oz	531	429
Vegetarian Tacos	6 oz	295	265
Tacos Dinner	16 oz	560	525
Veggie Taco Salad			
Large	17 oz	647	670
Small	10 oz	379	425
Yogurt, Nonfat	1 oz	15	22

McDONALD'S

FOOD	PORTION	CALORIES	SODIUM
BEVERAGES			
Apple Juice	6 oz	90	5
Coca-Cola Classic	16 oz	190	20
Diet Coke	16 oz	1	40
Grapefruit Juice	6 oz	80	0
Milk 1%	8 oz	110	130
Milk Shake			
Lowfat Chocolate	10.4 oz	320	240
Lowfat Strawberry	10.4 oz	320	170
Lowfat Vanilla	10.4 oz	290	170
Orange Drink	16 oz	177	20
Orange Juice	6 oz	80	0
Sprite	16 oz	190	20

FOOD	PORTION	CALORIES	SODIUM
BREAKFAST SELECTIONS			
Biscuit			
w/ Bacon, Egg & Cheese	1	440	1215
w/ Sausage	1	420	1040
w/ Sausage & Egg	1	505	1210
w/ Spread	1	260	730
Breakfast Burrito	1	280	580
Cheerios	¾ cup	80	210
Egg McMuffin	1	280	710
English Muffin w/ Spread	1	170	285
Fat-Free			
Apple Bran Muffin	1	180	200
Blueberry Muffin	1	170	220
Hash Brown Potatoes	1 serving	130	330
Hotcakes w/ Margarine & Syrup	1 portion	440	685
Sausage	1	160	310
Sausage McMuffin	1	345	770
Sausage McMuffin w/ Egg	1	430	920
Scrambled Eggs	1 portion	140	290
Wheaties	¾ cup	90	220
DESSERTS			
Apple Pie	1 (3 oz)	260	240
Cone, Lowfat Frozen Yogurt, Vanilla	1 (3 oz)	105	80
Cookies			
Chocolaty Chip	1 pkg (2 oz)	330	280
McDonaldland	1 pkg (2 oz)	290	300
Danish			
Apple	1	390	370
Cinnamon Raisin	1	440	430
Iced Cheese	1	390	420
Raspberry	1	410	310

FOOD	PORTION	CALORIES	SODIUM
Sundae, Lowfat Frozen Yogurt			
Hot Caramel	1 (6 oz)	270	180
Hot Fudge	1 (6 oz)	240	170
Strawberry	1 (6 oz)	210	95
MAIN MENU SELECTIONS			
Big Mac	1	500	890
Cheeseburger	1	305	725
Chicken Fajita	1	185	310
Chicken McNuggets	6	270	580
Filet-O-Fish	1	370	730
French Fries	1 lg	400	200
French Fries	1 med	320	150
French Fries	1 sm	220	110
Hamburger	1	255	490
McChicken	1	415	830
McLean Deluxe	1	320	670
w/ Cheese	1	370	890
Quarter Pounder	1	410	645
w/ Cheese	1	510	1110
SALADS, DRESSINGS & SAUCES			
1000 Island Dressing	1 pkg	225	500
Bacon Bits	.1 oz	15	95
Bleu Cheese Dressing	1 pkg	250	750
Chef Salad	1 serving	170	400
Chunky Chicken Salad	1 serving	150	230
Croutons	.3 oz	50	140
Garden Salad	1	50	70
Lite Vinaigrette Dressing	1 pkg	48	240
McNuggets Sauce			
Barbeque	1.12 oz	50	340

FOOD	PORTION	CALORIES	SODIUM
Honey	.5 oz	45	0
Hot Mustard	1.05 oz	70	250
Sweet 'N Sour	1.12 oz	60	190
Ranch Dressing	1 pkg	220	520
Red French Reduced Calorie Dressing	1 pkg	160	460
Side Salad	1 serving	30	35

NATHAN'S

French Fries	1 (7 oz)	550	151
Hot Dog & Roll	1	290	675

PIZZA HUT

HAND TOSSED MEDIUM			
Cheese	2 slices	518	1276
Pepperoni	2 slices	500	1267
Super Supreme	2 slices	556	1648
Supreme	2 slices	540	1470
PAN PIZZA MEDIUM			
Cheese	2 slices	492	940
Pepperoni	2 slices	540	1127
Super Supreme	2 slices	563	1447
Supreme	2 slices	589	1363
PERSONAL PAN PIZZA			
Pepperoni	1 pie	675	1335
Supreme	1 pie	647	1313
THIN 'N CRISPY MEDIUM			
Cheese	2 slices	398	867
Pepperoni	2 slices	413	986
Super Supreme	2 slices	463	1336

FOOD	PORTION	CALORIES	SODIUM
Supreme	2 slices	459	1328

PONDEROSA

BEVERAGES

Cherry Coke	6 oz	77	4
Chocolate Milk	8 oz	208	149
Coca-Cola	6 oz	72	7
Coffee, Black	6 oz	2	26
Diet Coke	6 oz	tr	8
Caffeine Free	6 oz	tr	8
Diet Sprite	6 oz	2	4
Dr Pepper	6 oz	72	14
Lemonade	6 oz	68	50
Milk	8 oz	159	122
Mr Pibb	6 oz	71	10
Orange Soda	6 oz	82	0
Root Beer	6 oz	80	9
Sprite	6 oz	72	16
Tea	6 oz	2	0

DESSERTS
Ice Milk

Chocolate	3.5 oz	152	70
Vanilla	3.5 oz	150	58

Topping

Caramel	1 oz	100	72
Chocolate	1 oz	89	37
Strawberry	1 oz	71	29
Whipped	1 oz	80	16

MAIN MENU SELECTIONS

BBQ Sauce	1 tbsp	25	260

FOOD	PORTION	CALORIES	SODIUM
Bake 'R Broil Fish	1 serving (5.2 oz)	230	330
Baked Potato	1	145	6
Beans Baked	1 serving (4 oz)	170	330
Beans Green	1 serving (3.5 oz)	20	391
Breaded			
Cauliflower	1 serving (4 oz)	115	446
Okra	1 serving (4 oz)	124	483
Onion Rings	1 serving (4 oz)	213	620
Zucchini	1 serving (4 oz)	102	584
Carrots	1 serving (3.5 oz)	31	33
Cheese Herb Garlic Spread	1 tbsp	100	120
Cheese Sauce	2 oz	52	355
Chicken			
Breast	1 serving (5.5 oz)	90	400
Wings	2	213	610
Chopped Steak	4 oz	225	150
Chopped Steak	5.3 oz	296	296
Corn	1 serving (3.5 oz)	90	5
Fish Fried	1 serving (3.2 oz)	190	170
Fish Nuggets	1	31	52
French Fries	1 serving	120	39
Gravy			
Brown	2 oz	25	167
Turkey	2 oz	25	228
Halibut, Broiled	1 serving (6 oz)	170	68
Hot Dog	1	144	460
Italian Breadsticks	1	100	200

FOOD	PORTION	CALORIES	SODIUM
Kansas City Strip	5 oz	138	850
Macaroni And Cheese	4 oz	67	320
Margarine, Liquid	1 tbsp	100	110
Mashed Potatoes	1 serving (4 oz)	62	191
Meatballs	1	58	8
Mini Shrimp	6	47	125
New York Strip, Choice	10 oz	314	1420
New York Strip, Choice	8 oz	384	570
Pasta Shells, Plain	2 oz	78	tr
Peas	1 serving (3.5 oz)	67	120
Porterhouse	13 oz	441	1844
Choice	16 oz	640	1130
Potato Wedges	1 serving (3.5 oz)	130	171
Ribeye	5 oz	219	1130
Choice	6 oz	281	570
Rice Pilaf	1 serving (4 oz)	160	450
Roll			
Dinner	1	184	311
Sourdough	1	110	230
Roughy, Broiled	1 serving (5 oz)	139	88
Salmon, Broiled	1 serving (6 oz)	192	72
Sandwich Steak	4 oz	408	850
Scrod, Baked	1 serving (7 oz)	120	80
Shrimp, Fried	7 pieces	231	612
Sirloin			
Choice	7 oz	241	570
Tips, Choice	5 oz	473	280
Spaghetti Plain	2 oz	78	tr
Spaghetti Sauce	4 oz	110	520

FOOD	PORTION	CALORIES	SODIUM
Steak Kabobs, Meat Only	3 oz	153	280
Stuffing	4 oz	230	800
Sweet/Sour Sauce	1 oz	37	80
Swordfish, Broiled	1 serving (6 oz)	271	0
T-Bone	8 oz	176	850
Choice	10 oz	444	850
Teriyaki Steak	5 oz	174	1420
Tortilla Chips	1 oz	150	80
Trout, Broiled	1 serving (5 oz)	228	51
Winter Mix	1 serving (3.5 oz)	25	33
SALAD BAR			
Alfalfa Sprouts	1 oz	10	0
Apple	1	80	1
Apples, Canned	4 oz	90	15
Applesauce	4 oz	80	20
Banana	1	87	1
Banana Chips	.2 oz	25	tr
Banana Pudding	1 oz	52	29
Bean Sprouts	1 oz	10	1
Beets, Diced	4 oz	55	307
Breadsticks, Sesame	2	35	60
Broccoli	1 oz	9	4
Cabbage			
Green	1 oz	9	7
Red	1 oz	1	1
Cantaloupe	1 wedge	13	5
Carrots	1 oz	12	13
Cauliflower	1 oz	8	4
Celery	1 oz	4	36

FOOD	PORTION	CALORIES	SODIUM
Cheese Imitation, Shredded	1 oz	90	420
Cheese Spread	1 oz	98	188
Cherry Peppers	2 pieces	7	415
Chicken Salad	3.5 oz	212	335
Chow Mein Noodles	.2 oz	25	42
Cocktail Sauce	1 oz	34	453
Coconut, Shredded	.2 oz	25	14
Cottage Cheese	4 oz	120	330
Croutons	1 oz	115	351
Cucumber	1 oz	4	2
Eggs, Diced	2 oz	94	75
Fruit Cocktail	4 oz	97	7
Garbanzo Beans	1 oz	102	7
Gelatin, Plain	4 oz	71	73
Grapes	10	34	2
Green Onion	1	7	1
Green Pepper	1 oz	6	4
Ham, Diced	2 oz	120	780
Honeydew	1 wedge	24	9
Lemon	1 wedge	3	0
Lettuce	1 oz	5	5
Macaroni Salad	3.5 oz	335	431
Margarine, Whipped	1 tbsp	34	65
Meal Mates Sesame Crackers	2	45	95
Melba Snacks	2	18	60
Mousse			
Chocolate	1 oz	78	18
Strawberry	1 oz	74	17
Mushrooms	1 oz	8	4

FOOD	PORTION	CALORIES	SODIUM
Olives			
Black	1	4	24
Green	1	3	69
Onions, Red & Yellow	1 oz	11	3
Orange	1	45	1
Pasta Salad	3.5 oz	269	441
Peaches, Canned	4 oz	70	10
Pears, Canned	4 oz	98	7
Pickles			
Dill Spears	.14 oz	tr	54
Sweet Chips	.14 oz	4	tr
Pineapple			
Fresh	1 wedge	11	tr
Tidbits	4 oz	95	2
Potato Salad	3.5 oz	126	300
Radishes	1 oz	4	5
Ritz	2	40	50
Saltine Crackers	2	25	38
Spiced Apple Rings	4 oz	100	20
Spinach	1 oz	7	20
Strawberries	2 oz	14	61
Strawberry Glaze	1 oz	37	4
Tartar Sauce	1 oz	85	477
Tomatoes	1 oz	6	1
Turkey Ham Salad	3.5 oz	186	655
Turkey Julienne	1 oz	29	192
Vanilla Wafer	2	35	25
Watermelon	1 wedge	111	4
Yogurt			
Fruit	4 oz	115	70
Vanilla	4 oz	110	75

FOOD	PORTION	CALORIES	SODIUM
Zucchini	1 oz	5	tr
SALAD DRESSINGS			
Blue Cheese	1 oz	130	266
Cole Slaw	1 oz	150	284
Creamy Italian	1 oz	103	373
Cucumber Reduced Calorie	1 oz	69	315
Italian Reduced Calorie	1 oz	31	371
Parmesan Pepper	1 oz	150	282
Ranch	1 oz	147	298
Salad Oil	1 tbsp	120	0
Sour Cream	1 tbsp	26	6
Sweet-N-Tangy	1 oz	122	347
Thousand Island	1 oz	113	405

RAX

FOOD	PORTION	CALORIES	SODIUM
BEVERAGES AND DESSERTS			
Chocolate Chip Cookie	1	262	192
Chocolate Shake	11 oz	445	248
Coke	16 oz	205	11
Diet Coke	16 oz	1	21
MAIN MENU SELECTIONS			
Bacon	1 slice	14	40
Baked Potato	1	264	15
w/ 1 Tbsp Margarine	1	364	115
Barbecue Sauce	1 pkg	11	158
Beef Bacon 'N Cheddar	1	523	1042
Cheddar Cheese Sauce	1 oz	29	225
Country Fried Chicken Breast Sandwich	1	618	1078
Deluxe Roast Beef	1	498	864

FOOD	PORTION	CALORIES	SODIUM
French Dressing	2 oz	275	442
French Fries	1 reg	282	75
Gourmet Garden Salad			
w/ French Dressing	1	409	792
w/ Lite Italian Dressing	1	305	643
w/o Dressing	1	134	350
Grilled Chicken Breast Sandwich	1	402	872
Grilled Chicken Garden Salad			
w/ French Dressing	1	477	1189
w/ Lite Italian Dressing	1	264	1040
w/o Dressing	1	202	747
Lite Italian Dressing	2 oz	63	294
Mushroom Sauce	1 oz	16	113
Philly Melt	1	396	1055
Regular Rax	1	262	707
Swiss Slice	1 slice	42	157

RED LOBSTER

All of the following are for a cooked portion unless otherwise noted.

FOOD	PORTION	CALORIES	SODIUM
Atlantic Cod	1 lunch serving	100	200
Atlantic Ocean Perch	1 lunch serving	130	190
Blacktip Shark	1 lunch serving	150	90
Calamari, breaded & fried	1 lunch serving	360	30
Calico Scallops	1 lunch serving	180	60
Catfish	1 lunch serving	170	50
Chicken Breast, Skinless	4 oz	140	60
Deep Sea Scallops	1 lunch serving	130	260
Filet Mignon Steak	8 oz	350	105
Flounder	1 lunch serving	100	95
Grouper	1 lunch serving	110	70

FOOD	PORTION	CALORIES	SODIUM
Haddock	1 lunch serving	110	180
Halibut	1 lunch serving	110	105
Hamburger	5 oz	410	115
King Crab Legs	1 lb	170	900
Langostino	1 lunch serving	120	410
Lemon Sole	1 lunch serving	120	90
Mackerel	1 lunch serving	190	250
Maine Lobster	18 oz	240	550
Mako Shark	1 lunch serving	140	60
Monkfish	1 lunch serving	110	95
Norwegian Salmon	1 lunch serving	230	60
Pollack	1 lunch serving	120	90
Rainbow Trout	1 lunch serving	170	90
Red Rockfish	1 lunch serving	90	95
Red Snapper	1 lunch serving	110	140
Rib Eye Steak	12 oz	980	150
Rock Lobster	1 tail (13 oz)	230	1090
Shrimp	8 to 12 pieces (7 oz)	120	110
Sirloin Steak	8 oz	350	110
Snow Crab Legs	1 lb	150	1630
Sockeye Salmon	1 lunch serving	160	60
Strip Steak	9 oz	560	115
Swordfish	1 lunch serving	100	140
Tilefish	1 lunch serving	100	60
Yellowfin Tuna	1 lunch serving	180	70

SHONEY'S

BEVERAGES

Clear Soda	1 lg	105	21

FOOD	PORTION	CALORIES	SODIUM
Clear Soda	1 sm	52	10
Coffee, Regular & Decaf	1 cup	8	8
Cola	1 lg	139	10
Cola	1 sm	69	5
Creamer	⅜ oz	14	8
Hot Chocolate	1 cup	110	154
Hot Tea	1 cup	0	19
Milk 2%	1 cup	121	122
Orange Juice	4 oz	54	1
Sugar	1 pkg	13	0
BREAKFAST SELECTIONS			
100% Natural	½ cup	244	45
Ambrosia Salad	¼ cup	75	167
Apple	1	81	1
Apple Butter	1 tbsp	37	0
Apple Grape Surprise	¼ cup	19	2
Apple Ring	1	15	0
Apple sliced	1 slice	13	0
Bacon	1 strip	36	101
Beef Stick	1	43	17
Biscuit	1	170	364
Blueberries	¼ cup	21	2
Blueberry Muffin	1	107	1
Bread Pudding	1 sq	305	409
Breakfast Ham	1 slice	26	263
Brunch Cake			
Apple	1 sq	160	150
Banana	1 sq	152	120
Carrot	1 sq	150	159
Pineapple	1 sq	147	120

FOOD	PORTION	CALORIES	SODIUM
Brunch Cake (cont.)			
Sour Cream	1 sq	160	135
Buttered Toast	2 slices	163	296
Cantaloupe			
Diced	½ cup	28	7
Sliced	1 slice	8	2
Captain Crunch Berry	½ cup	73	122
Cheese Sauce	1 ladle	26	166
Chicken Pieces	1 piece	40	28
Chocolate Pudding	¼ cup	81	81
Cinnamon Honey Bun	1	344	169
Donut, Mini Cinnamon	1	56	65
Cottage Cheese	1 tbsp	12	66
Cottage Fries	¼ cup	62	124
Country Gravy	¼ cup	82	255
Croissant	1	260	260
DoughNugget	1	157	194
Egg, Fried	1	159	69
Egg, Scrambled	¼ cup	95	155
English Muffin w/ Margarine	1	140	1
Fluff	¼ cup	16	0
French Toast	1 slice	69	157
Fruit Delight	¼ cup	54	2
Fruit Topping All Flavors	1 tbsp	24	3
Glaced Fruit	¼ cup	51	5
Golden Pound Cake	1 slice	134	144
Grape Jelly	1 tbsp	60	0
Grapefruit, Canned	¼ cup	24	5
Grapes	25	57	2
Grits	¼ cup	57	62

FOOD	PORTION	CALORIES	SODIUM
Hashbrowns	¼ cup	43	24
Home Fries	¼ cup	53	24
Honey Bun	1	265	33
Honeydew, Sliced	1 slice	13	4
Jelly Packet	1	40	2
Jr. Bun			
Chocolate	1	141	70
Honey	1	141	70
Maple	1	141	70
Kiwi, Sliced	1 slice	11	1
Marble Cake w/ Icing	1 slice	136	149
Mixed Fruit	¼ cup	37	3
Mushroom Topping	1 oz	25	323
Oleo, Whipped	1 tbsp	70	97
Omelette Topping	1 spoonful	23	99
Orange	1 med	65	2
Sections	1 section	7	0
Oriental Salad	¼ cup	79	32
Pancake	1	41	238
Pear	1	98	1
Pineapple			
Bits	1 tbsp	9	2
Fresh, Sliced	1 slice	10	0
Pistachio Pineapple Salad	¼ cup	98	39
Prunes	1 tbsp	19	0
Raisin Bran	½ cup	87	185
Raisin English Muffin w/ Margarine	1	158	280
Sausage			
Link	1	91	291
Patty	1	136	48

FOOD	PORTION	CALORIES	SODIUM
Sausage Rice	¼ cup	110	211
Shortcake	1	60	90
Sirloin Steak, Charbroiled	6 oz	357	160
Smoked Sausage	1	103	39
Snow Salad	¼ cup	72	18
Strawberries	5	23	1
Syrup			
Light	1 ladle	60	0
Low-Cal	2.2 oz	98	0
Tangerine	1	37	1
Trix	½ cup	54	89
Waldorf Salad	¼ cup	81	68
Watermelon			
Diced	½ cup	50	3
Sliced	1 slice	9	1
Whipped Topping	1 scoop	10	3
CHILDREN'S MENU SELECTIONS			
Jr. Burger All-American	1 serving	234	543
Kid's Chicken Dinner (fried)	1 serving	244	151
Kid's Fish N' Chips (includes fries)	1 serving	337	467
Kid's Fried Shrimp	1 serving	194	633
Kid's Spaghetti	1 serving	247	193
DESSERTS			
Apple Pie A La Mode	1 slice	492	574
Carrot Cake	1 slice	500	476
Hot Fudge Cake	1 slice	522	485
Hot Fudge Sundae	1	451	226
Strawberry Pie	1 slice	332	247
Strawberry Sundae	1	380	145
Walnut Brownie A La Mode	1	576	435

FOOD	PORTION	CALORIES	SODIUM
MAIN MENU SELECTIONS			
All-American Burger	1	501	597
BBQ Sauce	1 souffle cup	41	232
Bacon Burger	1	591	801
Baked Fish	1 serving	170	1641
Baked Fish Light	1 serving	170	1641
Baked Ham Sandwich	1	290	1263
Baked Potato	10 oz	264	16
Beef Patty Light	1 serving	289	187
Charbroiled Chicken	1 serving	239	592
Charbroiled Chicken Sandwich	1	451	1002
Chicken Fillet Sandwich	1	464	585
Chicken Tenders	1 serving	388	239
Cocktail Sauce	1 souffle cup	36	260
Country Fried Sandwich	1	588	1501
Country Fried Steak	1 serving	449	1177
Fish N' Chips (includes fries)	1 serving	639	873
Fish N' Shrimp	1 serving	487	644
Fish Sandwich	1	323	740
French Fries	3 oz	189	273
French Fries	4 oz	252	364
Fried Fish, Light	1 serving	297	536
Grecian Bread	1 slice	80	94
Grilled Bacon & Cheese Sandwich	1	440	1200
Grilled Cheese Sandwich	1	302	880
Half o'Pound	1 serving	435	280
Ham Club On Whole Wheat	1	642	2105
Hawaiian Chicken	1 serving	262	593
Italian Feast	1 serving	500	369
Lasagna	1 serving	297	870

FOOD	PORTION	CALORIES	SODIUM
Liver N' Onions	1 serving	411	321
Mushroom Swiss Burger	1	616	1135
Old-Fashioned Burger	1	470	681
Onion Rings	1	52	102
Patty Melt	1	640	826
Philly Steak Sandwich	1	673	1242
Reuben Sandwich	1	596	3873
Ribeye	6 oz	605	141
Rice	3.5 oz	137	765
Sauteed Mushrooms	3 oz	75	968
Sauteed Onions	2.5 oz	37	221
Seafood Platter	1 serving	566	893
Shoney Burger	1	498	782
Shrimp Bite-Size	1 serving	387	1266
Shrimp Broiled	1 serving	93	210
Shrimp Charbroiled	1 serving	138	170
Shrimp Sampler	1 serving	412	783
Shrimper's Feast	1 serving	383	216
Large	1 serving	575	324
Sirloin	6 oz	357	160
Slim Jim Sandwich	1	484	1620
Spaghetti	1 serving	496	387
Steak N' Shrimp (charbroiled shrimp)	1 serving	361	198
(fried shrimp)	1 serving	507	249
Sweet N' Sour Sauce	1 souffle cup	58	5
Tartar Sauce	1 souffle cup	84	177
Turkey Club On Whole Wheat	1	635	1289
SALAD BAR Ambrosia Salad	¼ cup	75	167

FOOD	PORTION	CALORIES	SODIUM
Apple Grape Surprise	¼ cup	19	2
Apple Ring	1	15	3
Beet Onion Salad	¼ cup	25	167
Broccoli	¼ cup	4	4
Broccoli & Cauliflower	¼ cup	98	478
Broccoli Cauliflower Carrot Salad	¼ cup	53	193
Broccoli Cauliflower Ranch	¼ cup	65	12
Carrot	¼ cup	10	8
Carrot Apple Salad	¼ cup	99	10
Cauliflower	¼ cup	8	5
Celery	1 tbsp	5	7
Cheese, Shredded	1 tbsp	21	112
Chocolate Pudding	¼ cup	81	81
Chow Mein Noodles	1 spoonful	13	0
Cole Slaw	¼ cup	69	106
Cottage Cheese	1 tbsp	12	66
Croutons	1 spoonful	13	38
Cucumber	1 tbsp	1	0
Cucumber Lite	¼ cup	12	344
Don's Pasta	¼ cup	82	223
Egg, Diced	1 tbsp	15	14
Fruit Delight	¼ cup	54	2
Fruit Topping All Flavors	¼ cup	64	8
Glaced Fruit	¼ cup	51	5
Grapefruit	¼ cup	24	5
Green Pepper	1 tbsp	1	0
Italian Vegetable	¼ cup	11	110
Jello	¼ cup	40	26
Jello Fluff	¼ cup	16	0

FOOD	PORTION	CALORIES	SODIUM
Kidney Bean Salad	¼ cup	55	154
Lettuce	1.8 oz	7	5
Macaroni Salad	¼ cup	207	382
Margarine, Whipped	1 tsp	23	32
Melba Toast	2	20	45
Mixed Fruit Salad	¼ cup	37	3
Mixed Squash	¼ cup	49	230
Mushrooms	1 tbsp	1	0
Oil	1 tsp	45	0
Olives			
Black	2	10	38
Green	2	8	162
Onion, Sliced	1 tbsp	1	0
Oriental Salad	¼ cup	79	31
Pea Salad	¼ cup	73	89
Pepperoni	1 tbsp	30	81
Pickle			
Chips	1 slice	5	30
Spear	1 spear	2	271
Pineapple Bits	1 tbsp	9	2
Pistachio Pineapple Salad	¼ cup	98	39
Prunes	1 tbsp	19	0
Radish	1 tbsp	1	1
Raisins	1 spoonful	26	1
Rotelli Pasta	¼ cup	78	82
Seign Salad	¼ cup	72	122
Snow Delight	¼ cup	72	18
Spaghetti Salad	¼ cup	81	20
Spinach	¼ cup	1	4
Spring Pasta	¼ cup	38	162
Summer Salad	¼ cup	114	233

FOOD	PORTION	CALORIES	SODIUM
Sunflower Seeds	1 spoonful	40	2
Three Bean Salad	¼ cup	96	189
Trail Mix	1 spoonful	30	0
Turkey Ham	1 tbsp	12	121
Waldorf	¼ cup	81	68
Wheat Bread	1 slice	71	150
SALAD DRESSINGS			
Biscayne Lo-Cal	2 tbsp	62	334
Blue Cheese	2 tbsp	113	109
Creamy Italian	2 tbsp	135	454
French	2 tbsp	124	204
Golden Italian	2 tbsp	141	302
Honey Mustard	2 tbsp	165	5
Ranch	2 tbsp	95	10
Rue French	2 tbsp	122	364
Thousand Island	2 tbsp	130	179
W.W. Italian	2 tbsp	10	615
SOUP			
Bean	6 oz	63	479
Beef Cabbage	6 oz	86	503
Broccoli Cauliflower	6 oz	124	560
Cheddar Chowder	6 oz	91	948
Cheese Florentine Ham	6 oz	110	890
Chicken			
Gumbo	6 oz	60	1050
Noodle	6 oz	62	127
Rice	6 oz	72	117
Clam Chowder	6 oz	94	66
Corn Chowder	6 oz	148	510
Cream Of Broccoli	6 oz	75	415

FOOD	PORTION	CALORIES	SODIUM
Cream Of Chicken	6 oz	136	1164
Cream Of Chicken Vegetable	6 oz	79	714
Onion	6 oz	29	88
Potato	6 oz	102	335
Tomato			
Florentine	6 oz	63	683
Vegetable	6 oz	46	314
Vegetable Beef	6 oz	82	1254

T.J. CINNAMONS

FOOD	PORTION	CALORIES	SODIUM
Doughnuts			
Cake	2	454	582
Raised	2	352	198
Mini-Cinn			
Plain	1	75	89
With Icing	1	80	89
Original Gourmet Cinnamon Roll			
Plain	1	630	712
With Icing	1	686	712
Petite Cinnamon Roll			
Plain	1	185	214
With Icing	1	202	214
Sticky Bun			
Cinnamon Pecan	1	607	589
Petite Cinnamon Pecan	1	255	241
Triple Chocolate Classic Roll			
Plain	1	412	543
With Icing	1	462	563

TCBY

FOOD	PORTION	CALORIES	SODIUM
Nonfat			
All Flavors	1 giant	869	356
All Flavors	1 kiddie size	88	36

FOOD	PORTION	CALORIES	SODIUM
All Flavors	1 lg	289	118
All Flavors	1 reg	226	92
All Flavors	1 sm	162	66
All Flavors	1 super	418	171
Regular			
All Flavors	1 giant	1027	474
All Flavors	1 kiddie size	104	48
All Flavors	1 lg	341	158
All Flavors	1 sm	192	89
All Flavors	1 super	494	228
Sugar Free			
All Flavors	1 giant	632	316
All Flavors	1 kiddie size	64	32
All Flavors	1 lg	210	105
All Flavors	1 reg	164	82
All Flavors	1 sm	118	59
All Flavors	1 super	304	152

TACO BELL

FOOD	PORTION	CALORIES	SODIUM
Burrito			
Bean	1	447	1148
Beef	1	493	1311
Chicken	1	334	880
Combo	1	407	1136
Fiesta Bean	1	226	652
Supreme	1	503	1181
Chilito	1	383	893
Cinnamon Twists	1 order	171	234
Enchirito	1	382	1243
Green Sauce	1 oz	4	136
Guacamole	⅔ oz	34	113

FOOD	PORTION	CALORIES	SODIUM
Jalapeno Peppers	3.5 oz	20	1370
MexiMelt			
Beef	1	266	689
Chicken	1	257	779
Mexican Pizza	1	575	1031
Nacho Cheese Sauce	2 oz	105	393
Nachos	1	346	399
Bellgrande	1	649	997
Supreme	1	367	471
Pico De Gallo	1	8	80
Pintos 'N Cheese	1	190	642
Ranch Dressing	2.5 oz	236	571
Red Sauce	1 oz	10	261
Salsa	⅓ oz	18	376
Sour Cream	⅔ oz	46	0
Taco	1	183	276
Taco Bellgrande	1	335	472
Taco Fiesta	1	127	139
Taco Salad	1	905	910
Taco Salad w/o Shell	1	484	680
Taco Sauce	1 pkg	2	126
Taco Sauce, Hot	1 pkg	3	82
Taco Soft	1	225	554
Chicken	1	213	615
Fiesta	1	147	361
Steak	1	218	456
Supreme	1	272	554
Taco Supreme	1	230	276
Tostada	1	243	596
Tostada Fiesta	1	167	324

FOOD	PORTION	CALORIES	SODIUM
TACO JOHN'S			
Bean Burrito	1	197	636
Beef Burrito	1	303	666
Chicken Burrito w/ Green Chili	1	344	986
Chicken Super Taco Salad			
w/ Dressing	1	507	1232
w/o Dressing	1	377	882
Chimichanga	1	464	1246
w/ Chicken	1 serving	441	1234
Combo Burrito	1	250	651
Mexican Rice	1 serving	340	1280
Nachos	1 serving	468	444
Potato Olé	1 lg	414	1595
Smothered Burrito			
w/ Green Chili	1	367	998
w/ Texas Chili	1	455	1217
Softshell	1	140	506
w/ Chicken	1	180	490
Super Burrito	1	389	856
w/ Chicken	1	366	844
Super Nachos	1 serving	669	994
Super Taco			
Bravo	1	361	826
Salad w/ 2 oz Dressing	1	558	1250
Salad w/o Dressing	1	428	900
Taco	1	178	348
Bravo	1	319	658
Taco Burger	1	281	660
Taco Salad			
w/ 2 oz Dressing	1	359	790
w/o Dressing	1	228	440

FOOD	PORTION	CALORIES	SODIUM

WENDY'S

BEVERAGES

FOOD	PORTION	CALORIES	SODIUM
Chocolate Milk	8 oz	160	140
Coffee			
Black	6 oz	2	5
Decaffeinated Black	6 oz	2	tr
Cola	8 oz	100	10
Diet Cola	8 oz	1	20
Hot Chocolate	6 oz	110	115
Lemon-Lime	8 oz	100	20
Lemonade	8 oz	90	tr
Milk 2%	8 oz	110	115
Tea			
Hot	6 oz	1	5
Iced	12 oz	2	10

CHILDREN'S MENU SELECTIONS

FOOD	PORTION	CALORIES	SODIUM
Kid's Meal			
Cheeseburger	1	300	770
Hamburger	1	260	570

DESSERTS

FOOD	PORTION	CALORIES	SODIUM
Chocolate Chip Cookie	1	275	256
Frosty Dairy Dessert	1 sm	340	200

MAIN MENU SELECTIONS

FOOD	PORTION	CALORIES	SODIUM
¼ lb Hamburger Patty, no bun	1	180	210
American Cheese	1 slice	70	260
Bacon	1 strip	30	100
Big Classic	1	570	1085
Cheddar Cheese, Shredded	1 oz	110	175
Chicken Breast Fillet	1	220	400
Chicken Club Sandwich	1	506	930
Chicken Sandwich	1	440	725

FOOD	PORTION	CALORIES	SODIUM
Chili	1 reg	220	750
Country Fried Steak Sandwich	1	440	870
Crispy Chicken Nuggets	6 pieces	280	600
Fish Fillet Sandwich	1	460	780
French Fries	1 sm	240	145
Grilled Chicken Fillet	1	100	330
Grilled Chicken Sandwich	1	340	815
Honey Mustard	1 tbsp	71	170
Hot Stuffed Potato			
Bacon & Cheese	1	520	1460
Broccoli & Cheese	1	400	455
Cheese	1	420	310
Chili & Cheese	1	500	630
Plain	1	250	20
Sour Cream & Chives	1	500	135
Jr. Bacon Cheeseburger	1	430	840
Jr. Cheeseburger	1	310	770
Jr. Hamburger	1	260	570
Jr. Swiss Deluxe	1	360	765
Kaiser Bun	1	200	350
Ketchup	1 tbsp	17	145
Lettuce	1 leaf	1	tr
Mayonnaise	1 tbsp	90	60
Mustard	1 tsp	4	45
Nuggets Sauce			
Barbecue	1 pkg	50	100
Honey	1 pkg	45	tr
Sweet & Sour	1 pkg	45	55
Sweet Mustard	1 pkg	50	140
Onion	6 rings	4	tr
Pickles	½ oz	2	200

FOOD	PORTION	CALORIES	SODIUM
Plain Single	1	340	500
Sandwich Bun	1	160	290
Single With Everything	1	420	890
Sour Cream	1 oz	60	15
Tartar Sauce	⅔ oz	120	115
Tomatoes	2 slices	4	tr
SALAD/SUPER BAR			
Alfalfa Sprouts	1 oz	8	tr
Alfredo Sauce	2 oz	36	300
Applesauce Chunky	1 oz	22	tr
Bacon & Tomato Dressing, Reduced Calorie	1 tbsp	45	190
Bacon Bits	1 tbsp	40	400
Bananas	1 oz	26	tr
Blue Cheese Dressing	1 tbsp	90	105
Breadsticks	2	30	30
Broccoli	½ cup	12	10
Cantaloupe	2 oz	20	5
Carrots	¼ cup	12	10
Cauliflower	½ cup	14	10
Celery Seed Dressing	1 tbsp	70	65
Cheddar Chips	1 oz	160	445
Cheese Ravioli In Spaghetti Sauce	2 oz	45	290
Cheese Sauce	2 oz	39	305
Cheese Shredded, Imitation	1 oz	80	125
Cheese Tortellini In Spaghetti Sauce	2 oz	60	280
Chef Salad	1 (9 oz)	130	460
Chicken Salad	2 oz	120	215
Chives	1 oz	71	20

FOOD	PORTION	CALORIES	SODIUM
Chow Mein Noodles	½ oz	64	60
Cole Slaw	2 oz	70	130
Cottage Cheese	½ cup	108	425
Croutons	½ oz	60	155
Cucumbers	4 slices	2	tr
Eggs, hard cooked, chopped	1 tbsp	30	25
Fettucini	2 oz	190	3
Flour Tortilla	1	110	220
French Style Dressing	1 tbsp	60	178
French Sweet Red Dressing	1 tbsp	70	125
Garbanzo Beans	1 oz	46	5
Garden Salad	1 (8 oz)	70	60
Garlic Toast	1	70	65
Green Peas	1 oz	21	30
Green Peppers	¼ cup	10	tr
Hidden Valley Ranch Dressing	1 tbsp	50	95
Honeydew Melon	2 oz	20	5
Italian Caesar Dressing	1 tbsp	80	140
Italian Golden Dressing	1 tbsp	45	250
Jalapeno Peppers	1 tbsp	2	190
Lettuce			
Iceberg	1 cup	8	5
Romaine	1 cup	9	5
Mushrooms	¼ cup	4	tr
Oil	2 tbsp	250	0
Olives, Black	1 oz	35	245
Oranges	2 oz	26	0
Parmesan Cheese	1 oz	130	525
Imitation	1 oz	80	410

FOOD	PORTION	CALORIES	SODIUM
Pasta			
Medley	2 oz	60	5
Salad	¼ cup	35	120
Peaches	2 pieces	31	5
Pepperoni, Sliced	1 oz	140	435
Picante Sauce	2 oz	18	5
Pineapple Chunks	3 oz	60	tr
Potato Salad	2 oz	125	90
Pudding			
Butterscotch	2 oz	90	85
Chocolate	2 oz	90	70
Red Onions	3 rings	2	tr
Reduced Calorie Italian Dressing	1 tbsp	25	185
Refried Beans	2 oz	70	215
Rotini	2 oz	90	tr
Seafood Salad	2 oz	110	455
Sour Topping	1 oz	58	30
Spaghetti Meat Sauce	2 oz	60	315
Spaghetti Sauce	2 oz	28	345
Spanish Rice	2 oz	70	440
Strawberries	2 oz	17	tr
Sunflower Seeds and Raisins	1 oz	140	5
Taco Chips	1⅓ oz	260	20
Taco Meat	2 oz	110	300
Taco Salad	1 (17 oz)	530	825
Taco Sauce	1 oz	16	140
Taco Shell	1	45	45
Thousand Island Dressing	1 tbsp	70	105
Three Bean Salad	2 oz	60	15
Tomatoes	1 oz	6	5

FOOD	PORTION	CALORIES	SODIUM
Tuna Salad	2 oz	100	290
Turkey Ham	1 oz	35	275
Watermelon	2 oz	18	tr
Wine Vinegar	1 tbsp	2	5

THE
IRON
COUNTER

MONITOR YOUR IRON INTAKE, AND REDUCE YOUR RISK OF HEART DISEASE

OVER 8,000 ENTRIES IDENTIFYING KEY SOURCES OF IRON IN BRAND NAME, GENERIC, AND FAST FOODS

Annette Natow, Ph.D., R.D., and Jo-Ann Heslin, M.A., R.D.

Bestselling Authors of
The Fat Counter and *The Cholesterol Counter*

POCKET
BOOKS

Available from Pocket Books

647-01